MEDICAL TERMINOLOGY

Active Learning Through Case Studies

Joan-Beth Gow
Anna Maria College

Arne Christensen
Westfield State University

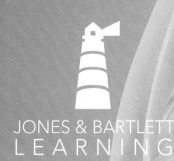

JONES & BARTLETT
LEARNING

World Headquarters
Jones & Bartlett Learning
25 Mall Road
Burlington, MA 01803
978-443-5000
info@jblearning.com
www.jblearning.com

Jones & Bartlett Learning books and products are available through most bookstores and online booksellers. To contact Jones & Bartlett Learning directly, call 800-832-0034, fax 978-443-8000, or visit our website, www.jblearning.com.

21075-0

Production Credits

Vice President, Product Management: Marisa Urbano
Vice President, Product Operations: Christine Emerton
Director, Product Management: Cathy Esperti
Product Manager: Bill Lawrensen
Content Strategist: Ashley Malone
Content Coordinator: Elena Sorrentino
Director, Project Management and Content Services: Karen Scott
Project Manager: Kristen Rogers
Project Specialist: Janet Vail
Digital Project Specialist: Rachel DiMaggio
Marketing Manager: Mark Adamiak
Content Services Manager: Colleen Lamy
VP, Manufacturing and Inventory Control: Therese Connell
Composition: Exela Technologies
Project Management: Exela Technologies
Cover Design: Briana Yates
Text Design: Briana Yates
Media Development Editor: Faith Brosnan
Rights & Permissions Manager: John Rusk
Rights Specialist: Liz Kincaid
Cover Image, Chaper Opener: © Yevhen Vitte/Shutterstock
Printing and Binding: LSC Communications

Library of Congress Cataloging-in-Publication Data

Names: Gow, Joan-Beth, author. | Christensen, Arne (Arne K.), author.
Title: Medical terminology : active learning through case studies / Joan-Beth Gow, Arne Christensen.
Description: First edition. | Burlington, MA : Jones & Bartlett Learning, [2023] | Includes bibliographical references and index.
Identifiers: LCCN 2021034105 | ISBN 9781284210668 (paperback)
Subjects: MESH: Medicine | Terminology | Case Reports
Classification: LCC R123 | NLM W 15 | DDC 610.1/4–dc23
LC record available at https://lccn.loc.gov/2021034105

6048

Printed in the United States of America
25 24 23 22   10 9 8 7 6 5 4 3 2 1

This text is dedicated to the healthcare professionals that cared for patients during the SARS-2 pandemic.

Brief Contents

Contents

Preface

Medical Terminology: Active Learning Through Case Studies is a new type of medical terminology textbook that invites you to become more actively engaged in the learning process. Active learning promotes deeper thought and cognitive processing than passive learning, or by having information simply presented in a lecture. Academic research has clearly demonstrated that active learning is more effective than passive learning in building knowledge and putting knowledge into practice.

This text stands apart from the others through the emphasis on interpreting and using medical terms in a clinical context, which more readily translates to using terms in the real world. It offers a rich learning experience that will help you prepare to use medical terms with confidence in any health-related field.

Organization

This textbook is generally organized by individual body systems. Chapters 2 through 11 are each dedicated to a different body system. Chapter 12 focuses on the special senses of vision and hearing, and Chapter 13 is a special topics chapter covering medical specialties such as psychology, oncology, pharmacology, and rehabilitative medicine. Each chapter provides an overview of the anatomy and physiology of that body system and defines the relevant terminology, before presenting 10 clinical case studies that provide the framework to read, interpret, deconstruct, and construct medical terms. The cases have narratives that use a variety of different formats; some of the cases are short and technical whereas others are more involved and humanized. Some cases ask you to interpret laboratory values or consider specific disease signs or symptoms. Each case is followed by a set of questions that are also varied in their format. Some questions ask you to break down complex terms into their parts (e.g., prefixes, roots, and suffixes) to reveal their meaning; others are open-ended, probing for a more in-depth understanding of processes and mechanisms. You may be asked to predict or build your own terms based on your understanding of medical terms or

their parts, using different strategies to approach the varied styles of cases and questions throughout this study of medical terminology.

Each chapter introduction provides a foundation for interpreting the cases and answering the questions. The introductions include medical illustrations of the relevant anatomy to support visual learning and key terms that are defined in the glossary.

Case Studies

With the grounding provided by each chapter introduction, students will interpret and answer questions for cases organized by increasing complexity from Standard to Advanced. The cases have been written to provide broad coverage of each body system. The student will find that the more common terms and word parts are used across many cases studies, whereas more specialized terms are limited to the more unique cases. The cases present signs, symptoms, and diagnostics that are clinically accurate and are supported by additional figures and references for further reading. The fictional patients and practitioners have been created to reflect the diversity in race, ethnicity, sex, sexual orientation, and socioeconomic status that are encountered in a real-life clinical setting.

Note From the Authors

The book has been written to provide students and instructors with a framework to interpret, apply, and actively engage with medical terminology as part of the learning process. The authors are strong advocates for student-centered instruction and frequently use case studies as a method of instruction in their own classrooms, making this text a standout against others on the market. Overwhelming evidence has demonstrated the efficacy of active learning, one of the most robust trends presently affecting teaching and education. Students learn by doing; it engages and motivates them, and this text offers students the opportunity to do this in medical terminology.

Each chapter includes 10 cases that are organized by increasing narrative length, technical detail, and/or question depth. The cases focus on pathologies from the body systems, and the word parts and case questions span different body systems, reflecting interconnectedness of the body's organs and organ systems. Although all 10 cases may be used during the course of instruction, the case studies work on their own to best suit the student's background and the course learning objectives.

Slide-based teaching presentations include each case narrative and seven key terms and word parts. Seven was chosen as it is the *magical number* for working memory capacity, giving students a refresher of key terms before working through case questions. The teaching presentations also include an *origins* slide, which focuses on the etymology of highly relevant, unique, or complicated terms to provide students with additional context to support their learning.

Resources

Additional resources to support the text are available in the accompanying Navigate course. Resources include:

- Bonus Case Studies to promote active learning
- Case Study Answer Keys for both the in-text cases and the bonus cases
- Slides in PowerPoint format for additional pedagogical support
- Anatomy & Physiology Review Module

About the Authors

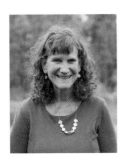

Joan-Beth Gow is a professor of biology in the Health Science Program at Anna Maria College in Paxton, MA. She has more than 20 years of experience teaching courses such as biology, microbiology, medical terminology, and genetics to science and non-science majors. Dr. Gow received her B.A. in biology from Colby College in Waterville, ME, and a Ph.D. in biology from Clark University in Worcester, MA. She is passionate about using engaging pedagogies in the classroom and relies heavily on case-based teaching to support active learning. She has been an author and co-author on several case studies published with the National Center for Case Study Teaching in the Sciences and has presented at multiple conferences promoting active learning.

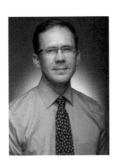

Arne Christensen is an assistant professor in the Department of Biology at Westfield State University in Westfield, MA. Dr. Christensen received his B.S. in biology and Ph.D. in molecular and cellular biology from the University of Massachusetts Amherst. Following graduate school, he spent several years doing postdoctoral research in the area of osmoregulatory physiology at the Conte Anadromous Fish Research Center. His research background is in physiology and cell biology, and he has 11 years of experience teaching human anatomy and physiology, cell biology, and other courses in the biological sciences.

Reviewers

Muhammad Amjad, PhD
Marshall University

Cynthia Blanton, PhD, RDN
Idaho State University

Nancy L. Cox, PTA, MS
Ivy Tech Community College

Tracy Davis, PhD
Rutgers University

Carol Jean Dorough, EdD, MSN, RN, MTASCP
Mount Vernon Nazarene University

Judy Dudley, MA, RHIA
Mercy College of Ohio

Christy Jackson, CPC, CPC-I, CCVTC, CEMC
Cuyahoga Community College

Robert Kulesher, PhD, MHA, FACHE
East Carolina University

Sharon Lawrence, DHSc, PTA
Southwestern Oklahoma State University

Jelena Malogajski, MD, PhD
LIU Brooklyn

Cherri D. McClain, BA, MAA, CCS, RHIT
Miami Dade College

Erin M. McKinley, PhD, RD, LDN, CLC, CHES
Louisiana State University

Lora Murphy, ART, MOTC
Illinois Central College

Susan M. Nava-Whitehead, PhD
Becker College

Yovanna Pomarico, CMBA, CMA
Rosalind Franklin University of Medicine and
    Science

Karen Robertson, RN, MSN, MBA
Rock Valley University

Nancy Simpson, MSN, RN-BC, CNE
Westbrook College of Health Professions

Marilyn Westerhoff, BA
Elgin Community College

CHAPTER 1

Introduction

KEY TERMS

Atom	Hydrogen	Potassium
Calcium	Macromolecule	Protein
Cardiac muscle	Molecules	RNA
Cell	Muscle tissue	Skeletal muscle
Connective tissue	Nervous tissue	Smooth muscle
DNA	Organ system	Sodium
Electrolyte	Organelles	Tissue
Epithelial tissue	Organ	

▶ Introduction to Medical Terminology

The language of medicine is based on medical terms, which are constructed in a way that communicates specific details of anatomy, physiology, procedures,

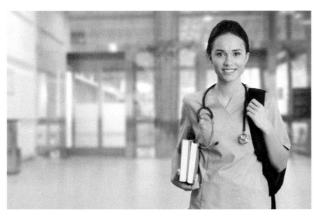

FIGURE 1.1 A student of medical terminology

injury, or disease. Many medical terms appear highly technical at first glance, and some of them are quite long, but there are patterns in their complexity and a logic to the way they are constructed. Once you have cracked the code of medical terminology, the study of medical terms, you will find that most terms are not difficult to interpret or understand. Indeed, they are helpful for thinking, and talking, about medicine. Cracking the code will take guidance and practice, the purpose of this text is to help provide you with both.

It is important to have a solid grasp of medical terminology in an allied health profession, because it will ensure that you can communicate with other healthcare professionals using a shared vocabulary. The vocabulary in this text is medical English, it is used consistently across medical fields and medical English is the language of choice for most international medical journals and conferences. The English terms tend to derive from ancient Greek or Latin. Effective use of medical terms fosters consistency in documenting, diagnosing, and treating patients' illnesses. Having this common language increases patient safety and decreases medical errors.

There are thousands of medical terms; *Taber's Cyclopedic Medical Dictionary* has more than 30,000 of them. Memorizing the meaning of each would be impossible, and pulling the dictionary out to look up each term in the middle of a conversation would be cumbersome and awkward. Fortunately, most medical terms are created by combining frequently used word parts, and if you learn the parts and how to combine them, you will have the ability to build terms, and dissect them to ascertain their meanings. It is like having an array of articles of clothing that you can mix and match into many different outfits. Let us take a closer look at the component parts and how they can be mixed and matched to construct the words of the language of medicine

The foundation of most medical terms is the root. Roots are often derived from Greek or Latin and may apply to a particular cell, tissue, or organ. For example, the root *nephr* means kidney and it is derived from *nephros*, which is Greek for kidney. There are numerous medical terms using this one root, and if you know its meaning, you know what tissue or organ the term is referring to. Roots have other word parts added to them to enhance their meaning. These word parts may be additional roots, suffixes, or prefixes. All medical terms have suffixes, which are added at the end of roots, and often denote a condition or procedure. In this text, suffixes will be denoted with a hyphen preceding them, as in *-ectomy* and *-osis*. The suffix *-ectomy* means surgical removal and *-osis* means abnormal condition. A *nephrectomy* would be the surgical removal of a kidney and *nephrosis* is an abnormal condition of the kidney.

The suffixes *-ectomy* and *-osis* begin with vowels, so when they are added to the root *nephr*, they form terms that are easy to pronounce. Many suffixes, however, do not begin with vowels, which presents a problem with pronunciation. Consider, for example, the suffix *-megaly*, which means enlarged. Adding it to nephr would produce, *nephrmegaly*, which would be difficult to pronounce. To facilitate pronunciation, a combining vowel is used with a root to make a combining form. The combining vowel is nearly always the vowel *o*. Thus, the combining form for kidney would be *nephr/o*. Roots are typically written as their combining form to make pronunciation easier. Using this combining form, the correct term for an enlarged kidney would be *nephromegaly* (nephr/o + -megaly). Combining forms are used whenever a suffix begins with a consonant.

Some common roots, as combining forms, that refer to body organs are in the table below. Note that some medical terms have multiple meanings, *cervic/o* can mean cervix or neck. Some terms have multiple meanings that are similar, *orchid/o* means testicle and testis, which refer to the same structure, but both names are commonly used. Multiple terms may also have the same meaning, for example, the combining forms *pneum/o* and *pulmon/o* both refer to the lung.

TABLE 1.1
Common Roots as Combining Forms
arthr/o: joint
cardi/o: heart
ceric/o: cervix; neck
col/o: colon
cyst/o: urinary bladder; sac
dent/o: tooth
derm/o: skin
encephal/o: brain
enter/o: small intestine
gastr/o: stomach
gloss/o: tongue
hemat/o: blood
hem/o: blood
hepat/o: liver
hyster/o: uterus
muscul/o: muscle
nephr/o: kidney
neur/o: nerve; neuron
onych/o: nail
orchid/o: testicle, testis

Common Roots as Combining Forms
oophor/o: ovary
oste/o: bone
pneum/o: lung; air
phleb/o: vein
proct/o: anus; rectum
pulmon/o: lung
ren/o: kidney
rhin/o: nose
ureter/o: ureter

Combining forms are also used when two roots are used together in a term, as in the combination of *nephr/o, py/o*, which means pus, and *-osis* to form *nephropyosis*, or an abnormal condition of pus in the kidney. If the second root begins with a vowel, the combining form of the first root is still used. For example, *nephr/o, ureter/o* (means ureter), and *-ectomy* are combined to make the term *nephro-ureterectomy*, which means the surgical removal of a kidney and ureter.

Prefixes are added to the front of medical terms and often provide information about location, number, or time. In this text, prefixes will be denoted with a hyphen following them, as in *hemi-*, which means half. A *heminephrectomy* can be broken down into the following word parts; hemi-, nephr/o, and -ectomy, and means the surgical removal of half a kidney. Notice how multiple terms were made using the root *nephr* by combining it with prefixes and suffixes to add to its meaning, and describe medical procedures and conditions. Thus, many seemingly long and unintelligible medical terms can be broken apart and then defined by learning a list of commonly used combining forms, prefixes and suffixes.

▸ Body Organization

The size and location of a body structure can be embedded in a medical term. For the purposes of medical terminology, the size of structures that are discussed range from the level of an atom or molecule up to the organ or organ system. The way a location is described can be based on body region, body cavity, or relative position.

Levels of Organization

Atoms are the smallest stable units of matter; all of the materials that compose the human body are made of atoms. **Atoms** are composed of three types of subatomic particles: neutrons, protons, and electrons. Protons have a charge, it is positive; electrons have a negative charge; and neutrons have no charge, they are neutral. Hydrogen, carbon, nitrogen, oxygen, sodium, calcium, and potassium are all examples of types of atoms. Some atoms carry a charge when they gain, or lose, electrons; these atoms are called ions. The concentrations of specific ions in body fluids are tightly regulated because they have an enormous influence on critical body processes, like neuron communication and muscle contraction. **Hydrogen** (H^+), **sodium** ions (Na^+), **potassium** ions (K^+), and **calcium** ions (Ca^{2+}), are among the most impactful in this regard. **Electrolytes** are chemicals that break apart into ions when dissolved in water. Groups of atoms that share a strong bond, called a covalent bond, are called **molecules**. Pure water is made of molecules that contain an atom of oxygen covalently bound to two atoms of hydrogen. Large molecules, like **proteins**, **RNA**, and **DNA**, are classified as **macromolecules**. **Cells** are the building blocks of all life, similar to the way atoms are the building blocks of all matter. All living things are composed of one, or more, cells. In a human adult, there are tens of trillions of cells, each containing proteins that provide support and motility and drive metabolic reactions. Cells contain **organelles**, which typically include a nucleus, endoplasmic reticulum, and Golgi apparatus, among many other organelles, that provide compartments within the cell to perform particular tasks. Groups of cells that share a similar function are called **tissues**, the study of tissues is histology. Tissues are categorized as epithelial, connective, muscular, or nervous. **Epithelial tissues** are sheets of cells that cover and line organs. **Connective tissues** include bone, tendon, cartilage, fat, and blood. Connective tissues support and connect organs. **Muscle tissue** allows organs to move because it is composed of cells that contract, or shorten. It is classified as cardiac, smooth, or skeletal muscle. **Cardiac muscle** is found only in the heart, its contractions drive the heartbeat. **Smooth muscle** is found in the walls of hollow organs, like

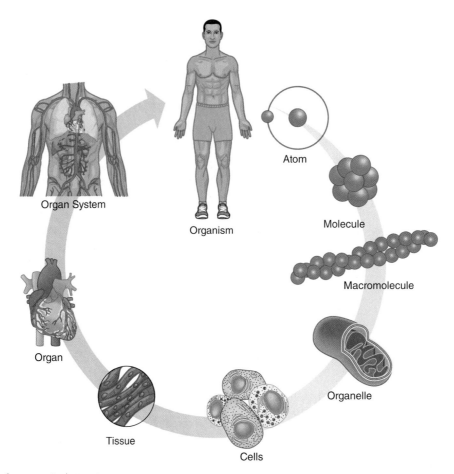

FIGURE 1.2 Scale of anatomical structures

The Membrane-bound Organelles of an Animal Cell

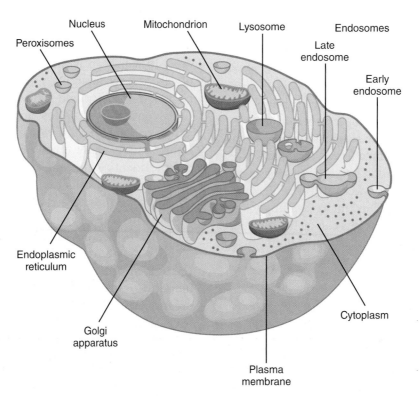

FIGURE 1.3 Cell organelles

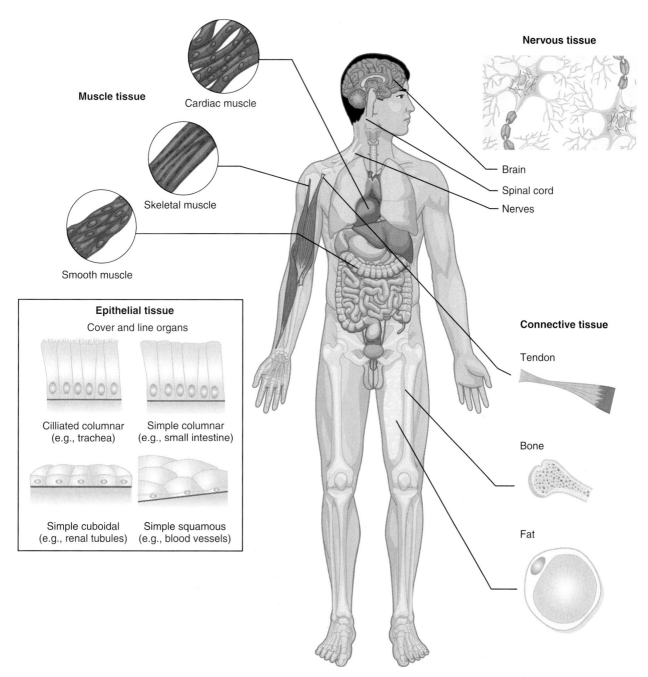

FIGURE 1.4 Some examples of types of tissues found in the body

blood vessels, the intestine, and the airways of the respiratory tract. Smooth muscle contraction tends to influence the movement of contents through the hollow tube. **Skeletal muscle** is the only muscle type that can be controlled voluntarily; it attaches to bone through tendons and allows movement of body parts. **Nervous tissue** is found in the brain, spinal cord, and nerves throughout the body. The primary functional cells of nervous tissue are neurons, which can transmit electrical impulse signals to other cells. **Organs** are composed of one, or more, tissue and perform special functions; the heart, brain, and stomach are examples of organs of the cardiovascular, nervous,

and digestive systems, respectively. **Organ systems**, like the cardiovascular system, work together to perform very complex functions. The heart pumps blood through the blood vessels of the cardiovascular system. The cardiovascular system provides all body cells, directly or indirectly, with nutrients and oxygen, while removing wastes and carbon dioxide. There are 12 body, or organ, systems; integumentary, muscular, skeletal, cardiovascular, lymphatic, respiratory, digestive, urinary, female reproductive, male reproductive, endocrine, and nervous. The systems are covered in more detail in the subsequent chapters of this text.

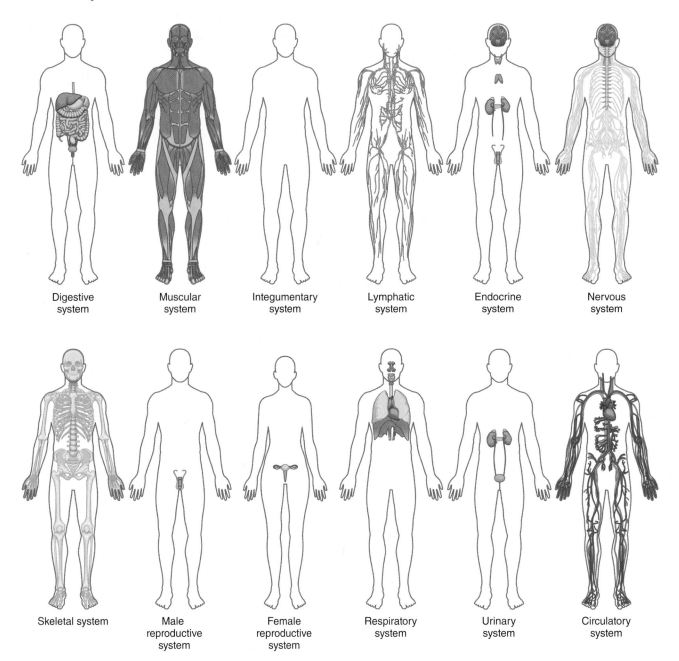

FIGURE 1.5 The organ systems

Body Regions

The body can be broken down into regions, or landmarks, that can be used to describe external locations, when referring to internal or external anatomy. Spending time to learn these landmarks and their names early in your study of medical terminology will be an invaluable asset as you progress through the body systems. The landmarks are frequently encountered when discussing anatomy, physiology, procedures, and diseases.

Body Cavities

The human body has four major cavities, which house specific organs. Two cavities are along the dorsal, or posterior, surface of the body. Two are ventral, located more anteriorly. The dorsal cavities include the cranial and spinal cavities, which enclose the brain and spinal cord. The ventral cavities are the thoracic and abdominopelvic cavities. The thoracic cavity contains the lungs, heart, esophagus, and thymus gland. The abdominopelvic cavity contains a wide range of

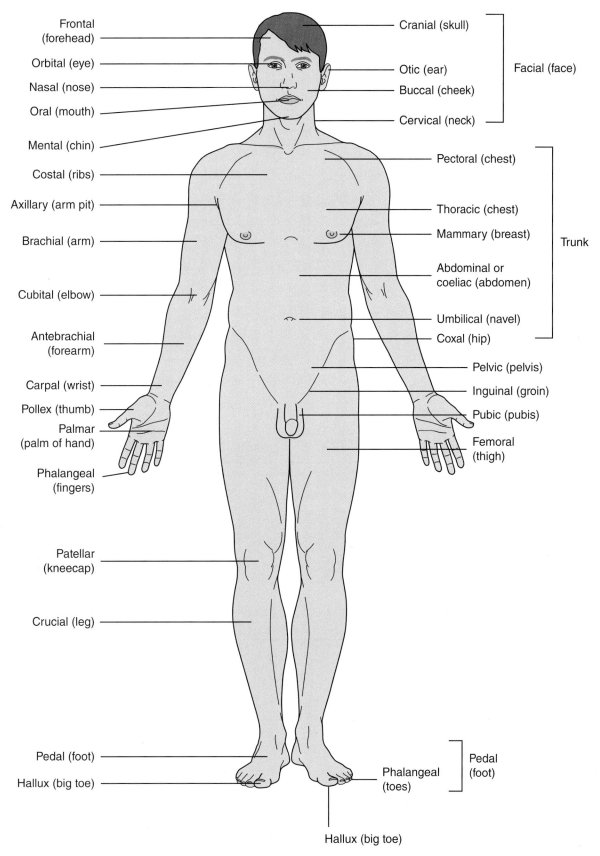

Frontal (forehead)
Orbital (eye)
Nasal (nose)
Oral (mouth)
Mental (chin)
Costal (ribs)
Axillary (arm pit)
Brachial (arm)
Cubital (elbow)
Antebrachial (forearm)
Carpal (wrist)
Pollex (thumb)
Palmar (palm of hand)
Phalangeal (fingers)
Patellar (kneecap)
Crucial (leg)
Pedal (foot)
Hallux (big toe)

Cranial (skull)
Otic (ear)
Buccal (cheek)
Cervical (neck)
Facial (face)
Pectoral (chest)
Thoracic (chest)
Mammary (breast)
Abdominal or coeliac (abdomen)
Umbilical (navel)
Coxal (hip)
Trunk
Pelvic (pelvis)
Inguinal (groin)
Pubic (pubis)
Femoral (thigh)
Pedal (foot)
Phalangeal (toes)
Hallux (big toe)

FIGURE 1.6 Anterior view of the body regions

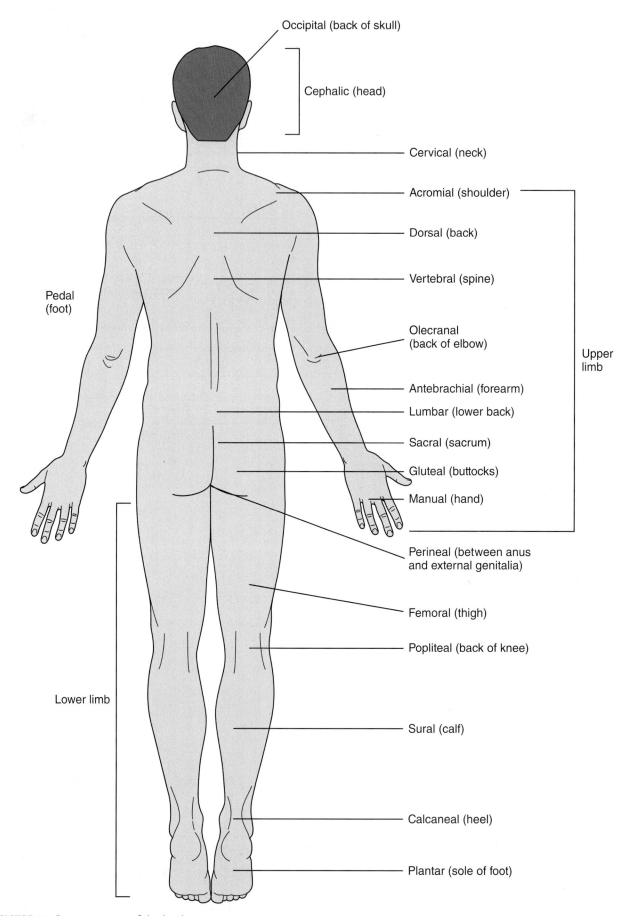

FIGURE 1.7 Posterior view of the body regions

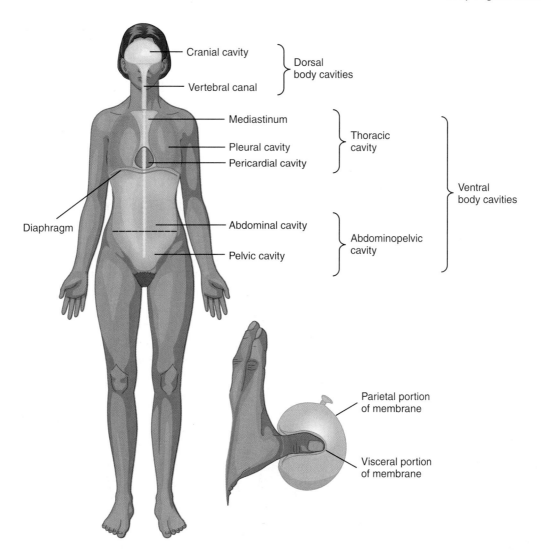

FIGURE 1.8 Body cavities

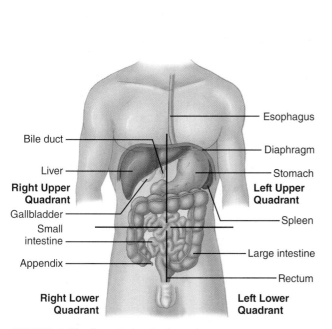

FIGURE 1.9 The four abdominal quadrants

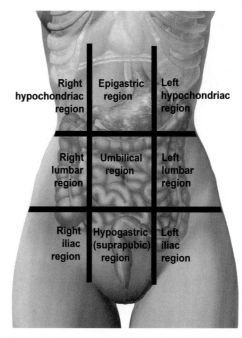

FIGURE 1.10 The nine abdominal regions

organs of the digestive, urinary, and reproductive systems. This cavity can be divided, from an anterior perspective, into four quadrants or nine regions. This facilitates describing, in greater detail, the location of an organ or symptom relating to an organ.

Body Planes

Planes through the body, organs, or other structures separate them into two parts. This is useful when explaining the position of one structure relative to another, or when describing a medical illustration that represents internal anatomy. To understand the planes, imagine cuts through the body or structure at a particular angle. The planes can be sagittal (or medial), frontal (or coronal), or transverse (or horizontal). A diagonal section is called oblique. A sagittal section produces left and right parts. It is important to recognize that when referring to anatomical left and right, it is always from the perspective of the patient or the medical illustration.

Although the left and right side of the body appear to be fairly similar, albeit opposite, reflections of each other, there are some profound anatomical differences between the two. A frontal section produces anterior and posterior parts, and a transverse section produces superior (top) and inferior (bottom) parts.

Directional Terms

Directional terms are used to describe anatomical structures relative to one another. A sagittal plane directly down the midline of the body is called a midsagittal section. Medial structures are closer to the midline whereas lateral structures are farther away from it. The left eye is medial to the left ear because it is closer to the midline; the left eye is also lateral to the left nostril because, in this pairing, it is farther from the midline. Proximal structures are closer to the attachment to the body; distal structures are farther away. Anterior structures are more toward

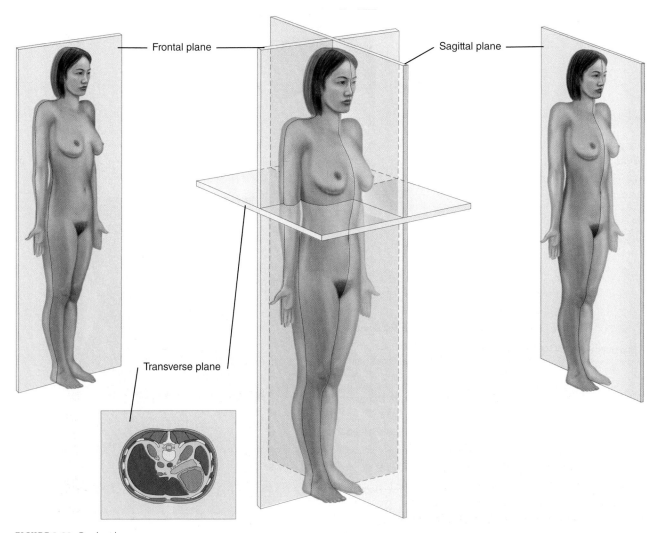

Frontal plane — Sagittal plane — Transverse plane

FIGURE 1.11 Body planes

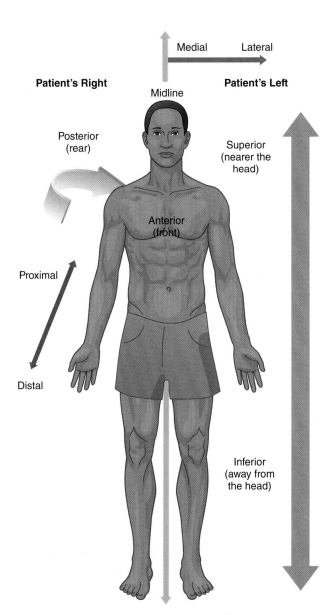

Medial   Lateral

Patient's Right   **Patient's Left**

Midline

Posterior (rear)

Superior (nearer the head)

Anterior (front)

Proximal

Distal

Inferior (away from the head)

FIGURE 1.12 Directional terms

the front, or belly, whereas posterior structures are more toward the back. Superior is closer to the head, or above another structure. Inferior is closer to the feet, or below another structure. Superficial structures are near the surface of the body or an organ, whereas underlying structures are described as deep.

▶ A Deeper Look at Medical Terminology

Now that you have been introduced to the basics of medical terminology and have considered the way the human body is organized, a more extensive list of word parts (i.e., prefixes, combining forms, and suffixes), many of which are used in multiple organ systems, will be presented. This will allow you to build a richer

TABLE 1.2 Word Parts That Describe Location or Position

Word parts in this category tend to be prefixes or combining forms

Prefixes	Combining Forms
anti-: against	anter/o: front
co-: together, with	cortic/o: outer layer
contra-: against, opposite	dist/o: away from
ecto-: out, outside	dors/o: back
endo-: within	infer/o: below
epi-: above	later/o: side
exo-: outward	medi/o: middle
extra-: outside of	medull/o: inner region
in-: inward; not	peripher/o: away from center
infra-: below, beneath	poster/o: back
inter-: between	proxim/o: near to
intra-: within	super/o: above
ipsi-: same	ventr/o: belly
meso-: middle	
peri-: around	
post-: after	
pre-: before	
re-: back; again	
retro-: behind	
sub-: under	
supra-: above, upper	
sym-: together, with	
trans-: across, through	

TABLE 1.3 Word Parts That Describe Amount, Quantity, or Speed

Word parts in this category tend to be prefixes, but a few are combining forms.

Prefixes	Combining Forms
a-: without, not	dipl/o: double
bi-: two	is/o: same, equal
brady-: slow	
de-: without	
di-: two, aside	
hemi-: half	
hyper-: above, excessive	
hypo-: below, deficient, insufficient	
macro-: large	
micro-: small	
mono-: one	
multi-: many	
non-: not	
pan-: all	
poly-: many, much	
quadri-: four	
tachy-: fast	
tetra-: four	
tri-: three	
un-: not	
uni-: one	

TABLE 1.4 Word Parts That Describe Color

The parts in this category are combining forms.

Combining Forms
albin/o: white
chlor/o: green
chrom/o: color
chromat/o: color
cirrh/o: yellow-orange
cyan/o: blue
eosin/o: rosy
erythr/o: red
glauc/o: gray
leuk/o: white
melan/o: black
xanth/o: yellow

TABLE 1.5 Word Parts That Describe Procedures

The word parts in this category are suffixes.

Suffixes
-centesis: puncture to withdraw fluid
-clast: to break
-desis: surgical fusion
-ectomy: surgical removal
-gram: record or picture
-graphy: recording
-lysis: to break down, destroy

Suffixes
-lytic: destruction
-manometer: instrument to measure pressure
-meter: instrument to measure
-metric: pertaining to measuring
-metry: measuring
-opsy: view of
-ostomy: surgically create an opening
-otomy: cutting into
-pexy: surgical fixation
-plasty: surgical repair
-rrhaphy: surgical suturing
-scope: instrument for viewing
-scopic: pertaining to visually examining
-scopy: visually examining
-therapy: treatment
-tripsy: surgical crushing

catalog of terms and dissect more complex ones. The tables below contain word parts organized by category, and each list within a table is separated by prefix, combining form, and suffix and are ordered alphabetically.

With the concepts and word parts covered thus far in this chapter, you can start breaking down terms to understand their meaning, even if you are unfamiliar with them. Use the medical term hemicolectomy as an example and two steps to reveal the meaning. Step 1 is to divide the term into its component parts: *hemi-*; *col/o*; *-ectomy*. Step 2 is to define each of the component parts. *Hemi-* you already learned means half. *Col/o* is the combining form for colon and *-ectomy* you already learned means surgical removal. The conventional way to put these together into a complete definition is to start with the suffix, move to the prefix, and end with the root. A patient who is scheduled for a *hemicolectomy* will undergo the surgical removal of half of the colon.

Think about the following two terms, *polyarthritis* and *onychopathology*. Try the two steps to see if you can determine their meaning and then continue. For *polyarthritis*, in Step 1, we will divide the term into its component parts: *poly-*; *arthr/o*; *-itis*. *Poly-* is a common prefix meaning many, *arthr/o* means joint, and *-itis* is a common suffix indicating inflammation. A patient with *polyarthritis* has an inflammation of many joints. *Onychopathology* is a term that is a combination of two roots with a suffix, and no prefix. *Onych/o* means nail (as in fingernail or toenail), *path/o* means disease, and *-logy* indicates the study of. The term refers to the study of nail diseases. Not every medical term

TABLE 1.6 Word Parts That Describe Conditions

The parts in this category tend to be suffixes, but a few are prefixes or combining forms.

Prefixes	Combining Forms	Suffixes
auto-: self	alges/o: sense of pain	-algesia: sensitivity to pain
dys-: painful; abnormal; difficult	dips/o: thirst	-algia: pain
eu-: normal	esthesi/o: sensation, feeling	-asthenia: weakness
hetero-: different	isch/o: to hold back	-chezia: defecation, elimination of waste
homeo-: same, unchanging	odyn/o: pain	-constriction: narrowing
homo-: same	path/o: disease	-dynia: pain

(continues)

TABLE 1.6 Word Parts That Describe Conditions		*(continued)*
Prefixes	**Combining Forms**	**Suffixes**
mal-: bad		-edema: swelling
pseudo-: false		-emesis: vomiting
		-esthesia: nervous condition
		-eurysm: widening
		-iasis: abnormal condition
		-itis: inflammation
		-malacia: softening
		-megaly: enlarged
		-osis: abnormal condition
		-pathy: disease
		-penia: abnormal decrease
		-phil: attracted to
		-phobia: irrational fear
		-phoria: feeling
		-ptosis: drooping, drooping eyelid
		-ptysis: spitting
		-rrhage: abnormal flow
		-rrhagia: abnormal flow condition
		-rrhea: discharge
		-rrhexis: rupture
		-sclerosis: hardening
		-spasm: sudden contraction
		-static: pertaining to stopping, standing still
		-stasis: standing still
		-uria: urine condition

TABLE 1.7 Word Parts That Refer to Practitioners or Specialists

The parts in this category tend to be suffixes.

Combining Forms	Suffixes
iatr/o: physician, medicine, treatment	-iatric: pertaining to medical treatment
	-iatrist: physician
	-iatry: medical treatment
	-ician: specialist
	-ist: specialist
	-istry: specialty of; pertaining to
	-logic: pertaining to study of
	-logist: one who studies
	-logy: study of'
	-metrist: specialist in measuring
	-or: one that is; condition of

TABLE 1.8 Word Parts That Refer to Proteins, Cells, or Tissues

Word parts in this category tend to be suffixes or combining forms.

Combining Forms	Suffixes
adip/o: fat	-blast: immature
blast/o: immature	-cyte: cell
carcin/o: cancer	-cytic: pertaining to cells
crin/o: secreting	-cytosis: more than the normal number of cells
cyt/o: cell	-gen: that which produces
histi/o: tissue	-genesis: producing, forming
hist/o: tissue	-genic: produced by or in
lip/o: fat	-genous: producing

(continues)

TABLE 1.8 Word Parts That Refer to Proteins, Cells, or Tissues	*(continued)*

Word parts in this category tend to be suffixes or combining forms.

Combining Forms	Suffixes
myomat/o: muscular tumor	-globin: protein
necr/o: death	-nuclear: nucleus
onc/o: tumor	-oid: resembling
troph/o: nourishment	-oma: tumor, mass
	-plasia: development; formation of cells
	-plasm: growth, formation
	-poiesis: formation
	-trophic: pertaining to development; stimulation
	-tropin: to stimulate
	-trophy: development

can be broken down in this way and some will require looking them up in a medical dictionary or other reliable resource, but the vast majority of terms can be dissected and translated once you have memorized a list of common prefixes and suffixes and learned the combining forms presented in each chapter.

TABLE 1.9 Other Commonly Used Suffixes	
General Suffixes	**General Suffixes to Form Adjectives**
-arity: relating to	-a: pertaining to
-ated: process, condition	-ac: pertaining to
-ation: process, condition	-al: pertaining to
-esis: condition, state of	-an: pertaining to
-ia: condition	-ar: pertaining to
-ice: condition	-ary: pertaining to
-ification: process of becoming	-atic: pertaining to
-ion: process	-atory: pertaining to
-ism: condition of	-eal: pertaining to

General Suffixes	General Suffixes to Form Adjectives
-ity: condition	-iac: pertaining to
-ive: tendency	-ic: pertaining to
-ization: process of making	-ical: pertaining to
-nymous: name	-id: pertaining to
-or: condition of	-ile: pertaining to
-um: structure	-ine: pertaining to
-us: structure, thing	-ior: pertaining to
-y: condition, process	-istry: pertaining to
	-nic: pertaining to
	-ory: pertaining to
	-ose: pertaining to
	-ous: pertaining to
	-tic: pertaining to
	-tory: pertaining to
	-tous: pertaining to

▶ Exceptions to the Rules

As you continue to learn about medical terminology, you will find that, like most complex systems that are built on rules, there are exceptions to the rules. A few examples include prefixes embedded in a term and imperfect combinations. An example of a prefix embedded in a term is neuroendocrinologist, which can be broken down into *neur/o*; *endo-*; *crin/o*; and *-logist*. *Neur/o* means neuron or nerve, *endo-* means within, *crin/o* means secreting, and *-logist* means one who studies. A neuroendocrinologist is one who studies secretions, in this case hormones, within the brain. Note that *endo-* is a prefix, but it is found embedded in the term. An example of an imperfect combination is the term monozygotic, which can be broken down into mono-; zygote; and -tic. The prefix *mono-* means one, a zygote is an egg that has been fertilized by a sperm cell, and -tic means pertaining to. Monozygotic describes twins that have arisen from a single fertilized egg, or identical twins. Combining the word parts without modification produces monozygotetic, which is an invented word without meaning that is difficult to pronounce. Moreover, there is no accepted combining form for zygote. As a result, this is a case where the term does not directly follow the rules as described earlier in this chapter but is an imperfect combination of word parts.

▶ Plural Endings

There is no straightforward rule for making a singular noun plural in medical terminology. In some cases, the English rule of adding a "s" or "es" to a noun, or dropping a "y" and adding "ies," is used. For example, the plural of the noun nerve is nerves, vsinus is sinuses, and therapy is therapies. In other cases, Greek and Latin rules apply when changing the ending of a noun to make it plural.

For example:

a is changed to *ae*, as in vertebra to vertebrae

ax is changed to *aces*, as in pneumothorax to pneumothoraces

en is changed to *ina*, as in foramen to foramina

is is changed to *es*, as in metastasis to metastases

ix is changed to *ices*, as in cervix to cervices

ma is changed to *mata*, as in fibroma to fibromata

on is changed to *a*, as in ganglion to ganglia

um is changed to *a*, as in atrium to atria

us is changed to *i*, as in alveolus to alveoli

x is changed to *ges*, as in meninx to meninges

y is changed to *ies*, as in therapy to therapies

▶ Abbreviations

Many medical terms have generally accepted abbreviations, although the abbreviations should only be used if they are approved in a particular facility or setting. Some examples of common abbreviations are CBC for Complete Blood Count, BUN for Blood Urea Nitrogen, and BMI for Body Mass Index. An extensive list of abbreviations is provided as an appendix.

▶ Practice Exercises

To practice what you have learned in this chapter, define the word parts and meaning for the terms below. You may remember the word part definitions; if not, look for them in the tables. Once entered, use them to think about what the meaning of the term is. If you need assistance, refer to a medical dictionary or other online resource (see preface). This exercise will help prepare you for the active learning and deeper thought required in subsequent chapters, as you are guided through the body systems and use your knowledge and creativity to interpret case studies and medical terms.

1. Hypertrophic: Hyper- _____, -trophic _____,

       means _____.

2. Anesthesia: An- _____,

       esthesi/o _____, -ia _____,

       means _____.

3. Bilateral: Bi- _____,

       later/o _____, -al _____,

       means _____.

4. Arthralgia: Arthr/o _____, -algia _____,

       means _____.

5. Tachycardia: Tachy- _____,

       cardi/o _____, -ia _____,

       means _____.

6. Dizygotic: Di- _____, zygote _zygote_ , -ic _____,

       means _____.

7. Ischemia: Isch/o _____,

     hem/o _____, -ia _____,

     means _____.

8. Hematochezia: Hemat/o _____, -chezia _____,

     means _____.

9. Anuria: An- _____, -uria _____,

     means _____.

10. Pancytopenia: Pan- _____,

     cyt/o _____, -penia _____,

     means _____.

11. Polydipsia: Poly- _____,

     dips/o _____, -ia _____,

     means _____.

12. Gastroenterostomy: Gastr/o _____,

     enter/o _____, -ostomy _____,

     means _____.

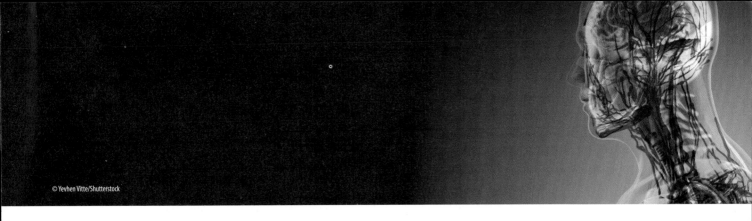

CHAPTER 2

Integumentary System

KEY TERMS

Arrector pili muscle
Cerumen
Ceruminous gland
Cyanotic
Dermis
Epidermis
Eponychium
Erythema
Free edge
Hair
Hair follicle

Hair shaft
Hypodermis
Hyponychium
Integument
Jaundice
Keratin
Keratinocyte
Langerhans cell
Lunula
Melanin
Melanocyte

Merkel cell
Nail body
Nail
Papilla of the hair
Sebaceous gland
Sebum
Skin
Striae
Subcutaneous layer
Sudoriferous gland

The **integument** is composed of the skin, the largest organ of the body, and accessory structures such as hair, fingernails and toenails, and sweat and oil glands. The word integument derives from the Latin *tegere*, which means "to cover"; the skin covers the body and without it the internal organs would be vulnerable to damage from ultraviolet (UV) light, noxious chemicals, dehydration, and infectious microbes. The skin is also an important structure for regulating body temperature, sensing touch and pain, and vitamin D production.

The **skin** is composed of two layers, a superficial epidermis and an underlying dermis. The **epidermis** is stratified squamous epithelium that is continuously renewed by a dedicated class of stem cells. Most epidermal cells are **keratinocytes** which produce the protein **keratin**, a fibrous structural protein that protects the underlying tissue from damage or stress. The epidermis also includes **Langerhans**

cells, which are responsible for identifying infectious microbes, and **melanocytes**, which produce a pigment called **melanin** that absorbs, and protects deeper tissues, from UV light. **Merkel cells** are located deep in the epidermis; these cells play a role in touch sensation.

The **dermis** contains dense irregular and areolar connective tissue and nervous, lymphatic, and vascular elements. The dermis provides both strength and flexibility due to the combination of collagen and elastic fibers. Dramatic changes in the dermis during pregnancy or extreme weight gain may be characterized by the appearance of dermal scarring called **striae**. Sweat glands in the dermis play a role in thermoregulation, and mechanoreceptors aid in sensation. Below the dermis is the **subcutaneous layer**, also called the **hypodermis**. This layer is not part of the skin but attaches it to underlying tissue and organs.

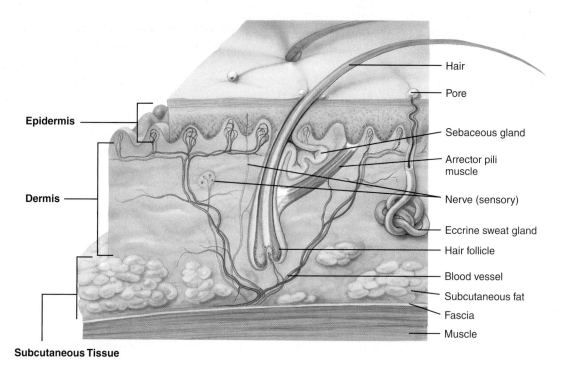

Epidermis

Dermis

Subcutaneous Tissue

Hair

Pore

Sebaceous gland

Arrector pili muscle

Nerve (sensory)

Eccrine sweat gland

Hair follicle

Blood vessel

Subcutaneous fat

Fascia

Muscle

FIGURE 2.1 The layers of the skin and accessory structures

The skin has many accessory structures. **Hair** is present on most of the skin's surfaces with the exception of the palms of the hands and the soles of the feet. Hair offers some protection from foreign particles and hair on the head decreases heat loss from the scalp. The root of a hair is located deep in the dermis. Surrounding the root is the **hair follicle**, which houses the **papilla of the hair**, the site of cell division responsible for hair growth. Bundles of smooth muscle cells called **arrector pili muscles** are attached to the follicle. These muscles respond to physiological or emotional stress by pulling the hairs perpendicular to the skin surface, causing

"goosebumps." Extending from the epidermal surface is the superficial portion of the hair called the **hair shaft**.

Nails are present on the dorsal surface of fingers and toes. These plates of keratinized epidermal cells protect the ends of digits, help in the grasp of small objects, and allow the scratching of body surfaces in response to itch. The parts of the nail are the free edge, the nail body, and the nail root. The **free edge** is what is seen extending past the distal end of fingers and toes. The thickened region of epithelial tissue, just beneath the free edge of a fingernail or toenail, is the **hyponychium**. The **nail body** is the

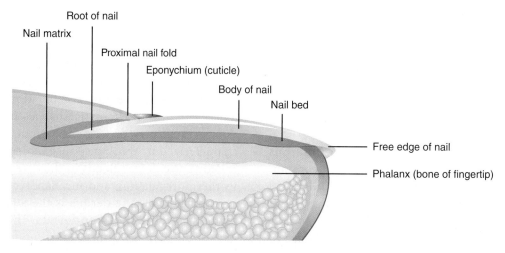

Root of nail

Nail matrix

Proximal nail fold

Eponychium (cuticle)

Body of nail

Nail bed

Free edge of nail

Phalanx (bone of fingertip)

FIGURE 2.2 Anatomy of the fingernail

visible portion of the nail proximal to the free edge. The root, responsible for growth of the nail, is buried in a fold of skin. The narrow band of epidermis that occupies the area between the proximal end of the nail and digit is called the **eponychium**, or the cuticle. The white crescent shaped area at the base of the nail is known as the **lunula**, meaning little moon. It appears white because the nail is thicker here, obscuring the view of the vascular tissue below it.

Glands are also accessory structures of the integument. **Sebaceous glands** secrete **sebum**, or oil. These glands are typically associated with hairs and help prevent them from drying out. Sebum also lubricates the skin, protecting it from friction and providing a moisture barrier. **Sudoriferous glands** secrete sweat into hair follicles or onto the skin through sweat pores. Sweat helps regulate body temperature through evaporation. **Ceruminous glands** secrete **cerumen** in the external ear. This earwax helps prevent the entrance of foreign substances.

The color of the skin can provide diagnostic clues to disease. **Cyanotic**, or blue skin can indicate inadequate oxygenation of the blood. **Jaundice**, or yellow skin can indicate liver disease. **Erythema** or red skin can indicate injury, infection, or inflammation.

TABLE 2.1
Key Integumentary System Prefixes
pachy-: heavy, thick

TABLE 2.2
Key Integumentary System Combining Forms
actin/o: ray
albin/o: white
cutane/o: skin
cyan/o: blue
dactyl/o: digit, finger, toe
derm/o: skin
dermat/o: skin
erythr/o: red
follicul/o: follicle
hidr/o: sweat
ichthy/o: scaly
kerat/o: horny tissue; cornea
leuk/o: white

Key Integumentary System Combining Forms
melan/o: black
muc/o: mucus
myc/o: fungus
myx/o: mucin, mucus
norm/o: normal
onych/o: nail
pedicul/o: lice
phot/o: light
poikil/o: varied, irregular
prurit/o: itchy
psor/o: itchy
pustul/o: pustules
scler/o: hard; sclera
seb/o: oil
squam/o: scales
ungu/o: nail
vesicul/o: vesicles
xanth/o: yellow
xer/o: dry

🔍 *STANDARD CASE STUDY*

2.1 Dermatophytic Fungus

A 36-year-old male presented to his primary care physician with discomfort and dystrophy of the toenail on the big toe of his left foot. Examination of the toenail revealed that it was yellowed, thickened, and chipped around the distal edge. A fungal culture from scrapings of the nail plate, nail bed, and subungual debris was positive for a dermatophytic fungus, *Trichophyton rubrum*.

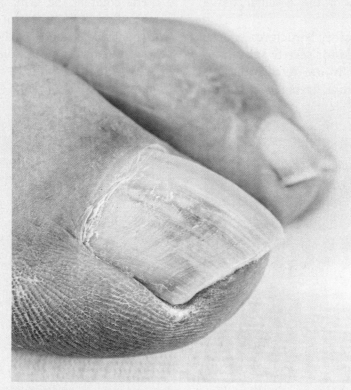

CASE FIGURE: Discolored toe nail

© Zlisjak/iStock/Getty Images Plus/Getty Images

1.   Define the word parts for subungal.

Subungal: Sub- _____, ungu/o _____ -al _____.

2.   Where is subungal debris collected from?

3.   Define the following word parts and then circle your diagnosis for this case study:

Onychomalacia: Onych/o _____, -malacia _____.

Onychomycosis: Onych/o _____, myc/o _____, -osis _____.

Dermatomycosis: Dermat/o _____, myc/o _____, -osis _____.

Onychocryptosis: Onych/o _____, crypt/o _____, -osis _____.

🔍 *STANDARD CASE STUDY*

2.2 Pachyonychia Congenita

A mother brings her 3-year-old girl to her pediatrician. The mother reports that once the child learned how to walk, she began developing painful blisters on the soles of her feet. The mother also reports that the child's palms and the soles of her feet frequently feel sweaty (i.e., palmar plantar hyperhidrosis). A physical examination reveals hypertrophic nail dystrophy on the hands and feet; the nails are normal in length but have distal prominent hyperkeratosis. The child also has oral leukokeratosis and follicular keratoses on the elbows, knees, and waistline.

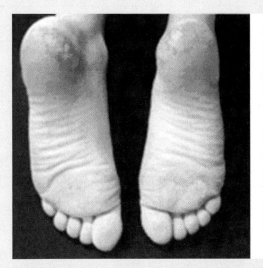 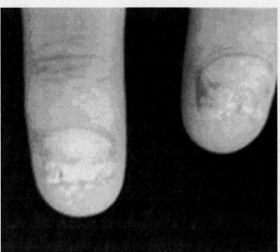

CASE FIGURE: Foot blisters and hypertrophic nail dystrophy

1. Define the word parts for *pediatrician*.

    Pediatrician: Ped/o _____, iatr/o _____, -ician _____.

2. Define the word parts and meaning for the following terms that relate to the infant's symptoms:

    Palmar plantar hyperhidrosis: Palmar _____, plantar _____,

    hyper- _____, hidr/o _____,

    -osis _____, means _____

    Hypertrophic: Hyper- _____, -trophic _____,

    means _____

    Dystrophy: Dys- _____, -trophy _____,

    means _____.

    Hyperkeratosis: Hyper- _____, kerat/o _____,

    -osis _____, means _____.

(continues)

🔍 *STANDARD CASE STUDY*   *(continued)*

Oral leukokeratosis: Or/o _____, -al _____, leuk/o _____,

kerat/o _____, -osis _____,

means _____.

Follicular keratosis: Follicul/o _____, -ar _____,

kerat/o _____, -osis _____,

means _____.

3. What do all of the infant's symptoms have in common?

4. Based on the symptoms, the pediatrician suspects that the infant has pachyonychia congenita and provides a referral to a disease specialist. Indicate the word parts for *pachyonychia* and define the term based on those parts.

5. Congenita means present at birth; describe what pachyonychia congenita is.

🔍 *STANDARD CASE STUDY*

2.3 A Question of Malignancy

A 35-year-old Caucasian female presents to a dermatologist with a chief complaint of a painless wart-like growth on her forehead above her left eye. The lesion has been present for more than 10 years and has not increased in size for several years. The lesion is uniformly light-brown, circular, 5 mm in diameter, has a well-defined border, and has a waxy appearance. The patient reports that she is not aware of any family history of cancer.

The patient will undergo local anesthesia and have the epidermal tumor excised and sent for histopathological examination.

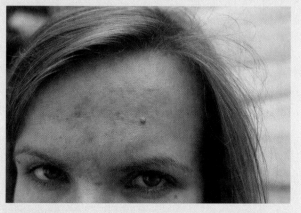

CASE FIGURE: A wart-like growth above the eye

© Only_NewPhoto/Shutterstock

1. Define the word parts for *dermatologist*.

   Dermatologist: Dermat/o _____, -logist _____.

2. Define the word parts for *anesthesia*.

   Anesthesia: An- _____, esthesi/o _____,

   -ia _____.

3. Define the following word parts of the following conditions:

   Malignant melanoma: Malign- _____, -ant _____,

   melan/ _____, -oma _____.

   Seborrheic keratosis: Seb/o _____, -rrhea _____,

   kerat/o _____, -osis _____.

4. Of two diagnoses, malignant melanoma and seborrheic keratosis, what do you think is more probable? Why?

🔍 STANDARD CASE STUDY

2.4 Severe Response to Sunburn

A 30-year-old male reports to the emergency room presenting with inflamed, fiery-red skin, severe itching, and moderate pain. The flare up has lasted several days and followed a mild sunburn. The patient reports that sunburns frequently trigger this skin reaction, but the symptoms are not typically as severe as this episode. The patient has a history of plaque psoriasis, a common skin condition characterized by well-defined regions of red papules and silvery plaques that are itchy and sometimes painful.

An examination revealed generalized findings of erythema involving 60% of the body surface area, desquamation, and pruritus. The patient was febrile and dehydrated. Further discussion with the patient reveals myalgia and insomnia. Based on the above observations, the attending physician made a clinical diagnosis that would need to be confirmed by histopathological study.

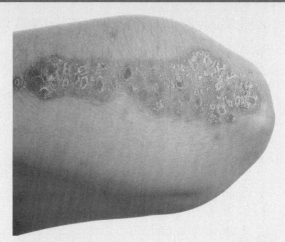

CASE FIGURE: The red papules and silvery plaques typical of psoriasis

© Petekarici/E+/Getty Images

(continues)

🔍 *STANDARD CASE STUDY* *(continued)*

1. There are five official types of psoriasis, and patients who are diagnosed with one type may also develop another. Define the word parts and meaning for *psoriasis*.

    Psoriasis: Psor/o_____, -iasis _____,

    means _____.

2. Complete the table below for the following terms:

Term	Word Parts	Meaning
erythema	*erythr/o; hem/o*	*blood red (refers to flushing of skin)*
desquamation		
febrile		
dehydrated		
myalgia		
insomnia		

3. The patient has plaques and papules. Explain these terms.

4. The diagnosis was confirmed by histopathological study. Indicate the word parts for *histopathological* and then define what type of study it is, based on the word parts.

5. Define the word parts of the following skin conditions, then circle your most likely diagnosis for this case study:

    Acrocyanosis: Acro-_____, cyan/o _____, -osis _____.

    Leukoderma: Leuk/o _____, -derma _____.

    Xanthoderma: Xanth/o _____, -derma _____.

    Erythrodermic psoriasis: Erythr/o _____, derm/o _____,

    -ic _____, psor/o _____,

    -iasis _____.

🔍 *STANDARD CASE STUDY*

2.5 Mosaic Epidermolytic Ichthyosis

A 25-year-old Korean female presents to her primary care physician with verrucous plaques, which have been present since 3 months of age. The lesions are hyperkeratotic, hyperchromic, malodorous, and are distributed in a whorled pattern on the left trunk and around joints of her left arm. She has no family history of ichthyosis. She has been diagnosed with mosaic epidermolytic ichthyosis resulting from a mutation in the *KRT1* gene, which encodes the keratin 1 protein. Her mutation was acquired sometime after conception, so not inherited from either parent. The lesions have been treated unsuccessfully. The patient is feeling depressed and hopeless and continues to pursue treatment options.

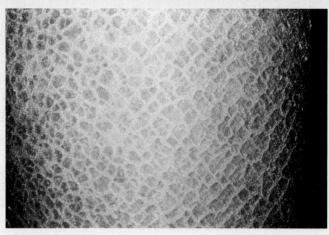

CASE FIGURE: Scaling from ichthyosis

Courtesy of Richard S. Hibbets/CDC

1. Define the word parts for *epidermolytic ichthyosis*.

   Epidermolytic: Epi- _____, derm/o _____,

   -lytic _____.

   Ichthyosis: Ichthy/o _____, -osis _____.

2. In the medical term mosaic epidermolytic ichthyosis, what does mosaic mean?

3. In the medical term mosaic epidermolytic ichthyosis, explain what epidermolytic means.

4. In the medical term mosaic epidermolytic ichthyosis, explain what ichthyosis means.

5. Define the following word parts of the following conditions:

   Hyperkeratotic: Hyper- _____, kerat/o _____,

   -tic _____.

(continues)

🔍 STANDARD CASE STUDY   *(continued)*

Hyperchromic: Hyper- _____, chrom/o _____,

-ic _____.

Malodorous: Mal- _____, odor _____

_____ *odor* _____, -ous _____.

🔍 ADVANCED CASE STUDY

2.6 Gustatory Hyperhidrosis

The last thing Alex, a 16-year-old male, remembered was the pitcher stepping up to the mound and winding up to throw a baseball, which struck the left side of Alex's head at the angle of the mandible. Alex fell to the ground and lost consciousness for several minutes before his teammates helped him up and walked him over to the bench. Several months after the injury, the left side of Alex's face would become flush and start sweating when he ate. Alex became increasingly concerned with these symptoms and made an appointment with his primary care physician, Dr. Pepple.

Dr. Pepple listened to Alex describe the baseball injury and subsequent symptoms. Dr. Pepple thought the probable diagnosis was Frey's syndrome, also known as gustatory hyperhidrosis, a rare disorder that can arise after surgery or injury to the area around the parotid glands. The parotid glands are the largest of the salivary glands and are located anterior and inferior to each ear. Trauma to a parotid gland and associated nerves can lead to unilateral hyperhidrosis and erythema occurring with gustatory stimulation.

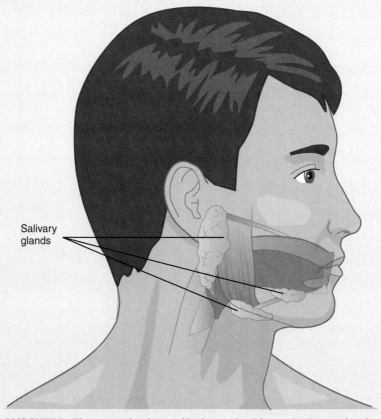

Salivary glands

CASE FIGURE: The parotid, submandibular, and sublingual salivary glands

1. Complete the table below for the following terms:

Term	Word Parts	Meaning
gustatory	*gustat/o; -ory*	*pertaining to taste*
hyperhidrosis		
parotid		
unilateral		
erythema	*erythr/o; hem/o*	

2. Hyperhidrosis is an abnormal condition of excessive sweating. What is the medical term for each of the following conditions that relate to sweat?

   Abnormal condition of insufficient sweat:

   Abnormal condition of no sweat:

3. Sweat glands are innervated by the sympathetic (fight-or-flight) division of the nervous system. Salivary glands secrete a watery saliva when stimulated by nerves of the parasympathetic (rest-and-digest) division of the nervous system. Trauma to the parotid region of the head can lead to damage of sympathetic and parasympathetic nerves; fortunately, these nerves can regenerate and remake connections to their target glands.

   Provide a hypothesis as to why nerve regrowth following trauma to the parotid region could lead to gustatory hyperhidrosis.

🔍 *ADVANCED CASE STUDY*

2.7 Scleromyxedema

Classification: Advanced

A 65-year-old African American man had a 2-year history of generalized papular lesions located on the face, ears, neck, trunk, arms, and dorsa of both hands. The papules were approximately 2 mm in diameter, waxy, normochromatic, and closely spaced, with some in a linear pattern. The patient had progressive induration, tightness, and infiltration of the skin, and sclerodactyly. The patient developed proximal and upper limb muscle weakness, arthralgia, dyspnea on exertion, and dysphagia to solids. Laboratory test results, including thyroid function, were normal except serum analysis revealed IgG λ paraproteinemia (i.e., excess immunoglobulins in the blood).

(continues)

🔍 ADVANCED CASE STUDY (continued)

A skin punch biopsy was obtained from the back and sent for histopathological analysis. The results showed dermal thickening and sclerosis, dermal deposition of mucin between abnormally thick collagen fibers, fibroblast proliferation, perivascular infiltration with lymphocytes, macrophages, and polymorphonuclear leukocytes. The histology findings were consistent with scleromyxedema. Based on clinical manifestations and histopathological and laboratory data, a diagnosis of scleromyxedema associated with gammopathy was made. Scleromyxedema is a rare cutaneous mucinosis, usually presenting with papular lesions and progressive sclerosis of the skin, systemic manifestations, and paraproteinemia.

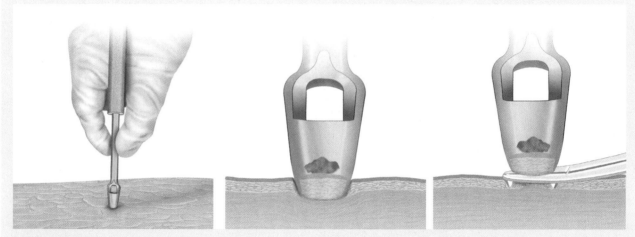

CASE FIGURE: Skin punch biopsy

© Ilusmedical/Shutterstock

1. Answer the following questions about the medical term *scleromyxedema*.

   Scleromyxedema is a type of cutaneous mucinosis, a group of conditions that is characterized by an accumulation of mucin in the skin. Mucin is a major constituent of mucus. Which word part of *scleromyxedema* refers to an accumulation of mucin in the skin?

   _____

   As scleromyxedema progresses, affected areas of skin become hardened and lose plasticity. Which word part of *scleromyxedema* refers to a hardening of the skin?

   _____

   As scleromyxedema progresses, soft tissues of affected areas of skin may swell. Which word part of *scleromyxedema* refers to a swelling of the skin?

   _____

2. What is meant by the term induration?

3. Complete the table below for the following terms:

Term	Word Parts	Meaning
normochromatic	*norm/o; chromat/o; -ic*	*pertaining to normal color*
sclerodactyly		
arthralgia		
dyspnea		
dysphagia		

4. Scleromyxedema is typically associated with paraproteinemia, or elevated levels of immunoglobulin in the blood. Define the word parts for *paraproteinemia*.

Paraproteinemia: Para- _____, protein _____ *protein* _____,

-emia _____.

Four cell types were identified during the histopathological analysis. Define the word parts for the four types of cells.

Fibroblast: Fibr/o _____, -blast _____.

Lymphocyte: Lymph/o _____, -cyte _____.

Macrophage: Macro- _____, -phage _____.

Polymorphonuclear leukocyte: Poly- _____, morph/o _____,

-nuclear _____, leuk/o _____,

-cyte _____.

🔎 ADVANCED CASE STUDY

2.8 Xeroderma Pigmentosum

An 8-year-old Iraqi girl is brought to her dermatologist for her three-month checkup; the girl requires frequent surveillance for skin cancer because she has been diagnosed with xeroderma pigmentosum (XP), a very rare skin disorder that results in cellular photohypersensitivity. Patients with XP have defects in the DNA repair system that typically corrects the mutations caused by ultraviolet light. If precautions are not taken to protect this child from ultraviolet light, she has a 10,000-fold increased risk of skin cancer and will experience premature aging of the skin and eyes. In patients with XP, exposure of the skin to ultraviolet light may result in xeroderma, hyperkeratosis, actinic keratosis, skin atrophy, and poikiloderma. In patients with XP, exposure of the eyes to ultraviolet light may result in photophobia, dry eye, and corneal keratitis, opacification, and vascularization. Precautions for protection from ultraviolet light include avoidance, protective clothing and glasses, and high-SPF suntan lotion.

(continues)

🔍 ADVANCED CASE STUDY (continued)

1. Describe what the medical term xeroderma pigmentosum means.

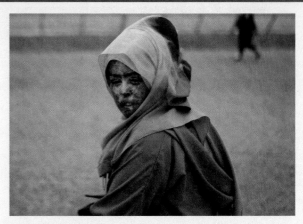

CASE FIGURE: Girl with xeroderma pigmentosum
© Mosa'ab Elshamy/AP/Shutterstock

2. Complete the table below for the following terms that relate to xeroderma pigmentosum symptoms of the skin:

Term	Word Parts	Meaning
xeroderma	xer/o; -derma	dry skin
hyperkeratosis		
actinic keratosis		
atrophy		
poikiloderma		

3. Complete the table below for the following terms that relate to xeroderma pigmentosum symptoms of the eye:

Term	Word Parts	Meaning
photophobia	phot/o; -phobia	irrational fear of light, in this case, sensitivity to light
keratitis		
opacification		
vascularization		

4. Ultraviolet light can induce damage to DNA. People with xeroderma pigmentosum carry a mutation in one of the genes responsible for repairing DNA mutations. Why are people with xeroderma pigmentosum prone to skin cancer?

🔍 *ADVANCED CASE STUDY*

2.9 Pediculosis Capitis

A 10-year-old girl, with a severe case of pediculosis capitis, is brought to her pediatrician. Visible nits and adults confirm an active *Pediculus humanus capitis* hyperinfestation. The patient's scalp is pruritic, reflective of an immune-mediated hypersensitivity reaction to enzymes in the louses' saliva. The child has missed several weeks of school due to the infestation, which the parents have been attempting to treat by applying mayonnaise to the scalp; the home remedy has not been effective. The parents report that this is the most recent in a series of infestations going back several months.

The child also has symptoms of iron-deficiency anemia; she is pale, fatigued, and she experiences exertional dyspnea. Upon examination her pulse was125 bpm (normal range: 58–90) and her blood pressure was 95/55 mm Hg (normal range: systolic 100–119, diastolic 65–76).

Laboratory values were normal except for the following notable blood test results:

Measured Value	Value	Normal Range
Hemoglobin	4.5 g/dL	11.2–16.5 g/dL (children)
Hematocrit	32%	30–43%
Mean Corpuscular Volume (MCV)	63.8 μm^3/RBC	86–98 μm^3/RBC
Serum iron	55 μg/dL	60–170 μg/dL
Serum ferritin	2.5 ng/mL	7.0–140.0 ng/mL

The laboratory values supported a likely diagnosis of iron-deficiency anemia. A fecal occult blood test was negative, indicating that there was no bleeding in her digestive tract, and a celiac screen was negative. Although no causal relationship has been established between chronic pediculosis capitis and iron-deficiency anemia, a number of cases have been reported that suggest the two may be related.

The child was treated with permethrin 1% cream and a hematologist was consulted to discuss treatment of the iron-deficient anemia.

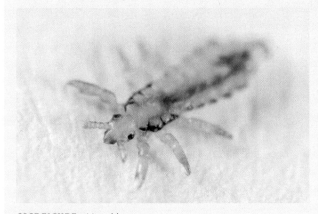

CASE FIGURE: Head louse
© Arlindo71/E+/Getty Images

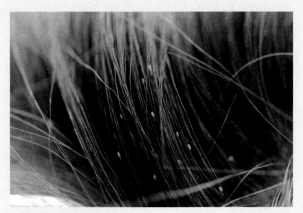

CASE FIGURE: Louse eggs
© Khunkorn/Shutterstock

(continues)

🔍 ADVANCED CASE STUDY   *(continued)*

1. Pediculosis capitis is a condition that results from infestation of the scalp by a species of louse, *Pediculus humanus capitis*. Define the word parts and meaning for *pediculosis capitis*.

   Pediculosis capitis: Pedicul/o _____, -osis _____,

   capitis ____*of the head*____, means _____.

2. Define the word parts for *pediatrician* and *hematologist*.

   Pediatrician: Ped/o _____, iatr/o _____,

   -ician _____.

   Hematologist: Hemat/o _____, -logist _____.

3. The terms systolic and diastolic refer to the arterial blood pressure when the heart muscles are contracted or relaxed, respectively. The keys to the terms are in the word parts systol/o and dia-, what do these word parts mean?

   Systol/o: _____.

   Dia-: _____.

4. Complete the table below for medical term word parts and meaning:

Term	Word Parts	Meaning
anemia	*an-; -emia*	*blood condition without (refers to reduction in red blood cells)*
dyspnea		
hemoglobin		
hematocrit		

5. The patient in the study had a mean corpuscular (or cell) volume of 63.8 µm^3, which refers to the mean volume of erythrocytes. Which condition does this value reflect (circle one)?

   Microcytosis
   Normocytosis
   Macrocytosis

6. What does occult mean and why do you think a fecal occult blood test and celiac screen were performed?

🔍 *ADVANCED CASE STUDY*

2.10 Herpes Zoster

A 55-year-old man presents to his primary care physician with a chief complaint of a pruritic rash on the lower right back. In areas where the rash is severe, vesiculopustular eruptions are present on an erythematous base. The rash is mostly limited to the lumbar region, correlating to dermatomes L2–L3. The patient is febrile and reports feeling lethargic and fatigued; prodromal symptoms include pain and paresthesia in the affected area. At the age of 5 years, the patient had a primary varicella infection (chickenpox), the present symptoms were consistent with a secondary infection, herpes zoster (shingles).

The physician explains, "Shingles is a reactivation of the virus that causes chickenpox. When the symptoms of chickenpox fade, the virus can settle into cells of the nervous system and become inactive for years. In your case, the awakened virus appears to have been dormant for about fifty years in specific spinal nerves. Part of this spinal nerve is dedicated to feeling sensations on the area of the skin that is affected by the rash. This is why you have the numb tingling sensations in this area, and as the infection progressed you developed a rash and eruptions on the skin."

The likely diagnosis is localized herpes zoster. The physician advises the patient to avoid people who are immunosuppressed, or who have not been vaccinated for varicella, until the lesions have dried and crusted over. Oral antiviral therapy is prescribed and a follow-up in one week is requested. The patient will be monitored for postherpetic neuralgia after lesions have healed.

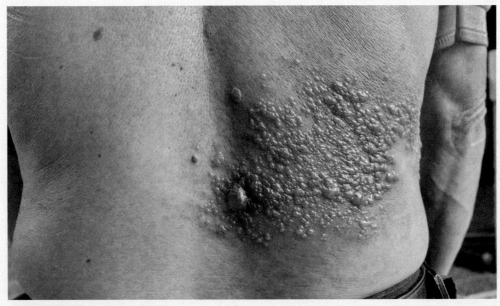

CASE FIGURE: Herpes zoster

© Anukool Manoton/Shutterstock

1. In Greek, dromos means to run, the prefix pro- means before. What do you think prodromal means when used to describe symptoms relating to the shingles rash?

(continues)

🔍 ADVANCED CASE STUDY   *(continued)*

2. Complete the table below for medical term word parts and meaning:

Term	Word Parts	Meaning
pruritic	*prurit/o; -ic*	*pertaining to itchiness*
vesiculopustular		
erythematous		
intercostal		
dermatome		
febrile		
paresthesia		

3. Why is it recommended that the patient avoid people who have not been vaccinated for chickenpox?

4. Patients with herpes zoster may experience postherpetic neuralgia in the affected dermatome. Define the word parts for *postherpetic neuralgia*.

Postherpetic: Post- _____, herpetic _____*pertaining to herpes*_____.

Neuralgia: Neur/o _____, -algia _____.

References

Chamisa, I. (2010). Frey's syndrome--unusually long delayed clinical onset postparotidectomy: A case report. *The Pan African Medical Journal, 5*(1), 1. https://doi.org/10.4314/pamj.v5i1.56198

Durand, R., Andriantsoanirina, V., Brun, S., Laroche, L., & Izri, A. (2018). A case of severe pediculosis capitis. *International Journal of Dermatology, 57*(2), e14–e15.

Fudman, E. J., Golbus, J., & Ike, K. W. (1986). Scleromyxedema with systemic involvement mimics rheumatic diseases. *Arthritis & Rheumatism, 29*(7), 913–917.

Hau, V., & Muhi-Iddin, N. (2014). A ghost covered in lice: A case of severe blood loss with long-standing heavy pediculosis capitis infestation. *BMJ Case Reports, 2014*, bcr2014206623. doi:10.1136/bcr-2014-206623

Megna, M., Gallo, L., Balato, N., & Balato, A. (2019). A case of erythrodermic psoriasis successfully treated with ixekizumab. *Dermatologic Therapy, 32*(2), e12825. https://doi.org/10.1111/dth.12825

Mendes, M. S., Kouzak, S. S., Aquino, T. A., Takano, G. H., & Lima, A. (2013). Mosaic epidermolytic ichthyosis - case report. *Anais Brasileiros de Dermatologia, 88*(6 Suppl 1), 116–119. https://doi.org/10.1590/abd1806-4841.20132203. Herpes zoster.

Mohan, R. P., Verma, S., Singh, U., & Agarwal, N. (2013). Herpes zoster. *BMJ Case Reports, 2013*, bcr2013010246. https://doi.org/10.1136/bcr-2013-010246

Park, S., & Dock, M. (2003). Xeroderma pigmentosum: A case report. *Pediatric Dentistry, 25*(4), 397–400.

Sala, A. C., Cunha, P. R., Pinto, C. A., Alves, C. A., Paiva, I. B., & Araujo, A. P. (2016). Scleromyxedema: Clinical diagnosis and autopsy findings. *Anais Brasileiros de Dermatologia, 91*(5 Suppl 1), 48–50. doi:10.1590/abd1806-4841.20164527

Stedman, T. L. (2005). Nath's *Stedman's medical terminology, 2e*. Philadelphia: Lippincott Williams & Wilkins.

Su, W. P., Chun, S., Hammond, D. E., & Gordon, H. (1990). Pachyonychia congenita: A clinical study of 12 cases and review of the literature. *Pediatric Dermatology, 7*(1), 33–38. https://doi.org/10.1111/j.1525-1470.1990.tb01070.x

Venes, D., & Taber, C. W. (2017). *Taber's Cyclopedic Medical Dictionary*. Ed. 23, illustrated in full color/Philadelphia: F.A. Davis.

Woodruff, C. M., & Chang, A. Y. (2019). More than skin deep: Severe iron deficiency anemia and eosinophilia associated with pediculosis capitis and corporis infestation. *JAAD Case Reports, 5*(5), 444–447.

CHAPTER 3

Musculoskeletal System

KEY TERMS

Actin
Appendicular skeleton
Articular cartilage
Axial skeleton
Cardiac muscle
Compact bone
Deep fascia
Diaphysis
Epiphysis
Fascia
Fascicle
Flat bone

Hyaline cartilage
Intercalcated disc
Irregular bone
Long bone
Medullary (marrow) cavity
Muscle fiber
Myofibril
Myosin
Periosteum
Red bone marrow
Sarcomere
Sesamoid bone

Short bone
Skeletal muscle
Smooth muscle
Spongy bone
Sprain
Strain
Striated muscle
Superficial fascia
Tendon
Thick filament
Thin filament
Yellow bone marrow

The musculoskeletal system is a combination of two body systems that are sometimes considered independently, the muscular system and the skeletal system. The muscular system is composed primarily of muscle tissue. The skeletal system contains tendons, ligaments, cartilage, and bones. Both work together to maintain body structure, drive body movement, and provide protection for organs.

Muscle tissue is classified as one of three types: skeletal muscle, smooth muscle, or cardiac muscle. **Skeletal muscle** is also referred to as **striated muscle** and is so named because alternating light and dark bands are visible when this tissue is examined microscopically. It accounts for almost 50% of the body's weight. It is controlled voluntarily and drives the body's movements by acting on the skeleton.

Skeletal muscle tissue is surrounded and protected by connective tissue called **fascia**. **Superficial fascia** separates muscle from skin. Through this layer of connective tissue and fat, nerves, blood vessels and lymphatic vessels are able to enter and leave muscle. This layer also provides insulation and protects muscles from damage. A layer of tough fibrous connective tissue called **deep fascia** holds muscles with similar functions together and lines the body wall. This fascia surrounds groups of individual muscle cells, or **muscle fibers** to assemble them in units called **fascicles**. The muscle fibers contain microscopic

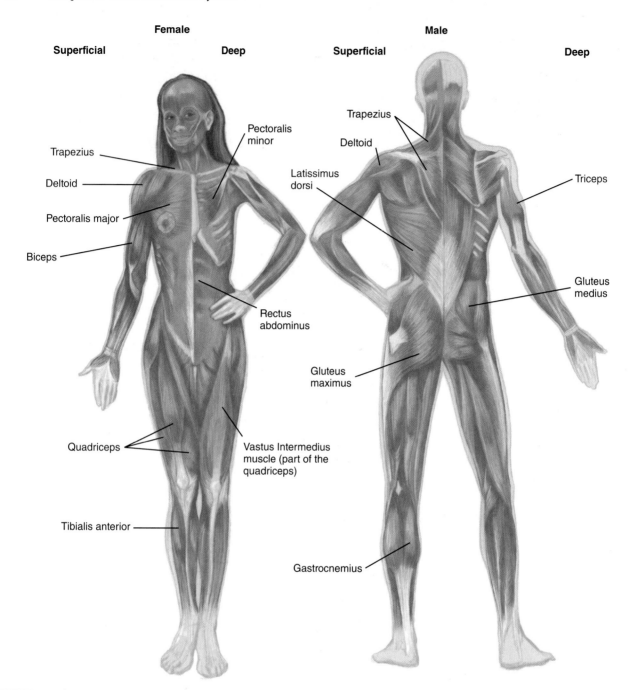

FIGURE 3.1 The major muscles of the muscular system

structures called **myofibrils**. These are the contractile organelles of skeletal muscle. The myofibrils are made up of **thin filaments** containing **actin** and **thick filaments** containing **myosin**. These are the contractile proteins of muscle. Overlapping groups of these filaments are called **sarcomeres** and it is these groups that give skeletal muscle its classic striations under the microscope.

Cardiac muscle constitutes the walls of the heart, the muscular pump that propels blood through the cardiovascular system. Its movement cannot be consciously controlled. Cardiac muscle fibers have the same arrangement of sarcomeres as skeletal muscle; however, the ends of these muscle fibers are connected by double layers of membrane that form **intercalated discs**. These discs help bind the muscle cells together and ensure coordinated signaling between the cells, which are necessary for heart muscle cells to contract in unison.

The movement of **smooth muscle**, also referred to as visceral muscle, is involuntary. This muscle type surrounds tube-like organs of the body, such as blood vessels and the digestive tract, and regulates the movements of tube contents. Smooth muscle looks

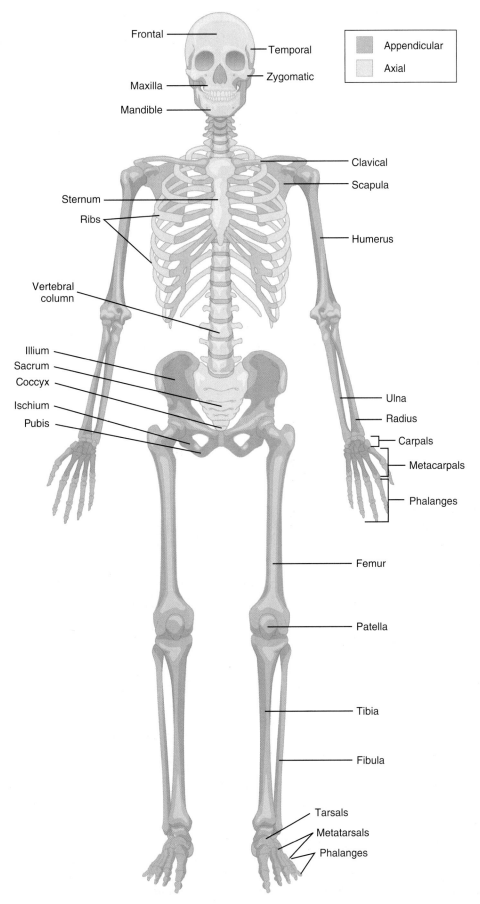

FIGURE 3.2 The major bones of the skeletal system

Types of Muscle

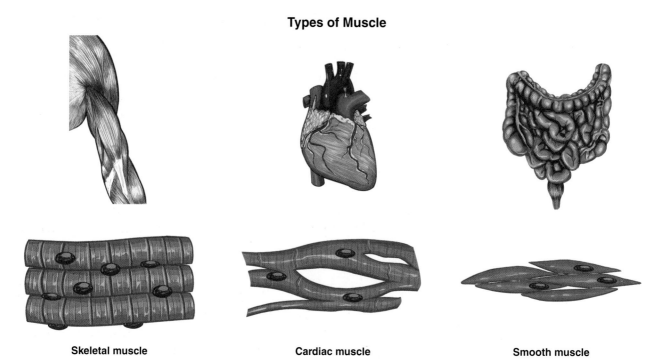

Skeletal muscle   **Cardiac muscle**   **Smooth muscle**

FIGURE 3.3 The three types of muscle tissue

© Drp8/Shutterstock

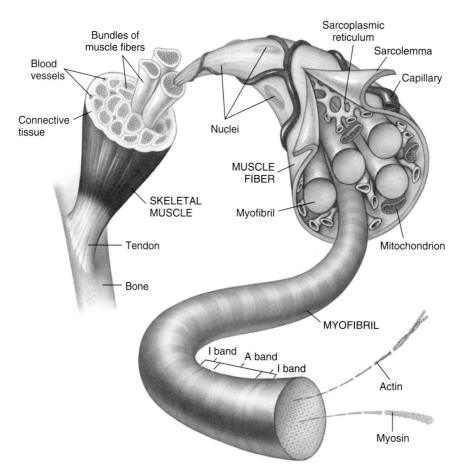

FIGURE 3.4 Skeletal muscle structure

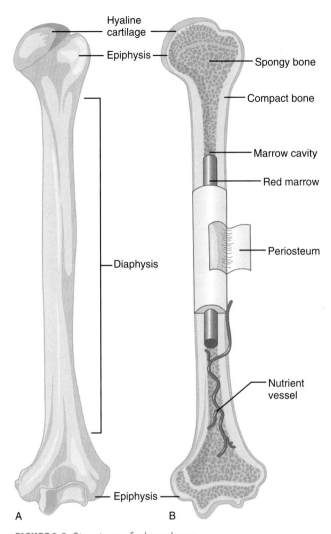

Hyaline cartilage

Epiphysis

Spongy bone

Compact bone

Marrow cavity

Red marrow

Diaphysis

Periosteum

Nutrient vessel

Epiphysis

A

B

FIGURE 3.5 Structure of a long bone

the spinal column. **Sesamoid bones** are shaped like a sesame seed (as their name implies). They can vary in number from person to person; however, an example that is present in everyone is the patella (kneecap). **Short bones** are roughly cubed shaped and are approximately equal in length and width. Examples are the carpals of the wrist and tarsals of the foot.

Most of the bones of the body are **long bones** consisting of a central shaft called a **diaphysis**, which widens at each end to an **epiphysis**. A tough sheath of dense connective tissue called the **periosteum** covers long bones. This protects the bone and assists in repairing fractures. The epiphyses of long bone are covered with **hyaline cartilage**, a glossy connective tissue made of collagen. Because it is found on the surface of the bone that articulates or joins with another bone, in this location, it is called **articular cartilage**; its role is to absorb shock and reduce friction.

Compact bone forms the hard walls of a long bone. This strong bone type is able to resist the stresses produced by weight and movement. Its hard matrix, composed of calcium and phosphate, can be extracted and transferred to systemic circulation when needed. **Spongy bone** lies deep to compact bone. Spongy bone is light to reduce the overall weight of a bone and it also supports and protects **red bone marrow**, which is the site of hematopoiesis or blood cell production. The cavity within the diaphysis is called the **medullary (marrow) cavity**, which contains **yellow bone marrow**, mostly composed of fat cells. Examples of long bones are the humerus of the arm and the femur of the leg.

considerably different from skeletal or cardiac muscle. These fibers have no striations and are tapered at each end. The speed of contraction of smooth muscle is slower than both skeletal and cardiac muscle. Muscle tissue provides motive forces as a result of muscle cell contraction, which contributes to the ability of the body to generate heat and to thermoregulate.

Bones come together at joints to form the skeleton, which provides structure and protection for the body and its organs. There are five main types of bone in the body, which are classified by shape. These are flat, irregular, sesamoid, short, and long. **Flat bones** are typically plate shaped. They provide significant protection and extensive area for muscle attachment. Examples are the sternum (breastbone) and ribs, which protect organs in the thorax such as the heart; and the cranial bones, which form part of the skull and protect the brain. **Irregular bones** have complex and irregular shapes. Examples are the maxilla and mandible, which form the jaw, and the vertebrae, which form

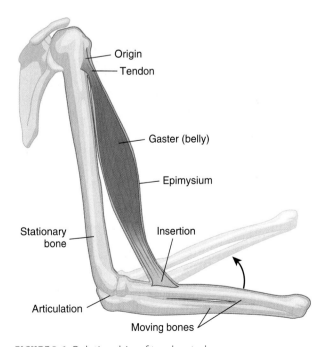

Origin

Tendon

Gaster (belly)

Epimysium

Stationary bone

Insertion

Articulation

Moving bones

FIGURE 3.6 Relationship of tendon to bone

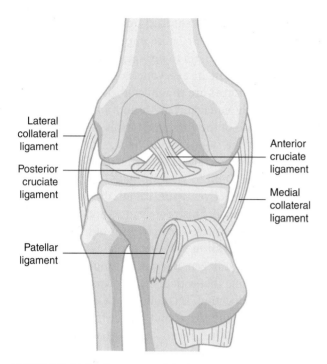

FIGURE 3.7 Major ligaments of the knee

There are approximately 206 bones in the adult human skeleton, most of which are paired on the left and right side of the body. These bones are grouped into two categories: the axial skeleton and the appendicular skeleton. The **axial skeleton** consists of the 80 bones that make up the head and trunk. The **appendicular skeleton** consists of the 126 bones that support the appendages. Individuals may have more or fewer bones due to anatomical variation. One example is the variation in the number of sesamoid bones among individuals.

Bones serve as attachment points for muscle, assisting body movement. Muscle attaches to bone with tough bands of fibrous connective tissue called **tendons**. Tendons also connect muscles to each other. Ligaments are also tough bands of fibrous connective tissue; they connect bones to other bones. When a joint is twisted forcibly enough to tear a ligament, it is called a **sprain**. Surrounding blood vessels, muscles, nerves, and tendons may also be damaged. Conversely, a **strain** is an overstretched or partially torn muscle.

TABLE 3.1
Key Musculoskeletal System Prefixes
ab-: away from
ad-: toward

TABLE 3.2
Key Musculoskeletal System Combining Forms
arthr/o: joint
auricul/o: ear
burs/o: sac
calcane/o: heel
carp/o: wrist
cervic/o: neck; cervix
cheil/o: lip
chondr/o: cartilage
cost/o: rib
crani/o: skull
dactyl/o: digit, finger, toe
dentin/o: teeth
duct/o: to bring; duct
extens/o: to stretch out
femor/o: femur
flex/o: to bend
gnath/o: jaw, mandible
kyph/o: hump
lord/o: curve
lumb/o: lower back
maxill/o: maxilla, upper jaw
metacarp/o: metacarpals, hand bones
muscul/o: muscle
my/o: muscle
ophthalm/o: eye
orth/o: straight

TABLE 3.2	*(conitnued)*
Key Musculoskeletal System Combining Forms	
oste/o: bone	
palat/o: palate	
phalang/o: phalange, finger, toe	
rhabdomy/o: skeletal muscle	
rheumat/o: watery flow	
roentgen/o: unit of X-ray exposure	
rotat/o: rotation	
sacr/o: sacrum	
scoli/o: crooked	
spondyl/o: vertebra	
stomat/o: mouth	
tend/o: tendon	
ten/o: tendon	
tendin/o: tendon	
vertebr/o: vertebra	

TABLE 3.3
Key Musculoskeletal System Suffixes
-asthenia: weakness
-desis: surgical fusion
-ion: process
-kinesis: movement
-listhesis: slipping
-malacia: softening
-ostosis: bone development
-paresis: paralysis
-penia: decrease
-phyte: plant-like growth
-plasia: development; formation of cells
-porosis: porous
-ptosis: drooping, drooping eyelid
-schisis: to split
-tonia: tone

STANDARD CASE STUDY

3.1 Spondylolysis
Current Complaint: Patient is a 15-year-old female gymnast presenting to the department of orthopedics with acute back pain in the lumbar region. On a scale of 1–10, the patient reports pain of 9.

Past History: Patient reports a yearlong history of low back pain that has recently become unmanageable.

Signs and Symptoms: Patient's pain extends to the buttocks and radiates downwards. Patient does not report tenderness on palpation. Patient's posture is hyperlordotic and she presents with exceptionally tight hamstrings. She reports a dull ache that has been present for the past year with significant pain increase after her last competition, where many of her moves required hyperextension. Upon examination, pain increases with lumbar extension and rotation, but not with flexion.

Diagnosis: Radiographic imaging confirms spondylolysis, a stress fracture of the pars interarticularis, which has progressed to spondylolisthesis, a condition in which a vertebra slips out of place.

Treatment: Conservative management with rest, refraining from sport until pain free, lumbar-sacral orthosis, and physical therapy. Rehabilitation exercises should focus on stabilization, flexibility, and building hip abduction and

(continues)

adduction strength. More aggressive treatments, including spondylosyndesis, will be discussed if patient does not respond to conservative treatment.

SPONDYLOLYSIS AND SPONDYLOLISTHESIS

PARS INTERARTICULARIS	SPONDYLOLYSIS	SPONDYLOLISTHESIS

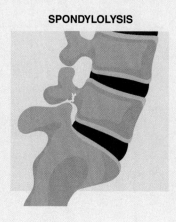
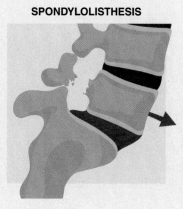

© Logika600/Shutterstock

1. The combining form spondyl/o means _____.

    Another combining form, not used in this case, also meaning this is _____.

    Contrast the difference in usage of these two combining terms.

2. The term in the case referring to the region of the low back is _____.

3. Define the word parts for *hyperlordotic*.

    Hyperlordotic: Hyper- _____, lord/o _____, -tic _____,

    means _____.

4. Complete the following table for the muscle action terms used in the case:

Term	Word Parts	Meaning
extension	*extens/o; -ion*	*action of stretching out*
flexion		
rotation		
abduction		
adduction		

5. Complete the following table for the pathologies and procedures in this case:

Term	Word Parts	Meaning
spondylolysis	*spondyl/o; -lysis*	*breakdown of a vertebra*
spondylolisthesis		
spondylosyndesis		

6. Define the word parts for *lumbar-sacral orthosis* and explain what is meant by this therapeutic term.

Lumbar-sacral orthosis: Lumb/o _____, -ar _____,

sacr/o _____ -al _____,

orth/o _____, -osis _____.

7. What is hyperextension and why are athletes, for example gymnasts, who frequently hyperextend, susceptible to spondylytic injuries?

🔍 *STANDARD CASE STUDY*

3.2 Meyenburg-Altherr-Uehlinger Syndrome

Mrs. Zavala, age 57, is seen by her rheumatologist for an acute painful inflammatory crisis of a previously diagnosed disease, Meyenburg-Altherr-Uehlinger syndrome, which is thought to be an autoimmune disease. Her current presenting symptom is bilateral auricular chondritis with erythematous edematous pinnae. Swelling and tenderness extend to both postauricular regions without associated mastoid tenderness. Additional complaints include polyarthralgia and polyarthritis, most severe in her metacarpophalangeal joints and knees. During examination, the rheumatologist notes nasal chondritis along with arthropathy of the costochondral joints that are attributed to costochondritis. Mrs. Zavala is prescribed corticosteroids to treat this most recent flare-up of her disease. She will continue to be monitored for systemic disease involvement and recurrent episodes of cartilage inflammation will be treated as they occur.

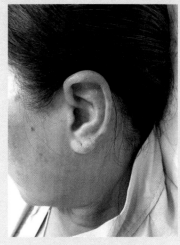

CASE FIGURE: Red swollen pinna
© Iweevy/Shutterstock

1. Define the word parts and meaning for the following terms that relate to the patient's symptoms:

Bilateral auricular chondritis: Bi- _____, later/o _____,

-al _____, auricul/o _____,

(continues)

-ar _____, chondr/o _____,

-itis _____, means _____.

Erythematous edematous pinnae: Erythr/o _____, hemat/o _____,

-ous _____, -edema _____,

-ous _____, pinnae ___*outer ears*___,

means _____.

2. Swelling and tenderness extend to the postauricular region without mastoid tenderness. Indicate word parts for *postauricular* and explain the location of the tenderness.

3. Define the word parts and meaning for the following joint regions related to the location of the patient's symptoms:

Metacarpophalangeal: Metacarp/o _____ phalang/o _____,

-al _____, means _____.

Costochondral: Cost/o _____, chondr/o _____, -al _____,

means _____.

4. Complete the following table for the pathologies in this case:

Term	Word Parts	Meaning
polyarthralgia	*poly-; arthr/o; -algia*	*pain of many joints*
polyarthritis		
arthropathy		
costochondritis		

5. Relapse means to fall back. Another name for the disease described in this case is relapsing polychondritis. Explain.

6. Recurrent inflammation in the tracheobronchial region can result in softening of cartilage in this area and can be a life-threatening complication of this disease. The medical term for softening of cartilage is

_____.

7. Inflammation of the outer part of the ear as described in this case is a classic symptom of the disease. Inflammation does not involve the earlobe, however. Why do you think that is true?

🔍 *STANDARD CASE STUDY*

3.3 Apert Syndrome
Craniofacial Surgery Consultation Report

Reason for Consultation: Discussion of upcoming endoscopic strip craniectomy.

History of Present Illness: Patient is a 3-month-old male with craniosynostosis resulting from Apert Syndrome, diagnosed at birth. The patient has multiple craniofacial deformities including acrocephaly, maxillary hypoplasia, and pseudoprognathism. Ocular manifestations include hypertelorism and exophthalmos. Bilateral syndactyly of hands and feet is also present.

Results of Physical Examination: Notwithstanding craniofacial deformities and syndactyly of digits, patient appears healthy with all vital signs within normal range. Patient is evaluated for possible respiratory, cardiac, and neurological manifestations of Apert Syndrome, which

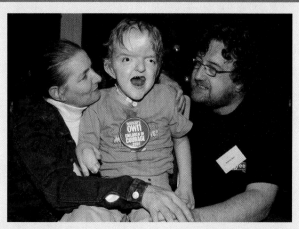

CASE FIGURE: A seven-year-old boy with Apert Syndrome
© Fiona Hanson - PA Images/Getty Images

appear not to be present at this time. Developmental milestones are age-appropriate.

Assessment: Patient and parents are prepared for scheduled surgery next month. Early endoscopic suture release by 4 months of age will give the brain adequate room to grow and will minimize risk of brain injury to the child.

Recommendation: Proceed with scheduled endoscopic strip craniectomy followed by helmet therapy to reduce skull shape deformity. Continue follow-up with multidisciplinary medical team in anticipation of future surgeries, possible hearing and speech problems, and dental issues related to jaw malformations.

1. Define the word parts for *acrocephalosyndactyly*, another term for Apert Syndrome:

    Acrocephalosyndactyly: Acr/o _____, cephal/o _____,

    syn- _____, dactyl/o _____,

    -y _____,

    means _____.

2. Indicate and define the component word parts for *endoscopic* and *craniectomy* and then describe what type of procedure an endoscopic strip craniectomy is.

(continues)

🔍 *STANDARD CASE STUDY*   *(continued)*

3. Complete the table below listing the symptoms of Apert Syndrome:

Term	Word Parts	Meaning
craniosynostosis	*crani/o ; syn-; -ostosis*	*bone condition of the skull together (occurs when the fibrous joints of the skull fuse prematurely)*
acrocephaly		
maxillary hypoplasia		
pseudoprognathism		
hypertelorism (ocular)		
exophthalmos		
bilateral syndactyly		

4. What does suture release refer to and why should it be performed when a child is still very young?

5. What do you think helmet therapy is and why would it be done after strip craniectomy?

🔍 *STANDARD CASE STUDY*

3.4 Osteoarthritis

S.A., a 77-year-old Caucasian woman, presented to her primary care physician (PCP) with a chief complaint of bilateral knee arthralgia. The patient's gait was mildly antalgic and her posture suggested reduced vertebral support. She had comorbid hypertension, hyperparathyroidism, and osteopenia. She reported that she staves off osteoporosis by eating a diet rich in calcium and vitamin D, taking long daily walks, and denies use of alcohol and tobacco. Despite these efforts, S.A. felt anxious about a loss of bone density and the pain that had developed in her knees. The PCP suspected that the cause of the knee arthralgia was osteoarthritis (OA), and was also concerned that the patient's osteopenia had progressed to osteoporosis. OA and osteoporosis are distinct but may occur together in older patients because the incidence of each increases with age. The PCP ordered knee X-rays for evidence of OA and a bone mineral density (BMD) test as a diagnostic for osteoporosis.

A knee X-ray can identify characteristics of osteoarthritis (OA), which is a degenerative disorder that presents with articular cartilage deterioration, osteophyte formation, subchondral sclerosis, and cysts. The knee X-ray identified roentgenographic signs of OA, including subchondral sclerosis and bony osteophytes, supporting a diagnosis of OA. The X-ray also ruled out bursitis, an inflammation of the sacs found in the vicinity of joints, that may present like OA.

A BMD test can provide information on bone health. The most common BMD test is central dual energy X-ray absorptiometry (DEXA), which measures bone density at the hip and lumbar spine. The test provides a BMD score that classifies bone density as normal, or diagnoses osteopenia or osteoporosis. The BMD test confirmed that the patient's osteopenia had progressed to osteoporosis.

S.A. was referred to a rheumatologist for treatment options for osteoporosis and OA.

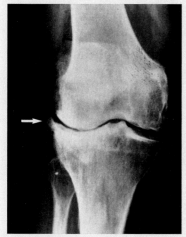

CASE FIGURE: Tibial osteophyte

OSTEOARTHRITIS

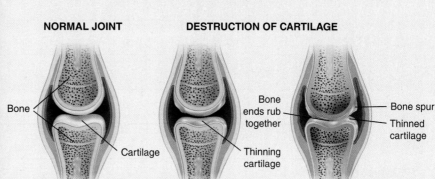

CASE FIGURE: Comparison of the articular cartilage in a normal joint to one with osteoarthritis

© Tefi/Shutterstock

1. The patient's chief complaint was bilateral knee arthralgia. Define the word parts for *bilateral* and *arthralgia* and then explain in general terms what is meant by bilateral knee arthralgia:

   Bilateral: Bi- _____, later/o _____, -al _____.

   Arthralgia: Arthr/o _____, -algia _____.

2. The term morbid means unhealthy or diseased. What does comorbid mean?

3. In this case, the patient presents with three comorbid diseases, presenting concurrent with the chief complaint of knee arthralgia. List the word parts, and a brief description, for the three comorbid diseases:

4. Define the word parts for *osteoporosis* and then explain how it is different from osteopenia.

   Osteoporosis: Oste/o _____, -porosis _____.

5. The knee X-rays produce roentgenographs of subchondral sclerosis and body osteophytes that are evidence of OA. The X-rays also rule out bursitis. Define the word parts and meaning for *roentgenograph*, *subchondral sclerosis*, *osteophyte,* and *bursitis.*

   Roentgenograph: Roentgen/o _____, -graph _____,

   means _____.

(continues)

🔍 *STANDARD CASE STUDY*   *(continued)*

Subchondral sclerosis: Sub- _____, chondr/o _____,

-al _____, scler/o _____, -osis _____,

means _____.

Osteophyte: Oste/o _____, -phyte _____,

means _____.

Bursitis: Burs/o _____, -itis _____,

means _____.

6. Define the word parts for *rheumatologist*, and what their specialty is.

Rheumatologist: Rheumat/o _____, -logist _____,

specializes in _____.

🔍 *STANDARD CASE STUDY*

3.5 Pierre Robin Sequence

A 4-year-old girl with Pierre Robin sequence, a constellation of congenital abnormalities that arise sequentially from mandibular hypotrophy, undergoes restorative surgery to correct a left-sided cleft lip, jaw, and palate. In addition to the craniofacial abnormality, the patient presented with typical symptoms of the disorder: retrognathia, micrognathia, glossoptosis, and associated dyspnea. The corrective surgery was undertaken to ameliorate complications with the patient's breathing and eating.

1. Why is Pierre Robin referred to as a sequence, not a syndrome, in this case?

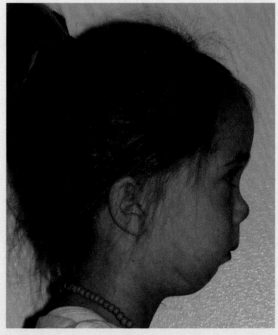

CASE FIGURE: A little girl with the facial abnormalities typical of Pierre Robin sequence

Courtesy of Cleft and Craniofacial Center at Cincinnati Children's Hospital Medical Center.

2. Define the word parts and meaning for *craniofacial*.

    Craniofacial: Crani/o _____, facial _____*facial*_____,

    means _____.

3. Define the following word parts and then circle the type of craniofacial abnormality in this case:

    Bilateral cheiloschisis: Bi- _____, later/o _____, -al _____,

    cheil/o _____, -schisis _____.

    Unilateral gnathoschisis: Uni- _____, later/o _____, -al _____,

    gnath/o _____, -schisis _____.

    Bilateral cheilognathoschisis: Bi- _____, later/o _____,

    -al _____, cheil/o _____,

    gnath/o _____, -schisis _____.

    Unilateral cheilognathopalatoschisis: Uni- _____, later/o _____,

    -al _____, cheil/o _____,

    gnath/o _____, palat/o _____,

    -schisis _____.

4. Complete the following table for the Pierre Robin sequence anomalies reported in the case:

Term	Word Parts	Meaning
retrognathia	*retro; gnath/o; -ia*	*condition of posterior position of the mandible*
micrognathia		
glossoptosis		
dyspnea		

5. Pierre Robin sequence is named after a French stomatologist who documented the disorder in 1923. Indicate the word parts for *stomatologist* and then describe the specialization of this professional.

(continues)

⌕ *STANDARD CASE STUDY* *(continued)*

6. Define the following word parts and then circle the type of corrective surgery in this case:

   Arthroplasty: Arthr/o _____, -plasty _____.

   Chondroplasty: Chondr/o _____, -plasty _____.

   Vertebroplasty: Vertebr/o _____, -plasty _____.

   Gnathoplasty: Gnath/o _____, -plasty _____.

   Femoroplasty: Femor/o _____, -plasty _____.

⌕ *ADVANCED CASE STUDY*

3.6 Osteogenesis Imperfecta

Cyrus and Hazel Mennas were beside themselves. This was the second fracture suffered by their 2-year-old daughter Lena who had fallen while playing in the yard with her brother. After her fall, Lena would not stop crying and refused to place any weight on her left leg. An X-ray of her leg revealed a spiral fracture of the tibial diaphysis, an injury that seemed out of proportion to the type of fall. Of additional concern were the fracture of her clavicle that Lena had suffered 6 months ago from a roll off of a low mattress, and the results from a radiographic skeletal survey revealing a previous humeral fracture, now healed. Child abuse is often suspected when repeated fractures are diagnosed in young children, but in this case, detailed interviews with the parents uncovered Hazel's history of frequent bone fractures when she was younger. The physician recognized the connection and after further testing, Lena was diagnosed with osteogenesis imperfecta (OI).

OI is also known as brittle bone disease and clinical presentation can range from mild to severe. In addition to frequent fractures of all types, signs and symptoms can include short stature, muscle weakness, ostealgia, osteopenia, scoliosis, kyphosis, and dentinogenesis imperfecta. Treatment focuses on minimizing fractures and managing them when they occur. Approaches include medication to increase bone mass, physical and occupational therapy, and surgery. Lena will be followed throughout her life by a multidisciplinary team with the goal of maximizing independent function.

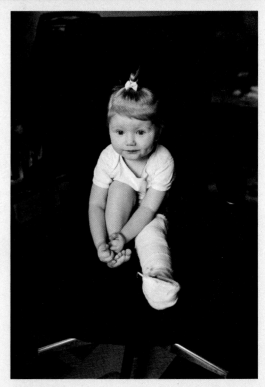

CASE FIGURE: Little girl with a fractured tibia

© Sergii Sobolevskyi/Shutterstock

1. Define the word parts for *osteogenesis* and explain what osteogenesis imperfecta is. Osteogenesis:

   Oste/o _____, -genesis _____.

2. Provide the common name for the location of fractures suffered by Lena.

   Tibial diaphysis:

Clavicle:

Humerus:

3. All types of fractures can occur with OI. Complete the following table describing fracture types. Use a medical dictionary if necessary:

Fracture Type	Description
spiral	*fracture line spirals around the shaft of the bone; often caused by a twisting injury*
comminuted	
transverse	
impacted	
greenstick	
closed	
compound	

4. Complete the following table for the signs and symptoms of OI:

Term	Word Parts	Meaning
ostealgia	*oste/o; -algia*	*pain of bone*
osteopenia		
scoliosis		
kyphosis		
dentinogenesis (imperfecta)		

5. Why do you think the signs of OI are often confused with child abuse?

🔍 *ADVANCED CASE STUDY*

3.7 Achilles Tendon Rupture

Nile Garcia was brought to the emergency department (ED) by his husband. He reported that he was playing a pick-up game of basketball with his young son when he heard a loud pop and felt a sudden severe pain in the back of his left ankle. His description of forced dorsiflexion of the ankle while landing a jump, and a physical examination, were consistent with a calcaneal tendon rupture. Ecchymosis and edema were present on the posterior portion of his ankle and tenodynia was noted. Using a contralateral comparison, a palpable defect of the left Achilles tendon was noted. Mr. Garcia was asked to lie in a prone position with his feet over the edge of the table. Squeezing of his calf muscle by the attending physician failed to elicit plantar flexion, a physical finding indicative of Achilles tendon rupture. A splint and crutches were provided, Mr. Garcia was instructed not to place weight on his left leg, and an appointment with an orthopedist was scheduled for the next day.

The orthopedist confirmed the diagnosis of an Achilles-tendon rupture and presented the patient with both surgical and nonsurgical treatment options. After learning that minimally invasive surgical management is associated with faster recovery time, quicker return to sports, and lower incidence of re-rupture, the patient opted for tendinoplasty as soon as possible. Following a successful tenorrhaphy of the proximal and distal ends of the damaged tendon, Mr. Garcia was placed in a cast. Full recovery is expected to take several months.

Calf Squeeze Test For Achilles Tendon Rupture

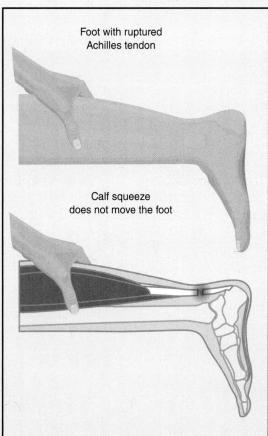
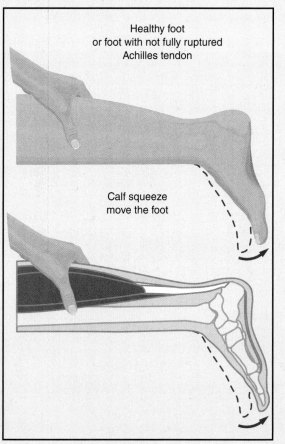

CASE FIGURE: Calf-test squeeze for ruptured Achilles tendon
© Aksanaku/Shutterstock

1. Define the word parts for *calcaneal*:

   Calcaneal: Calcane/o _____, -al _____.

2. Complete the following table for the muscle action and positional terms used in the case:

Term	Word Parts	Meaning
dorsiflexion	*dors/o; flex/o; -ion*	*process of bending backwards*
posterior		
contralateral		
prone	N/A	
plantar flexion		
proximal		
distal		

3. There are three different combining forms for the word tendon. List these.

4. List the words in the case pertaining to tendons, indicate their word parts, and define the terms.

🔍 *ADVANCED CASE STUDY*

3.8 Myasthenia Gravis

A 30-year-old woman presented to her primary care physician with ophthalmoparesis, ptosis, and binocular diplopia. She reported that the symptoms started a few months prior and tend to become more severe throughout the day. In the evening, she also experiences oropharyngeal muscle fatigue resulting in dysarthria and dysphagia. A cranial nerve examination showed near ophthalmoplegia. Applying a latex glove filled with crushed ice to the patient's eyes for 3 minutes improved ptosis, suggestive of myasthenia gravis, an autoimmune disorder of the neuromuscular junction that increases muscle fatigue. The patient was referred to a neurologist for consultation. A repetitive nerve stimulation test and a high titer of antibodies to the acetylcholine receptor confirmed a diagnosis of myasthenia gravis.

1. Define the word parts for *neurologist*.

Neurologist: Neur/o _____, -logist _____.

(continues)

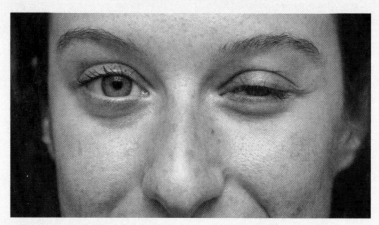

CASE FIGURE: Ptosis of the eye

© Sruilk/Shutterstock

2. Myasthenia gravis is an autoimmune neuromuscular disease. Communication between neurons and skeletal muscle cells is normally mediated by acetylcholine receptors on the muscle cells, which are attacked in patients with myasthenia gravis. Gravis is a Latin word that means serious, or grave. Define the following word parts for *neuromuscular* and *myasthenia*:

Neuromuscular: Neur/o _____, muscul/o _____,

        -ar _____.

Myasthenia: My/o- _____, -asthenia _____.

3. Explain what an autoimmune disease is. You may need to refer to a medical dictionary, or other resource, to complete your explanation.

4. Complete the table below for the following terms:

Term	Word Parts	Meaning
ophthalmoparesis	*ophthalm/o; -paresis*	*eye weakness (refers to the eye muscle)*
ophthalmoplegia		
ptosis (may also be used as a suffix, -ptosis)		
diplopia		
dysarthria		
dysphagia		

🔍 *ADVANCED CASE STUDY*

3.9 Tetanus

A mother brings her 10-year-old boy to the emergency department (ED) presenting with dyspnea; intermittent tonic spasms; and hypertonia of muscles in the mandibular, cervical, and dorsal body regions, resulting in risus sardonicus and trismus, and opisthotonus. The mother reports that the child was playing barefoot in their barn a week earlier and received a deep laceration on the sole of his left foot. The child was treated for the injury at home and then a few days later, he started to experience jaw discomfort, sialorrhea, anorexia, and drowsiness. The mother became concerned as the symptoms became progressively worse.

The child had not received any childhood vaccinations, including one to protect against tetanus. An infection of the foot injury by the bacterium *Clostridium tetani,* which produces the tetanus neurotoxin (tetanospasmin), was the suspected cause of the spasms. The child was sedated, intubated with an endotracheal tube, and mechanical ventilation was started prior to transfer to the pediatric intensive care unit. A necrectomy was performed on the foot injury to remove dead tissue. Tetanus immune globulin (antibody) was administered to bind to, and neutralize, circulating tetanospasmin. A high dose of intravenous antibiotic was administered to treat the *C. tetani* infection. The parent plans to give the child the tetanus vaccine once he has recovered.

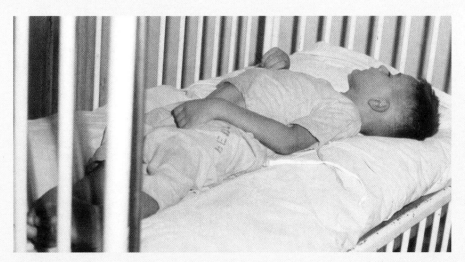

CASE FIGURE: The spasms typical of tetanus

Courtesy of Robert Krasner.

1. Indicate and define the component word parts for *hypertonia* and then use common terms to describe what is meant by hypertonia of muscles of the mandibular, cervical, and dorsal body regions.

2. The term *risus sardonicus* is Latin; it means a sardonic laugh. Using a medical dictionary, or other resource, explain what *risus* and *sardonicus* mean and how the term relates to the symptom.

(continues)

🔍 ADVANCED CASE STUDY *(continued)*

3. The term *trismus* is Greek; it means gnashing or grinding. Using a medical dictionary, or other resource, explain how the meaning of *trismus* relates to the symptom.

4. Complete the table below for the following terms that relate to the symptoms and treatment of tetanus in this case:

Term	Word Parts	Meaning
opisthotonous	*opisth/o; ton/o; -ous*	*pertaining to tension of backward/behind (back spasm)*
sialorrhea		
anorexia		
pediatric		
endotracheal		
necrectomy		

🔍 ADVANCED CASE STUDY

3.10 Crush Syndrome

Emergency Medical Services (EMS) were dispatched to a construction site at 9 a.m. for prehospital management and transport of a 45-year-old female with a crush injury to her lower right leg with tibial and fibular shaft fractures. The injury, resulting from a fallen steel beam, occurred several hours before her coworkers arrived at the site. Her coworkers found her trapped in the supine position by the beam and called 911. The dispatcher advised the coworkers to leave the patient and steel beam in place, nevertheless the coworkers removed the steel beam from the patient's leg and applied a tourniquet proximal to the injury.

The Emergency Medical Technicians (EMTs) found the patient alert and complaining of severe pain at the site of injury. Her vital signs suggested hypovolemia, hypotension (blood pressure 75/55 mmHg), tachycardia (heart rate 160 beats/min), and hyperpnea (respiratory rate 35 breaths/min). Paramedics attached a cardiac monitor and a 12-lead electrocardiogram revealed dysrhythmia characteristic of hyperkalemia. Analgesics were administered. Concerned that the patient had crush syndrome, the paramedics began aggressive fluid resuscitation with 0.9% saline and prepared the patient for transport to an emergency department.

Crush syndrome, also called traumatic rhabdomyolysis, occurs when skeletal muscle is subject to prolonged traumatic compression and then the compression is relieved and the tissue is reperfused. Compression may cause skeletal muscle ischemia and necrosis and cell lysis and dissolution. Reperfusion drives contents from damaged muscle cells (e.g., myoglobin, K⁺) into systemic circulation; plasma myoglobin may disrupt kidney function and lead to myoglobinuric renal failure. Impaired kidney function and lactic acid production by ischemic muscle tissue (anaerobic respiration) may result in metabolic acidosis. Moreover, damage to skeletal muscle tissue and increased capillary permeability shifts extracellular fluids into the site of injury, resulting in intravascular volume loss. Hypovolemia may be exacerbated by hemorrhagic volume loss. The most serious complication of crush syndrome is acute renal failure with a primary concern of dysrhythmia. A critical prehospital treatment is aggressive intravenous fluid resuscitation.

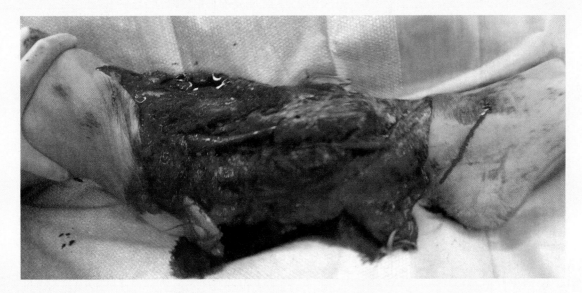

CASE FIGURE: Crush injury to lower leg

1. Which bones were fractured by the falling beam in this case?

2. The patient was found in the supine position. Describe this position.

3. Complete the table below for the following terms related to hypovolemia in this case:

Term	Word Parts	Meaning
hypovolemia	*hypo-; -volemia*	insufficient blood volume
hypotension		
tachycardia		
hyperpnea		

4. Define the word parts and meaning for *ischemia*, *dysrhythmia*, *hyperkalemia*, *analgesic*, and *hemorrhagic*:

   Ischemia: Isch/o _____, -emia _____,

   means _____.

(continues)

Dysrhythmia: Dys- _____, rhythm/o _____,

-ia _____,

means _____.

Hyperkalemia: Hyper- _____, kal/i _____,

-emia _____,

means _____.

Analgesic: An- _____, alges/o _____,

-ic _____,

means _____.

Hemorrhagic: Hem/o _____, -rrhage _____,

-ic _____,

means _____.

5. Define the word parts for *rhabdomyolysis*.

Rhabdomyolysis: Rhabdomy/o _____, -lysis _____.

6. Define the word parts for *myoglobinuric* and *renal* and then based on those word parts, explain what myoglobinuric renal failure is.

Myoglobinuric renal: My/o _____, globin/o _____,

ur/o _____, -ic _____,

ren/o _____, -al _____.

7. The 911 dispatcher advised the coworkers to leave the patient, and steel beam, in place. In the present case, why would it make sense to leave the patient where she was found, with the heavy beam compressing the leg muscles, in place?

References

Appendino, G., Pollastro, F., Verotta, L., Ballero, M., Romano, A., Wyrembek, P., Szczuraszek, K., Mozrzymas, J. W., & Taglialatela-Scafati, O. (2009). Polyacetylenes from Sardinian *Oenanthe fistulosa*: A molecular clue to *risus sardonicus*. *Journal of Natural Products, 72*(5), 962–965. doi:10.1021/np8007717

Bouras, T. & Korovessis, P. (2015). Management of spondylolysis and low-grade spondylolisthesis in fine athletes. A comprehensive review. *European Journal of Orthopaedic Surgery and Traumatology, 25*, 167–175. doi:10.1007/s00590-014-1560

Brucknerová, I., Dubovický, M., & Ujházy, E. (2017). How can the process of postnatal adaptation be changed by the presence of congenital abnormalities of lip and palate. *Interdisciplinary Toxicology, 10*(4), 168–171. doi:10.1515/intox-2017-0024

Carmont, M. R., Rossi, R., Scheffler, S., Mei-Dan, O., & Beaufils, P. (2011). Percutaneous & mini invasive Achilles tendon repair. *Sports Medicine, Arthroscopy, Rehabilitation, Therapy & Technology, 3*(28). doi:10.1186/1758-2555-3-28

de Jong, P. R., de Heer-Groen, T., Schröder, C. H. & Jansen, N. J. (2009). Generalized tetanus in a 4-year old boy presenting with dysphagia and trismus: A case report. *Cases Journal, 2*(7003). doi:10.1186/1757-1626-2-7003

Delye, H. H., Borstlap, W. A., & van Lindert, E. J. (2018). Endoscopy-assisted craniosynostosis surgery followed by helmet therapy. *Surgical Neurology International, 9*(59). doi:10.4103/sni.sni_17_18

Gangopadhyay, N., Mendonca, D. A., & Woo, A. S. (2012). Pierre Robin sequence. *Seminars in Plastic Surgery, 26*(2), 76–82. doi:10.1055/s-0032-1320065

Genthon, A. & Wilcox, S. R. (2014). Crush syndrome: A case report and review of the literature. *The Journal of Emergency Medicine, 46*(2), 313–319. https://doi.org/10.1016/j.jemermed.2013.08.052

Guzman-Cottrill, J. A., Lancioni, C., Eriksson, C., Cho, Y-J., & Liko, J. (2019). *Notes from the field*: Tetanus in an unvaccinated child — Oregon, 2017. *MMWR Morbidity and Mortality Weekly Report, 68*(9), 231–232. http://dx.doi.org/10.15585/mmwr.mm6809a3external icon

Jagodzinski, N. A., Weerasinghe, C., & Porter, K. (2010). Crush injuries and crush syndrome — a review. Part 1: The systemic injury. *Trauma, 12*(2), 69–88. doi:10.1177/1460408610372440

Kruse, D., & Lemmen, B. (2009). Spine injuries in the sport of gymnastics. *Current Sports Medicine Reports, 8*(1), 20–28. https://doi.org/10.1249/JSR.0b013e3181967ca6

Lespasio, M. J., Piuzzi N. S., Husni, M. E., Muschler, G. F., Guarino, A., & Mont, M. A. (2017). Knee osteoarthritis: A primer. *The Permanente Journal, 21*, 16–183. doi:10.7812/TPP/16-183

Pereira, E. M. (2015). Clinical perspectives on osteogenesis imperfecta versus non-accidental injury. *American Journal of Medical Genetics Part C Seminars in Medical Genetics, 169*(4), 302–306. doi:10.1002/ajmg.c.31463

Stedman, T. L. (2005). Nath's *Stedman's medical terminology, 2e*. Philadelphia: Lippincott Williams & Wilkins.

Venes, D., & Taber, C. W. (2017). *Taber's Cyclopedic Medical Dictionary*. Ed. 23, illustrated in full color/Philadelphia: F.A. Davis.

Vitale, A., Sota. J., Rigante, E., Lopalco, G., Molinaro, F., Messina, M., Iannone, F., & Cantarini, L. (2016). Relapsing polychondritis: An update on pathogenesis, clinical features, diagnostic tools, and therapeutic perspectives. *Current Rheumatology Reports, 18*(3), 2–12. doi:10.1007/s11926-015-0549-5

CHAPTER 4

Cardiovascular System

The cardiovascular system, also called the **circulatory system**, ensures that a constant supply of blood, rich in oxygen and nutrients, is delivered to cells throughout the body. The cardiovascular system also collects carbon dioxide and other metabolic waste from cells and transports them to the lungs, liver, and kidneys for elimination from the body. The heart and blood vessels are the anatomical structures of this body system.

The heart is a muscular organ responsible for the pumping of blood toward the body tissues. It is located in the **mediastinum**, the central region of the thoracic cavity, and is just behind the sternum, or breastbone. It is shaped like an upside down pear and angles down, and to the left, of the mediastinum. It is about the size of a closed fist with an average mass of 300 g in an adult male and 250 g in an adult female.

There are three layers to the heart: the endocardium, the myocardium, and the epicardium. The innermost layer is the **endocardium**, which lines the chambers of the heart and covers its valves. The middle layer, the **myocardium**, is composed of cardiac muscle tissue and is responsible for the pumping action of the heart. The **epicardium** is the outermost layer and is also called the visceral layer of the serous pericardium. The **pericardium**, the membrane that surrounds and protects the heart, is composed of two layers, the superficial **fibrous pericardium** made of tough connective tissue with the role of protecting the heart and anchoring it to the mediastinum, and the deeper **serous pericardium**, itself composed of two layers. The outer layer of the serous pericardium is the **parietal layer**; it is fused to the fibrous pericardium. The inner visceral layer sticks tightly to the surface of the heart, and as stated

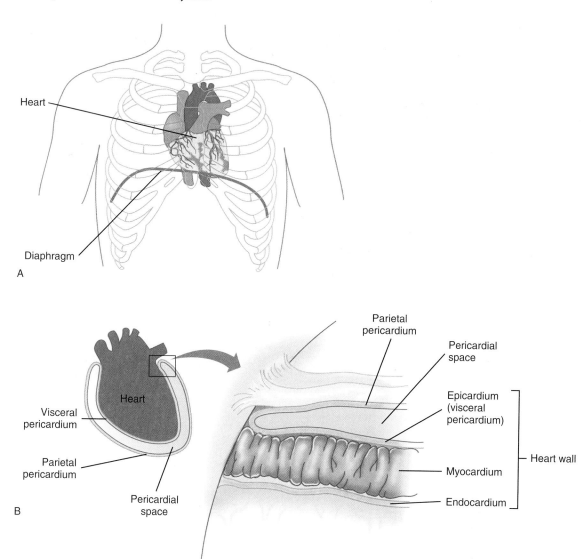

FIGURE 4.1 The heart and pericardium. (A) The relative position of the heart and diaphragm, (B) Structure of the pericardium, (C) The pericardium and wall of the heart

previously, is also called the epicardium. **Serous fluid** fills the **pericardial space** between the two pericardial layers; its role is to reduce friction as the heart moves.

The human heart has four chambers. The superior two chambers are the **atria**, which receive blood returning to the heart. The right **atrium** receives deoxygenated blood from tissues and cells of the body, delivered from the lower body by the **inferior vena cava** and from the upper body by the **superior vena cava**. The left atrium receives oxygenated blood from the lungs via the **pulmonary veins**. A thin partition called the **interatrial septum** divides these two chambers.

The inferior chambers are the **ventricles**, responsible for the pumping function of the heart. The right ventricle pumps deoxygenated blood through the **pulmonary artery** to the lungs for oxygenation and the left ventricle pumps oxygenated blood through the **aorta** to systemic arteries of the body. These chambers are divided by the **interventricular septum**.

Valves are important to prevent the backward flow of blood as it moves through the heart chambers. Between each atrium and ventricle is an **atrioventricular valve**, blood passes from the right atrium to the right ventricle through the **tricuspid valve** and from the left atrium to the left ventricle through the **mitral valve**, sometimes referred to as the bicuspid valve. The ventricles also have valves to ensure one-way flow of blood; these valves are called **semilunar valves** because of their crescent moon shape. Blood passes from the right ventricle through the **pulmonary valve** and from the left ventricle through the **aortic valve**.

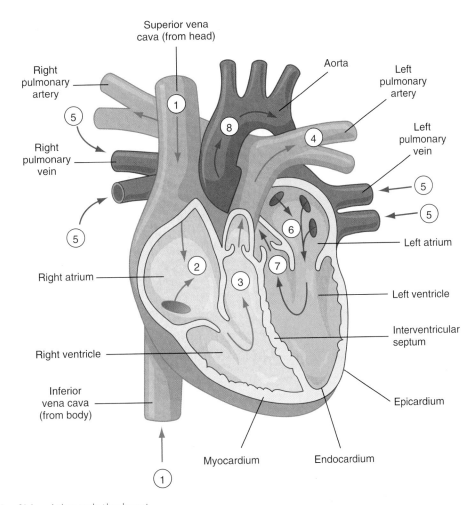

FIGURE 4.2 Path of blood through the heart

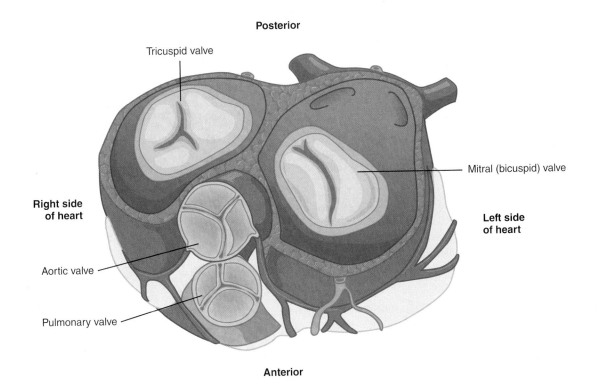

FIGURE 4.3 The valves of the heart

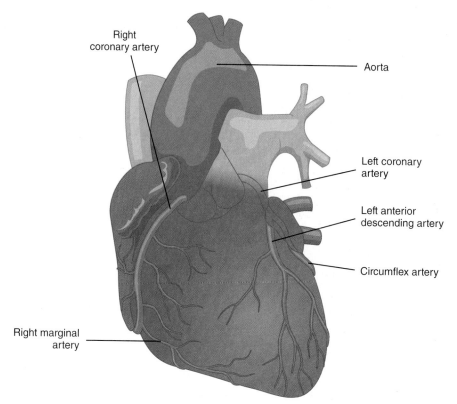

FIGURE 4.4 Major coronary arteries

The heart itself has its own network of blood vessels to supply it with blood. The right and left **coronary arteries** branch from the aorta, the main artery that carries oxygenated blood away from the heart. These vessels branch further to encircle the heart and supply the myocardium with oxygen and nutrients.

The blood vessels make up the transportation network of the cardiovascular system. The five general types of blood vessels are arteries, arterioles, veins, venules, and capillaries. **Arteries** are large and thick-walled and rich with elastic fibers, allowing them to stretch easily in response to pressure increases. Their role is to carry blood away from the heart. The pulmonary artery carries deoxygenated blood from the heart to the lungs, and the aorta, the largest artery of the body, carries oxygenated blood to all body systems. Arteries branch to smaller **arterioles**; these play a key role in regulating blood pressure. Arterioles branch to **capillaries**, the microscopic conduits between arteries and veins. The number of capillaries near various body tissues varies depending on metabolic requirements. Tissues such as tendons and ligaments have fewer capillaries due to their lower metabolic needs. Tissues such as muscle and nerve have high metabolic needs and, therefore, more capillaries. Some tissues, such as cartilage and the cornea of the eye, are avascular; these tissues lack capillaries entirely.

Gas exchange occurs in capillary beds, which are networks of tiny blood vessels. Oxygen passes through the single layer of cells that make up capillaries to body tissues and waste carbon dioxide passes from tissues to capillaries. Capillaries merge into **venules**, small veins carrying deoxygenated blood.

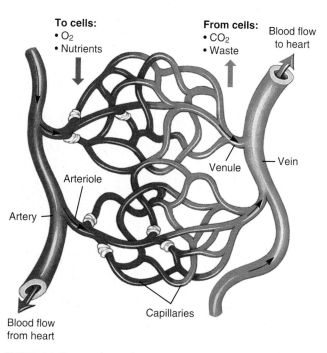

FIGURE 4.5 Types of vessels and their role in blood circulation

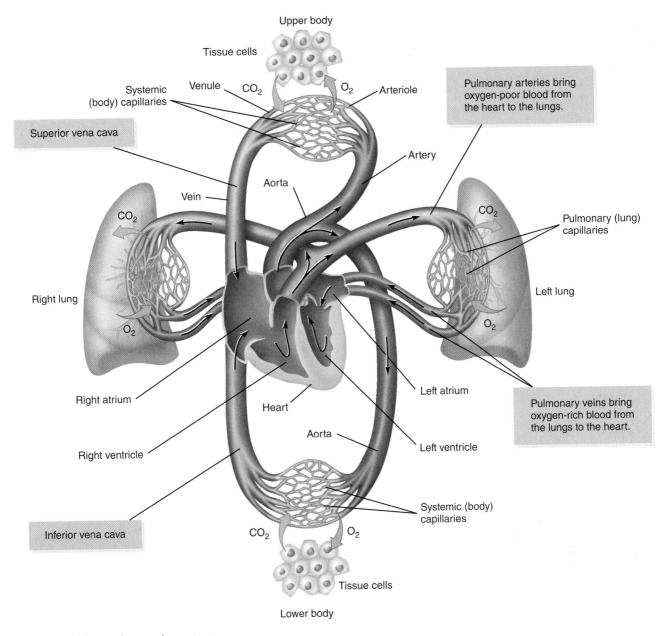

Upper body

Tissue cells

Systemic (body) capillaries   Venule CO_2 O_2 Arteriole

Superior vena cava

Pulmonary arteries bring oxygen-poor blood from the heart to the lungs.

Artery

Vein   Aorta

CO_2 Pulmonary (lung) capillaries

Right lung CO_2 Left lung

O_2 O_2

Right atrium   Left atrium

Heart   Pulmonary veins bring oxygen-rich blood from the lungs to the heart.

Right ventricle   Aorta   Left ventricle

Inferior vena cava CO_2 O_2 Systemic (body) capillaries

Tissue cells

Lower body

FIGURE 4.6 The cardiovascular system

Venules merge into larger **veins**, which are responsible for carrying blood back to the heart. Veins have thinner walls than arteries and lack their elastic fibers. Because of the lower pressure in veins compared to arteries, blood flows slower through them and may back up. Many contain valves to prevent the backflow of blood and aid in venous return. The vena cavae are the largest veins, responsible for collecting deoxygenated blood from smaller veins and carrying it to the heart. The pulmonary vein carries oxygenated blood from the lungs to the heart. **Pulse** and **blood pressure** are two of the vital signs and are measures of the health of the cardiovascular system.

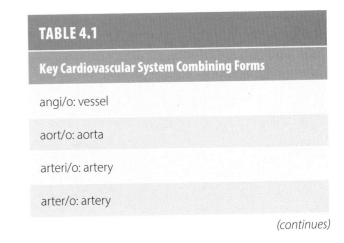

TABLE 4.1

Key Cardiovascular System Combining Forms

angi/o: vessel

aort/o: aorta

arteri/o: artery

arter/o: artery

(continues)

TABLE 4.1	(continued)
Key Cardiovascular System Combining Forms	
ather/o: fatty substance	
atri/o: atrium	
cardi/o: heart	
carotid/o: carotid artery	
coron/o: heart	
cholesterol/o: cholesterol	
embol/o: plug	
hemat/o: blood	
hem/o: blood	
isch/o: to hold back	
man/o: pressure	
myocardi/o: heart muscle, myocardium	
ox/i: oxygen	
ox/o: oxygen	
phleb/o: vein	
rrhythm/o: rhythm	
sept/o: wall	
sphygm/o: pulse	

Key Cardiovascular System Combining Forms
steth/o: chest
syncop/o: to cut off; faint
thromb/o: clot
thorac/o: chest
valv/o: valve
valvul/o: valve
varic/o: dilated vein
vascul/o: blood vessel
vas/o: vessel
ven/o: vein
ventricul/o: ventricle

TABLE 4.2
Key Cardiovascular System Suffixes
-cardia: heart condition
-emia: blood condition
-tension: pressure
-volemia: blood volume

🔍 STANDARD CASE STUDY

4.1 Bacterial Endocarditis

Current Complaint: A 45-year-old male was brought to the emergency department by ambulance for mental status changes. Upon admission, the patient complained of dyspnea, fever with shaking chills, night sweats, myalgia, anorexia, and general malaise.

Past History: Patient is a long-standing intravenous drug user (IDU). Past medical history was significant for previous hospitalization for bacteremia secondary to cellulitis resulting from repeated drug injection.

Signs and Symptoms: Physical examination was significant for temperature of 39.1 °C (102 °F), tachypnea, and tachycardia. Blood cultures were positive for *Staphylococcus aureus*. Transthoracic echocardiography revealed significant tricuspid valve vegetation.

Diagnosis: Bacterial infective endocarditis, causative agent *Staphylococcus aureus*.

Treatment: Antibiotic therapy for 4–6 weeks with oxacillin (8–12 g/day). If fever and bacteremia persist despite antimicrobial chemotherapy, valvectomy with eventual valve replacement or vegectomy with valvuloplasty will be considered. Continuing drug use carries a high risk of reinfection so the patient will be strongly counseled to attend a drug rehabilitation program.

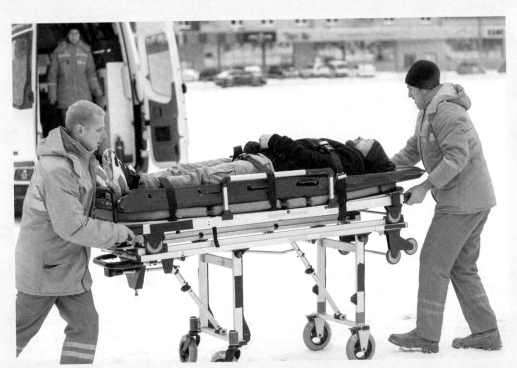

CASE FIGURE: A man on his way to the hospital by ambulance

© Pressmaster/Shutterstock

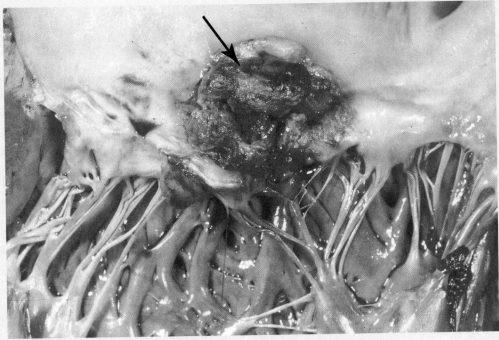

CASE FIGURE: Vegetations (arrow) on heart valve from endocarditis

Courtesy of Leonard V. Crowley, MD, Century College.

(continues)

⌕ STANDARD CASE STUDY   *(continued)*

1. Complete the table below for the symptoms related to the case:

Term	Word Parts	Meaning
dyspnea	*dys-; -pnea*	*breathing that is difficult*
anorexia		
myalgia		
malaise	N/A	
bacteremia		
tachypnea		
tachycardia		

2. Complete the table below for the procedures and treatments related to the case:

Term	Word Parts	Meaning
transthoracic echocardiography	*trans-; thorac/o; -ic echo-; cardi/o; -graphy*	*recording reflected sound of the heart pertaining to across the chest region*
antibiotic		
valvectomy		
valvuloplasty		

3. Vegetation means plant life in everyday use. What does vegetation mean when used as a medical term as in this case? Which term in the case means removal of these vegetations?

4. What is cellulitis and what is its relation to intravenous drug use?

5. Indicate and define the component word parts for *endocarditis*. Should the patient be offered surgical intervention if it becomes necessary because he continues to use drugs?

🔍 *STANDARD CASE STUDY*

4.2 Danon Disease

A 20-year-old female with a family history of sudden cardiac death was referred to a cardiologist for recurrent and frequent events of syncope. She also reported sporadic episodes when she felt like her heart was racing. Echocardiography revealed left ventricular hypertrophy. Supraventricular tachycardia was recorded with ambulatory monitoring. Due to her family history, she was referred for genetic testing. DNA analysis identified a gene mutation for an X-linked dominant disorder, Danon disease. Symptoms typical of Danon disease are cardiomyopathy, skeletal muscle myopathy, and intellectual disability. Males typically present early in life with all three symptoms; females typically present later in life, often with just cardiomyopathy. Due to the progressive course of ventricular arrhythmias in Danon disease, the patient was referred for cryoablation and subsequent implantation of an internal cardioverter defibrillator (ICD). Regular cardiac evaluations will occur every six months with possible discussion of cardiac transplant due to the expected cardiac progression from this disease.

Left ventricular hypertrophy

Normal heart

Right ventricle

Left ventricle

Thickening of the myocardium of the left ventricle

© Alila Medical Media/Shutterstock

1. Define the word parts for *cardiologist*.

   Cardiologist: Cardi/o _____, -logist _____.

2. Syncope comes from the root syncop/o, which means _____.

3. Define the word parts and meaning for the following terms that relate to the woman's symptoms:

   Ventricular hypertrophy: Ventricul/o _____, -ar _____,

   hyper- _____, -trophy _____,

   means _____.

(continues)

Supraventricular tachycardia: Supra- _____, ventricul/o _____,

-ar _____, tachy- _____,

cardi/o _____, -ia _____,

means _____.

Cardiomyopathy: Cardi/o _____, my/o _____,

-pathy _____,

means _____.

Myopathy: My/o _____, -pathy _____,

means _____.

Ventricular arrhythmia: Ventricul/o _____, -ar _____,

a- _____, rrhythm/o _____, -ia _____,

means _____.

4. Ventricular hypertrophy is also known as an enlarged heart. A medical term for enlarged heart is

_____

5. Indicate the word parts for *echocardiography* and explain the procedure based on those parts.

6. Explain what ambulatory monitoring means.

7. Provide a brief definition of cryoablation. How is this treatment supported by implantation of an internal cardioverter defibrillator (ICD)?

🔍 STANDARD CASE STUDY

4.3 Routine Physical

Hans, a 66-year-old Caucasian male, met with his primary care physician for his annual physical. Hans is 6 feet tall, weighs 190 lb (86 kg), and smokes about a pack of cigarettes a day. The patient reports a family history of cardiovascular disease. His vital signs are normal with the exception of blood pressure; systolic 130 mm Hg and diastolic 80 mm Hg. The chief complaint is angina pectoris with physical exertion. Based on the patient's history and blood pressure, the physician ordered an electrocardiogram, basic metabolic panel, lipid panel, and urinalysis. All tests were normal except lipid analysis revealed hyperlipidemia, specifically hypercholesterolemia, which can promote the formation of lipid plaques on the inner walls of arteries; angiocardiography was ordered and revealed coronary artery atherosclerosis. The patient was advised to make lifestyle changes, prescribed an ACE inhibitor drug to treat hypertension, and atorvastatin (Lipitor), an antilipidemic, to reduce plasma cholesterol. Depending on treatment efficacy, an atherectomy may have to be considered in the future.

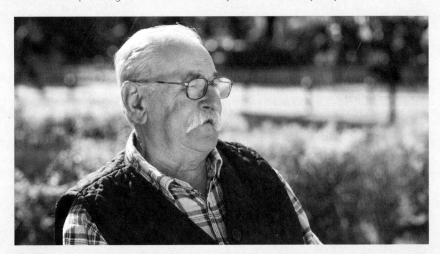

CASE FIGURE: Hans contemplating the advice of his physician following his annual physical

1. Blood pressure is generally represented as two values: systolic and diastolic pressures. One is the higher pressure when the heart ventricles contract whereas the other is the lower pressure when ventricles relax. Which is which?

   Systolic:

   Diastolic:

   Define the following word parts for each cardiovascular disorder and then circle the best choice for what describes Hans' condition. You may need to use an outside reference to check for normal values.

   Hypertension: Hyper- _____, -tension _____.

   Hypotension: Hypo- _____, - tension _____.

   Hypervolemia: Hyper-_____, -volemia _____.

   Hypovolemia: Hypo-_____, -volemia _____.

(continues)

⌕ STANDARD CASE STUDY   *(continued)*

2. Chronic elevated blood pressure can lead to changes in the myocardium, which can lead to ischemia. Angina pectoris can result from myocardial ischemia. Explain what *angina pectoris* is and then define the word parts and meaning for *ischemia*.

    Angina pectoris:

    Ischemia: Isch/o _____, hem/o _____, -ia _____,

    means _____.

3. Define the word parts and meaning for *hyperlipidemia*, *angiocardiography*, and *antilipidemic*.

    Hyperlipidemia: Hyper- _____, lip/o _____,

    -id _____, -emia _____,

    means _____.

    Hypercholesterolemia: Hyper- _____, cholesterol/o _____

    -emia _____, means _____.

    Angiocardiography: Angi/o _____, cardi/o _____,

    -graphy _____, means _____.

    Antilipidemic: Anti- _____, lip/o _____,

    -id _____, -emic _____,

    means _____.

4. Atherosclerosis is a type of arteriosclerosis. Indicate and define the component word parts for *atherosclerosis* and *arteriosclerosis* and then briefly describe each disorder.

5. Define the word parts, and meaning, for *atherectomy*.

    Atherectomy: Ather/o _____, -ectomy _____,

    means _____.

⚲ STANDARD CASE STUDY

4.4 Abdominal Aortic Aneurysm

A 65-year-old African American male presented in the emergency department with abdominal pain. Patient social history includes smoking. A significant medical history includes hypertension, hyperlipidemia, and previous cardiac events including myocardial infarction (MI) and angina. An abdominal computed tomography (CT) angiogram revealed an abdominal aortic aneurysm (AAA), which was surgically repaired by endovascular aneurysm repair (EVAR).

Four days following EVAR, the patient developed a fever, hematochezia, and anuria. The symptoms following AAA repair suggested embolism of mesenteric vasculature, which was decreasing colonic perfusion resulting in ischemic colitis. A sigmoidoscopy revealed necrosis of the sigmoid colon. A general surgeon performed a colorectal anastomosis and the patient was transferred to postoperative intensive care for recovery.

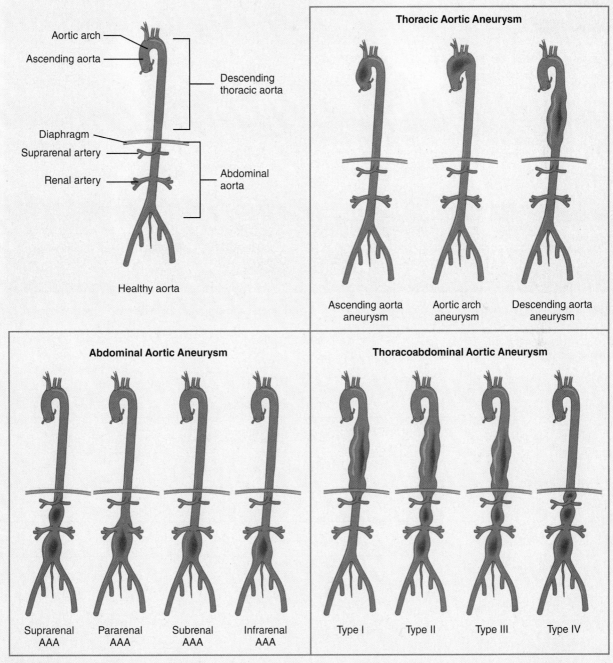

CASE FIGURE: Classification of aortic aneurysms

(continues)

⌕ STANDARD CASE STUDY   (continued)

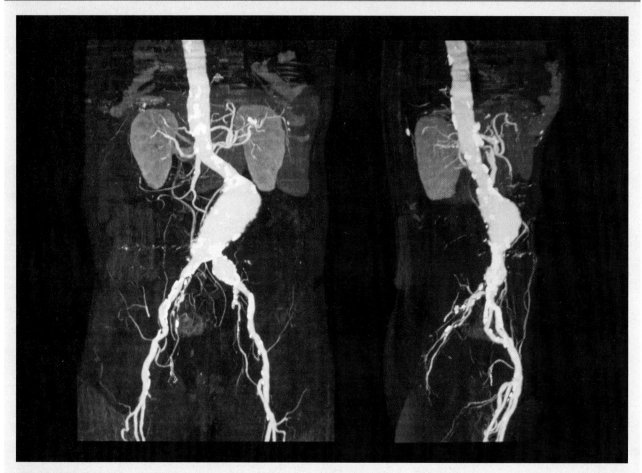

CASE FIGURE: Patient computed tomography angiography of abdominal aortic aneurysm, prone view (left) and lateral view (right)

© Suttha Burawonk/Shutterstock

1. Define the word parts and meaning for *hypertension* and *hyperlipidemia*.

   Hypertension: Hyper- _____, -tension _____,

   means _____.

   Hyperlipidemia: Hyper- _____, lip/o_____,

   -id _____, -emia _____,

   means _____.

2. Describe what a myocardial infarction (MI), angina, and aneurysm are.

   Myocardial infarction (MI):

Angina:

Aneurysm:

3. Define the word parts, and meaning, for *angiogram*.

    Angiogram: Angi/o _____, -gram _____,

    means _____.

4. An abdominal CT angiogram showed that the patient had an AAA. Looking at the case images, classify the patient's aneurysm.

5. Complete the table below for the symptoms and diagnostics following AAA repair:

Term	Word Parts	Meaning
hematochezia	*hemat/o; -chezia*	*bloody stool*
anuria		
embolization		
mesenteric	N/A	
ischemic colitis		
sigmoidoscopy		
necrosis		

6. Part of the patient's digestive tract became necrotic due to ischemia. The necrotic region is surgically removed by colorectal anastomosis, a procedure that joins two parts of a tube. What two parts of the digestive tract are joined by this procedure?

🔍 *STANDARD CASE STUDY*

4.5 Kawasaki Disease

A 6-year-old Native American male presents in the clinic with a five-day history of fever and 2 days of a palmar erythematous nonpruritic rash, periungual desquamation, bilateral conjunctivitis, cheilitis, and lymphadenopathy. The parents report that fever started about five days ago; the other symptoms started a few days ago and have become progressively worse. Laboratory tests were unremarkable for plasma, but urinalysis results included mild proteinuria. Based on patient history and symptoms, Kawasaki disease (KD) was given as the likely diagnosis. KD is a pediatric syndrome including vasculitis of small and medium arteries. Its etiology is unknown. It is normally self-limiting but can give rise to severe complications including coronary arteritis, myocarditis, and pericarditis. The typical course of treatment was followed: aspirin and intravenous gamma globulins (i.e., antibodies). The symptoms started to improve the following day and the child was discharged.

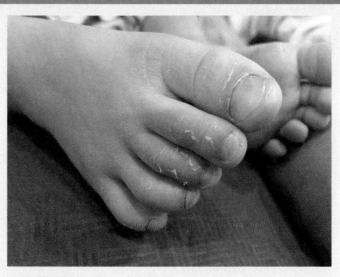

CASE FIGURE: Peeling of the toes seen in Kawasiki disease
© PJUTISIR/Shutterstock

1. Complete the table below for the terms relating to the patient's symptoms:

Term	Word Parts	Meaning
erythematous	*erythr/o; hemat/o; -ous*	*pertaining to blood red (refers to flushing of skin)*
nonpruritic		
bilateral		
conjunctivitis		
cheilitis		
periungual		
desquamation		
lymphadenophathy		

2. Define the word parts, and meaning, for the urinalysis and proteinuria.

Urinalysis: Urin/o _____, -lysis _____,

means _____.

Proteinuria: Protein/o _____, -uria _____,

means _____.

3. KD is a pediatric vasculitis disease. Define the words part for *pediatric* and *vasculitis*, then describe what *pediatric vasculitis* means.

    Pediatric: Ped/o _____, iatr/o _____, -ic _____.

    Vasculitis: Vascul/o _____, -itis _____.

4. Complications from KD include *coronary arteritis*, *myocarditis*, and *pericarditis*; define the word parts and meanings of these conditions.

    Coronary arteritis: Coron/o _____, -ary _____,

    arteri/o _____, -itis _____,

    means _____.

    Myocarditis: Myocardi/o _____, -itis _____,

    means _____.

    Pericarditis: Peri- _____, cardi/o _____,

    -itis _____, means _____.

ADVANCED CASE STUDY

4.6 Cardiac Tamponade

A 24-year-old man was brought to the emergency department approximately 30 minutes after colliding with a tree while snowboarding. He was conscious on admission but anxious and restless. Immediately after admission he developed hypotension and tachypnea. He reported pain in the abdominal and thoracic regions. Physical exam revealed significant thoracic-area bruising, cold, clammy extremities attributed to peripheral hypoperfusion, and venous distention of his jugular veins. CT scan revealed a large pericardial effusion contributing to cardiac tamponade. Emergency echocardiography-guided pericardiocentesis was performed to manage the effusion and the patient was transferred to the operating room. A thoracotomy was performed and a laceration of the right atrium at the junction of the superior vena cava was identified. Cardiorrhaphy was performed to repair the laceration and the patient was released 15 days later following an uncomplicated postoperative course of treatment.

1. Define the following word parts to the following conditions:

    Hypotension: Hypo- _____, -tension _____.

    Tachypnea: Tachy- _____, -pnea _____.

2. Indicate and define the component word parts for *peripheral hypoperfusion* and explain how this relates to cold clammy extremities.

(continues)

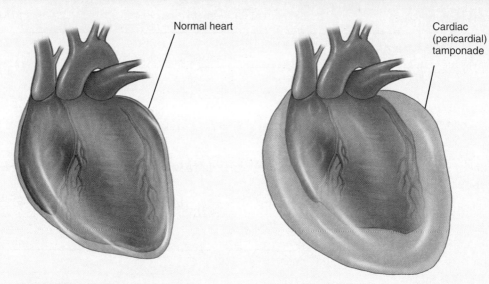

Normal heart

Cardiac (pericardial) tamponade

CASE FIGURE: Cardiac tamponade

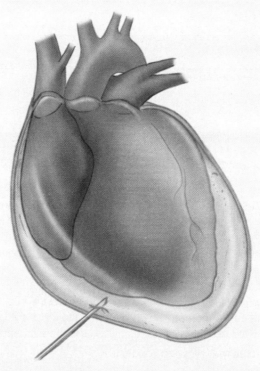

CASE FIGURE: Pericardiocentesis. Draining some of the pericardial fluid by pericardiocentesis is often an effective temporizing maneuver for cardiac tamponade

3. Effusion is the escape of fluid into a part. Define the word parts for *pericardial* and explain what is meant by a pericardial effusion and how it can lead to cardiac tamponade.

Pericardial: Peri- _____, cardi/o _____, -al _____

4. Distention means swelling or bulging. Explain what is meant by venous distention of the jugular veins and how this might be related to cardiac tamponade.

5. Complete the table below for the following procedural terms:

Term	Word Parts	Meaning
echocardiography	*echo-; cardi/o; -graphy*	*recording reflected sound of the heart*
pericardiocentesis		
thoracotomy		
cardiorrhaphy		

🔍 ADVANCED CASE STUDY

4.7 Chronic Venous Insufficiency

Elvera Danforth, a 60-year-old, heavy-set woman, presents to her primary care physician complaining of rope-like, dilated veins in both legs.

"They are so ugly," she says to her physician, "and they hurt. My legs ache and they feel so heavy. I've had varicose veins forever, but my legs bother me so much more now. The skin around my ankles is tight and itchy and my ankles swell at the end of the day."

Dr. Cortman examines Mrs. Danforth's legs. "The edema, xerosis, stasis dermatitis, and pruritus you are describing are all indicative of lipodermatosclerosis from poor venous return. Improving blood flow in your leg veins will prevent further complications such as leg ulcers and phlebitis and will help cosmetically with the varicose veins. We will schedule you for a lower limb venous ultrasonography, which will provide more information and better guide our treatment decisions and we will refer you to a vascular specialist. Some treatment options include endovenous laser ablation, sclerotherapy, and microphlebectomy. In the meantime, you should wear compression stockings and elevate your legs as much as possible. Here is a pamphlet for you to read with more information."

Mrs. Danforth books her appointment for an ultrasound and thanks Dr. Cortman. The doctor has told her that losing weight, implementing a regular exercise routine, and sitting less can all help improve her condition and she is determined to implement these lifestyle changes.

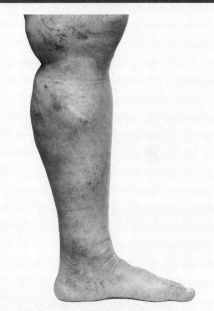

CASE FIGURE: Varicose veins on swollen leg from venous insufficiency

© Olga Aniven/Shutterstock

1. Indicate the word parts for *varicose* and define the term based on those parts. What signs indicate that Mrs. Danforth has varicose veins?

(continues)

Varicose Vein

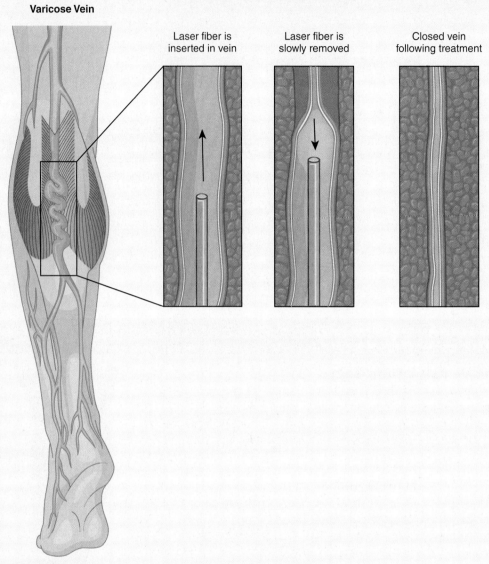

Laser fiber is inserted in vein

Laser fiber is slowly removed

Closed vein following treatment

CASE FIGURE: Endovenous laser treatment for varicose veins

2. Complete the table below for the signs and symptoms related to the case:

Term	Word Parts	Meaning
edema	*N/A*	*swelling*
xerosis		
stasis dermatitis		
pruritus		
lipodermatosclerosis		
phlebitis		

3. The patient was scheduled for a lower limb venous ultrasonography. Define the word parts and meaning for this procedure.

   Venous ultrasonography: Ven/o _____, -ous _____,

               ultra- _____, son/o _____,

               -graphy _____, means _____.

   Name and describe the treatment options presented to the patient. Use a medical dictionary for further information if necessary.

4. Define the word parts for *vascular*.

   Vascular: Vascul/o _____, -ar _____.

🔍 ADVANCED CASE STUDY

4.8 Takayasu's Arteritis

A 30-year-old woman of Asian descent presents to the emergency department for what she believes to be complications from a viral infection. For the past month she has felt generally unwell with fever, fatigue and malaise, myalgia, dyspnea, and orthopnea. Increasingly difficult breathing, right-arm claudication, and right-sided carotidodynia prompted her visit to the emergency department. Significant blood pressure discrepancy between the left and right arm were detected by sphygmomanometry during the physical exam. Right carotid, brachial, and radial pulses were barely palpable. CT angiography showed partial occlusion of the right common carotid artery, and dilation of the ascending and descending thoracic aorta. Evidence of large vessel vasculitis led to a diagnosis of occlusive thromboaortopathy, also known as Takayasu's arteritis. The patient was prescribed corticosteroids and immunosuppressive drugs to reduce inflammation. If the patient does not respond to this intervention or vascular complications escalate, surgical intervention may be necessary. Angioplasty, aortic valve replacement, and endarterectomy are procedures that may be considered if complications become severe.

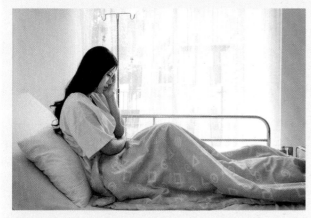

CASE FIGURE: A woman in a hospital bed feeling unwell

© Travelpixs/Shutterstock

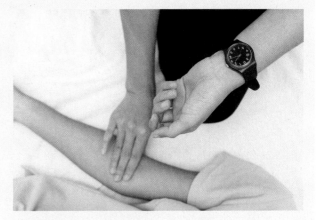

CASE FIGURE: Brachial pulse assessment

© Bangkoker/Shutterstock

(continues)

🔍 ADVANCED CASE STUDY *(continued)*

1. Complete the table below for symptoms and findings related to the case:

Term	Word Parts	Meaning
myalgia	*my/o; -algia*	*pain in muscles*
dyspnea		
orthopnea		
malaise	N/A	
carotidodynia		
vasculitis		
arteritis		
thromboaortopathy		

2. Give a short definition for the medical terms *claudication*, *occlusion*, *palpable*, and *dilation*.

   Claudication:

   Occlusion:

   Palpable:

   Dilation:

3. Define the word parts, and meaning, for *sphygmomanometry*.

   Sphygmomanometry: Sphygm/o _____, man/o _____,

   -metry _____, means _____.

4. Describe the location of the *carotid*, *radial*, and *brachial* pulses.

   Carotid:

Radial:

Brachial:

5. Define the following word parts to the following procedures:

Angiography: Angi/o _____, -graphy _____.

Angioplasty: Angi/o _____, -plasty _____.

Endarterectomy: Endo- _____, arteri/o _____,

-ectomy _____.

6. Where is the aortic valve found?

ADVANCED CASE STUDY

4.9 Atrial Septal Defect

Dennis, a 40-year-old Hispanic male, presented to the emergency department (ED) with complaints of dyspnea and acrocyanosis following intense physical exertion. The symptoms had become progressively worse over the preceding 2 weeks. Relevant patient history included pulmonary hypertension, and family history of cardiovascular disease. Auscultation of heart sounds with a stethoscope by the ED physician, Dr. Faust, revealed a heart murmur. Dr. Faust ordered an electrocardiograph (EKG), which did not detect any arrhythmias. He also requested an echocardiograph (ECHO), which revealed mitral valve stenosis (MVS), an atrial septal defect (ASD), and right atriomegaly.

"Wait, what? A hole in my heart! Is it serious?" Dennis asked.

Dr. Faust replied, "It could possibly become serious. I'll refer to you to a cardiologist for more tests. You have an abnormal opening between the upper two chambers of your heart, the atria. This is an opening that is present during fetal development, but it generally closes after birth."

Dennis listened intently, as Dr. Faust continued, "Normally, the right side of the heart pumps oxygen-poor blood to the pulmonary circuit, to become oxygenated by the lungs. The left side of the heart pumps oxygen-rich blood to the systemic circuit, to deliver oxygen to body tissues. Because gas exchange occurs at the placenta during fetal development, the fetus has some modifications causing circulation to largely bypass the lungs. These modifications are typically shut down after birth. One of these fetal modifications is an opening between the right and left atrium called the foramen ovale, and yours is still a little open. We call this patent foramen ovale, or an atrial septal defect. The cardiologist will help determine if the defect can be managed without surgery, but I suspect that closure will be recommended."

"In the meantime I'll take it easy?" Dennis asked.

"That certainly wouldn't hurt," replied Dr. Faust.

(continues)

⌕ ADVANCED CASE STUDY

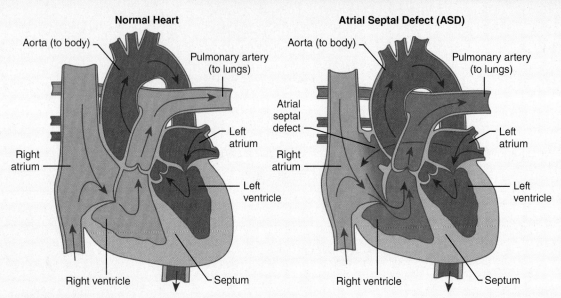

CASE FIGURE: Normal heart and heart with atrial septum defect

1. Complete the table below for symptoms and testing related to the case:

Term	Word Parts	Meaning
dyspnea	dys-; -pnea	difficult breathing
acrocyanosis		
auscultation	N/A	
stethoscope		
electrocardiograph		
echocardiograph		

2. Dennis had a history of pulmonary hypertension and family history of cardiovascular disease. Define the word parts, and meaning, for *pulmonary hypertension* and *cardiovascular*.

Pulmonary hypertension: Pulmon/o _____, -ary _____,

hyper-_____, -tension_____,

means _____.

Cardiovascular: Cardi/o _____, vascul/o _____, -ar _____,

means _____.

3. In this case, EKG did not detect any arrhythmias and ECHO revealed mitral valve stenosis (MVS), an atrial septal defect (ASD), and right atriomegaly. Describe what each condition is.

Arrhythmia:

Mitral valve stenosis:

Atrial septal defect:

Right atriomegaly:

4. What are heart murmurs? Which of the conditions described above can produce a heart murmur?

🔍 *ADVANCED CASE STUDY*

4.10 Transposition of the Great Vessels

A cyanotic neonate, gestational age 38 weeks, presents with arterial blood oxygen saturation of 89% (hypoxia), a breathing rate of 70 breath/min (tachypnea), and arterial blood pH 7.2 (acidosis). Echocardiography and chest X-ray show transposition of the great arteries (TGA). TGA is a pediatric congenital heart defect wherein the origin of the two large arteries of the heart, the pulmonary trunk and aorta, are reversed so that the right atrium empties into the aorta (instead of the pulmonary trunk) and the left atrium empties into the pulmonary trunk (instead of the aorta). As a result, most of the deoxygenated blood from the body that enters the right side of the heart is returned directly to the body tissues instead of to the lungs. Therefore, O_2 concentration is not increased and CO_2 concentration is not decreased, which means CO_2-rich blood is being circulated to body tissue rather than O_2-rich blood. Moreover, blood that is rich in oxygen, coming from the lungs, is returned directly to the lungs. The baby was administered prostaglandins to maintain a patent ductus arteriosus, a fetal structure that channels blood from the pulmonary trunk to the aorta but normally closes shortly after birth. Cardiac catherization and balloon atrial septostomy (BAS) were used to promote the mixing of blood between the sides of the heart, which improved systemic arterial oxygen saturation (95%). The following week, the baby underwent heart surgery for an arterial switch procedure, which entails transection and switching of the aorta and pulmonary trunk. This procedure restores normal ventriculoarterial connections.

(continues)

🔍 *ADVANCED CASE STUDY*   (continued)

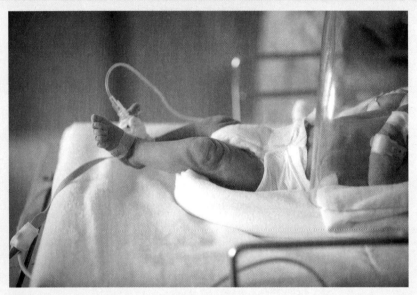

CASE FIGURE: A newborn in a hospital bed

© M.Moira/Shutterstock

1.   Define the word parts, and meaning, for the patient's symptoms: *cyanosis*, *hypoxia*, *tachypnea*, and *acidosis*.

Cyanosis: Cyan/o _____, -osis _____,

        means _____.

Hypoxia: Hypo- _____, ox/o _____, -ia _____,

        means _____.

Tachypnea: Tachy- _____, -pnea _____,

        means _____.

Acidosis: Acid- _____, -osis _____,

        means _____.

2.   Explain what the following anatomical structures of the heart are:

Atria:

Arial septum:

Ventricles:

Ventricular septum:

Pulmonary trunk:

Aorta:

Ductus arteriosus:

3. A balloon catheter was used in this patient to perform an atrial septostomy. This procedure promotes mixing of oxygenated and deoxygenated blood between the largely separated pulmonary and systemic circuit. Define the word parts, and meaning, for *atrial septostomy*.

Atrial septostomy: Atri/o _____, -al _____,

sept/o _____, -ostomy _____,

means _____

4. The baby had an arterial switch procedure performed to restore normal ventriculoarterial connections. Define the word parts for *ventriculoarterial* and then explain what is meant by normal ventriculoarterial connections.

Ventriculoarterial: Ventric/o _____, arteri/o _____, -al _____,

means _____

Normal ventriculoarterial connections:

References

Ji, Y., Kujtan, L., & Kershner, D. (2012). Acute endocarditis in intravenous drug users: A case report and literature review. *Journal of Community Hospital Internal Medicine Perspectives, 2*(1). doi:10.3402/jchimp.v2i1.11513

Kim, H., Kwon, T. W., Cho, Y. P., & Moon, K. M. (2012). Report of a case of ischemic colitis with bilaterally patent internal iliac arteries after endovascular abdominal aneurysm repair. *Journal of the Korean Surgical Society, 82*(3), 200–203. https://doi.org/10.4174/jkss.2012.82.3.200

Lee C-Y. (2018). Cardiac tamponade: A case series. *Clinics in Surgery, 3*(2051), 1–3.

Medical Advisory Secretariat. (2010). Endovascular laser therapy for varicose veins: An evidence-based analysis. *Ontario Health Technology Assessment Series, 10*(6), 1–92.

Leonardi, S., Barone, P., Gravina, G., Parisi, G. F., Di Stefano, V., Sciacca, P., & La Rosa, M. (2013). Severe Kawasaki disease in a 3-month-old patient: A case report. *BMC Research Notes, 6*(500). https://doi.org/10.1186/1756-0500-6-500

Mulder, B. A., Hoedemaekers, Y. M., van den Berg, M. P., van Loon, R. L., Wind, A. M., Jongbloed, J. D., & Wiesfeld, A. C. (2019). Three female patients with Danon disease presenting with predominant cardiac phenotype: A case series. *European*

Heart Journal -Case Reports, 3(3), ytz132. doi:10.1093/ehjcr/ytz132

Perera, A. H., Mason, J. C. & Wolfe, J. H. (2013). Takayasu Arteritis: Criteria for surgical intervention should not be ignored. *International Journal of Vascular Medicine*, Article ID 618910, 8 pages. doi:10.1155/2013/618910

Petit, C. J., Rome, J. J., Wernovsky, G., Mason, S. E., Shera, D. M., Nicolson, S. C., Montenegro, L. M., Tabbutt, S., Zimmerman, R. A., & Licht, D. J. (2009). Preoperative brain injury in transposition of the great arteries is associated with oxygenation and time to surgery, not balloon atrial septostomy. *Circulation, 119*(5), 709–716. https://doi.org/10.1161/CIRCULATIONAHA.107.760819

Radico, F., Cicchitti, V., Zimarino, M. & De Caterina, R. (2014). Angina pectoris and myocardial ischemia in the absence of obstructive coronary artery disease: Practical considerations for diagnostic tests. *Journal of the American College of Cardiovascular Interventions, 7*(5) 453–463.

Sears, C. R., Bosslet, G. T., & Hage, C. A. (2010). 51 year-old male with dyspnea and hypoxia. *Respiratory Medicine CME, 3*(3), 135–137.

Stedman, T. L. (2005). Nath's *Stedman's medical terminology, 2e.* Philadelphia: Lippincott Williams & Wilkins.

Tackling, G., & Borhade, M. B. Hypertensive heart disease. [Updated February 7, 2021]. In: Treasure Island (FL): StatPearls Publishing; Available from: https://www.ncbi.nlm.nih.gov/books/NBK539800/

Ultee, K. H., Zettervall, S. L., Soden, P. A., Darling, J., Bertges, D. J., Verhagen, H. J., Schermerhorn, M. L., & Vascular Study Group of New England (2016). Incidence of and risk factors for bowel ischemia after abdominal aortic aneurysm repair. *Journal of Vascular Surgery, 64*(5), 1384–1391. https://doi.org/10.1016/j.jvs.2016.05.045

Venes, D., & Taber, C. W. (2017). *Taber's Cyclopedic Medical Dictionary.* Ed. 23, illustrated in full color/Philadelphia: F.A. Davis.

Voulalas, G., & Maltezos, C. (2016). A case of acute ischemic colitis after endovascular abdominal aortic aneurysm repair. *Journal of Acute Disease. 5*(1), 79–82.

CHAPTER 5

Blood and Lymphatic System

KEY TERMS

Agranulocyte
Albumin
Basophil
Blood
Complete blood count (CBC)
Eosinophil
Erythrocyte
Fibrinogen
Globulin
Granulocyte
Hematocrit

Hematopoiesis
Hemoglobin
Interstitial fluid
Leukocyte
Lymph
Lymph node
Lymphatic capillary
Lymphatic duct
Lymphatic vessel
Lymphocyte
Macrophage

Monocyte
Mucosa associated lymphatic tissue
　(MALT)
Neutrophil
Plasma
Platelet
Spleen
Thrombocyte
Thymus
Tonsil

Blood and lymph are the two largest volumes of circulating fluid in the body. Blood transports materials to and from most cells, whereas lymph is composed of fluid that is cleared from body tissues and returned to systemic circulation. Blood and lymph contain a myriad of immune cells that perform immune surveillance, attack pathogens, neutralize toxins, and remove debris.

Blood transports nutrients and oxygen to most of the body's tens of trillions of cells. It also clears waste products and carbon dioxide from these cells and delivers them to the liver, kidney, and lungs for elimination. Blood is a key part of maintaining homeostasis as various body systems balance blood temperature and chemistry which, in turn, provides an optimal environment for cells, tissues, and organs that the blood supplies. Blood is a slightly sticky fluid with a temperature of approximately 38°C and a slightly alkaline pH (normal arterial blood pH is 7.35–7.45). The blood volume in an average-sized

adult female is 4 to 5 liters and, in an average-sized adult male, is 5 to 6 liters. Blood constitutes about 8% of total body mass.

Approximately 55% of blood is plasma and 45% is formed elements, which are cells and cell fragments. Blood **plasma**, the liquid component of blood, is about 92% water. The remainder is plasma proteins and other solutes. **Albumin** is the most abundant plasma protein, produced by the liver, with a role of transporting steroid hormones and fatty acids. **Globulins** are the second most abundant type of plasma protein; these proteins play a role in immunity. A third type of plasma protein, **fibrinogen**, plays an essential role in blood clotting. Other solutes present in low amounts include ions such as Na^+, K^+, and Cl^-, nutrients such as glucose, vitamins, and minerals, dissolved gasses such as CO_2 and O_2, enzymes, hormones, and waste products such as urea and ammonia.

Erythrocytes, also called red blood cells or RBCs, are the most abundant of the blood cells, making up

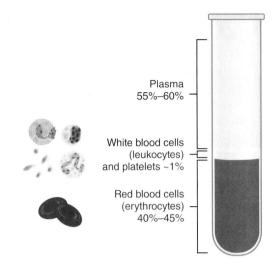

FIGURE 5.1 Composition of fractionated blood

approximately 99% of formed elements. Erythrocytes have a biconcave shape and do not have a nucleus; their primary function is to transport oxygen and carbon dioxide. Each red blood cell contains approximately 280 million molecules of the protein **hemoglobin**, responsible for most of the oxygen, and part of the carbon dioxide, transport in blood. RBCs have a life cycle of only 120 days and they are unable to divide.

Leukocytes, also called white blood cells or WBCs, make up less than 1% of the blood cells, but they have a critical role in protection from pathogens and toxins. There are five classes of leukocytes: lymphocytes, monocytes, neutrophils, eosinophils, and basophils. Two of these, lymphocytes and monocytes, are classified as **agranulocytes**, because of their lack of conspicuous cytoplasmic granules when

stained. The other three: neutrophils, eosinophils, and basophils, are considered **granulocytes** due to the visible presence of cytoplasmic granules when stained.

Lymphocytes are cells that fight infection and can raise an immune response after infection or vaccination. **Monocytes** are large cells that can enter body tissues and differentiate into **macrophages**, which are aggressive phagocytes, engulfing pathogens and cellular debris. **Neutrophils** are generally the most abundant of the leukocytes and like macrophages, they are phagocytic. Eosinophils and basophils are relatively rare. **Eosinophils** attack pathogens that have antibodies attached to them and become more abundant when fighting parasitic infections. **Basophils** secrete heparin, which prevents blood clotting, and histamine, a vasodilator. Formed elements also include **thrombocytes**, or **platelets**, which are cell fragments that play a major role in blood clotting. All formed elements in blood are produced by a process called **hematopoiesis**, which occurs in red bone marrow.

A valuable test to monitor health is the **complete blood count (CBC)**. Usually included in this is the number and type of WBCs, and the number of RBCs and platelets. Other common laboratory tests include a measure of the amount of blood hemoglobin; and a **hematocrit**, the percentage of RBCs in total blood volume. Low hemoglobin and hematocrit levels are reported as anemia.

The lymphatic system is composed of an extensive network of vessels and an array of lymphoid tissues and organs. The functions of the lymphatic system are to drain excess interstitial fluid from tissue spaces, to distribute lymphocytes and other

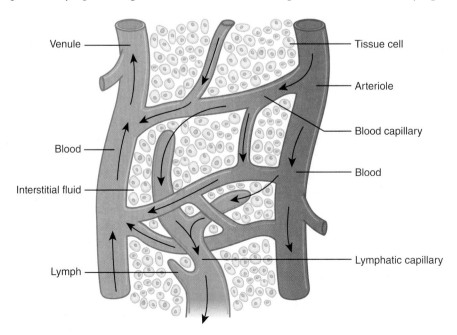

FIGURE 5.2 Blood and lymphatic vessels

cells of the immune system throughout the body, and to transport lipids and lipid-soluble vitamins. **Interstitial fluid** is the fluid found between cells; once it passes into lymphatic vessels, it is a clear-to-milky-white fluid called **lymph**.

Lymphatic vessels begin as **lymphatic capillaries**, which are slightly larger in diameter than blood capillaries with a unique blind-ended structure that collects fluid from between cells. Lymphatic capillaries drain to larger **lymphatic vessels** that contain lymph nodes, which drain into lymphatic trunks, then to **lymphatic ducts**. There are two lymphatic ducts that

deliver lymph to the bloodstream via the subclavian veins, which are near the clavicles (collar bones). All lymphatic vessels contain valves, which ensures a one-way flow of lymph. From a disease standpoint, cancer cells may exploit the lymphatic passageways to metastasize and spread to sites distant from the original, or primary, tumor.

The lymphoid organs include lymph nodes, the thymus, and the spleen. There are about 600 bean-shaped **lymph nodes** scattered throughout the body, usually clustered in groups. The **thymus** is located posterior to the sternum and is most active in youth; by the time a

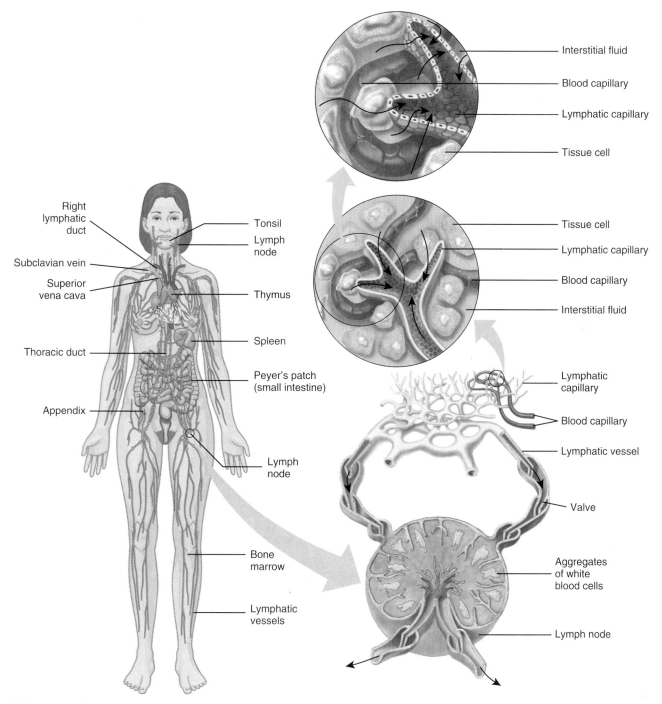

FIGURE 5.3 Major organs and tissues of the lymphatic system

person has reached maturity, the thymus has atrophied significantly. The **spleen** is the largest single mass of lymphatic tissue and is located to the upper left of the abdomen, protected by the ribcage.

Lymphoid tissues are regions of connective tissues that are rich in lymphocytes. These tissues include **tonsils**, which are found in the pharynx, and **mucosa associated lymphatic tissue (MALT)**, which is found in epithelia of the respiratory, digestive, urinary, and reproductive systems. The lymphoid organs and tissues are responsible for the maturation and maintenance of lymphocytes and stimulating an immune response to pathogens, toxins, or vaccines.

TABLE 5.1

Key Blood and Lymphatic System Combining Forms

adenotonsill/o: adenoids

agglutin/o: clumping

albumin/o: albumin

anis/o: unequal

capillar/o: capillary

coagul/o: clotting

constrict/o: narrow

dilat/o: widen

electr/o: electric

embol/o: plug

globin/o: protein

hem/o: blood

hemat/o: blood

immun/o: protection

inguin/o: groin

kal/i: potassium

ket/o: ketone

keton/o: ketone

leuk/o: white

lymphaden/o: lymph node

lymphangi/o: lymph vessel

lymph/o: lymph

morph/o: shape

myel/o: bone marrow; spinal cord

natr/o: sodium

phleb/o: vein

poikil/o: varied, irregular

reticul/o: network

scint/i: spark

splen/o: spleen

syncop/o: faint

thromb/o: clot

viscos/o: sticky

TABLE 5.2

Key Blood and Lymphatic System Suffixes

-apharesis: removal, carry away

-blast: immature

-crit: separation of

-cytosis: more than the normal number of cells

-emia: blood condition

-edema: swelling

-globin: protein

-globulin: protein

-penia: abnormal decrease

-phil: attracted to

-phoresis: carrying

-poietic: pertaining to formation

🔍 *STANDARD CASE STUDY*

5.1 Paroxysmal Nocturnal Hemoglobinuria

Marcus, a 24-year-old male training for his third marathon, had been concerned about his health for the past few months. He was a runner through all of his high school and college years and was used to fatigue and muscle aches from intense training regimens, but this was different. The overwhelming tiredness would not go away no matter how many recovery days he took; he had a constant nagging headache and he felt as though a vise was gripping his abdomen. In the morning he woke up with a fever and noticed an odd cola-like color to his urine, he made an appointment with his physician.

Dr. Zeitler listened to Marcus' history, performed a physical examination, and ordered some lab tests. The doctor noted that Marcus was febrile, tachycardic, and tachypneic. Hepatomegaly was noted following abdominal palpation. Marcus' lab results were of definite concern, indicating anemia, pancytopenia, hyperbilirubinemia, reticulocytosis, and coagulopathy. Dr. Zeitler referred Marcus to a hematologist for consultation.

After reviewing Marcus' lab results and medical history, the hematologist ordered some additional tests. The results led to a diagnosis of paroxysmal nocturnal hemoglobinuria (PNH). The hematologist explained that PNH is a rare acquired hematopoietic stem cell disorder that can have life-threatening complications. Affected individuals usually present with symptoms relating to hemolysis, thrombosis, and impaired bone marrow function. Disease progression and long-range outlook vary significantly but patients taking a newer drug, used to prevent destruction of red blood cells, have reported significant symptom abatement and improved quality of life.

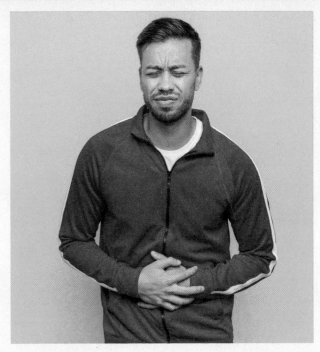

CASE FIGURE: Marcus with severe abdominal pain

© Asier Romero/Shutterstock

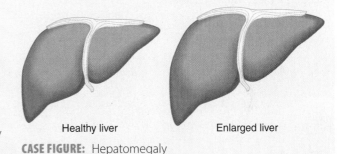

Healthy liver   Enlarged liver

CASE FIGURE: Hepatomegaly

Marcus was determined that this medical challenge would not take over his life. He joined a support group for patients with rare blood disorders and hopes to be cleared to return to running, the sport he loves, once his blood counts improve.

1. Complete the table below for the signs noted at Marcus' physical exam:

Term	Word Parts	Meaning
febrile	*febri-;-ile*	*pertaining to fever*
tachycardic		
tachypneic		
hepatomegaly		

(continues)

🔍 STANDARD CASE STUDY   (continued)

2. Complete the table below for Marcus' abnormal lab values:

Term	Word Parts	Meaning
anemia	*an-; -emia*	*blood condition without (refers to reduction in red blood cells)*
pancytopenia		
hyperbilirubinemia		
reticulocytosis		
coagulopathy		

3. The type of physician who specializes in blood disorders is a _____.

4. Marcus is diagnosed with paroxysmal nocturnal hemoglobinuria. Paroxysmal means a sudden recurrence. Define the word parts for *nocturnal* and *hemoglobinuria* and then explain how you think paroxysmal nocturnal hemoglobinuria is related to the cola-like color of Marcus' urine.

    Nocturnal: Nocturn/o _____, -al _____.

    Hemoglobinuria: Hem/o _____, globin/o _____, -uria _____.

5. Indicate and define the component word parts for *hemolysis* and *thrombosis*.

6. Define the word parts for *hematopoietic*. What are hematopoietic stem cells?

    Hematopoietic: Hemat/o _____, -poietic _____.

🔍 STANDARD CASE STUDY

5.2 Polycythemia Vera

Tallulah Calhoun, a 60-year-old female, arrives at the blood center for her therapeutic phlebotomy treatment. Tallulah has been coming about seven times a year for the past 5 years for this procedure since her diagnosis of polycythemia vera (PV). The years leading up to her diagnosis were challenging as she was constantly fatigued, had bouts of dizziness, and her skin was red and always itchy. She also had frequent headaches, stomach pain, and joint pain.

   Tallulah has learned a lot about PV. She knows that it is a myeloproliferative neoplasm resulting in erythremia (also called erythrocytosis) and hyperviscosity. Leukocytosis and thrombocytosis can also occur with this disease, but she has been spared these thus far and has not had splenomegaly or osteoalgia, which can also occur with PV. She has been good about keeping up with regular venesections to keep her hematocrit under control.

Patients over 60-years-old with PV have an increased risk of thrombosis and her doctor talks with her today about additional treatments. One option is cytoreductive drug therapy and another may be erythrocytapharesis. Her doctor conveys to her the risk that a thrombotic event will lead to a heart attack or stroke and Tallulah promises to consider her options. Unless her blood counts change dramatically, she will return in about 6 weeks for her next therapeutic phlebotomy appointment and to further discuss her treatment options.

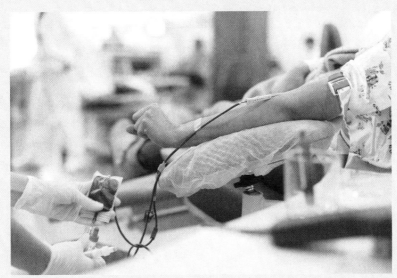

CASE FIGURE: Phlebotomy
© Matej Kastelic/Shutterstock

1. Fill in the component word parts as indicated and then put them together to build medical terms for symptoms used in the case.

   Headache: Head _____, pain _____, headache _____.

   Red skin (literally blood red): red _____, blood _____,

   red skin _____.

   Stomach pain: Stomach _____, pain _____,

   Stomach Pain _____.

   Joint pain: Joint _____, pain _____, joint pain _____.

   Itchiness: Itching _____, structure of _____,

   Itchiness _____.

2. Define the word parts and meaning for *polycythemia*.

   Polycythemia: Poly- _____, cyt/o _____,

   hem/o _____, -ia _____,

   means _____.

(continues)

STANDARD CASE STUDY (continued)

3. Proliferate means to reproduce rapidly. Define the following word parts and explain what is meant by *myeloproliferative neoplasm*.

   Myel/o _____, neo- _____,

   -plasm _____

4. Complete the table below for the following signs and symptoms of PV:

Term	Word Parts	Meaning
erythremia	*erythr/o; -emia*	*blood condition of red (refers to an increase in number of red blood cells)*
hyperviscosity		
erythrocytosis		
leukocytosis		
thrombocytosis		
splenomegaly		
ostealgia		
thrombosis		
hematocrit		

5. Complete the table below for some treatments of PV:

Term	Word Parts	Meaning
phlebotomy	*phleb/o; -otomy*	*process of cutting into a vein*
venesection		
cytoreductive (drug therapy)	*cyt/o; reductive (deceasing)*	
erythrocytapharesis		

6. Considering that PV is an abnormal increase in the number of red blood cells, explain how each of the above therapeutic procedures could be used to treat PV.

🔍 *STANDARD CASE STUDY*

5.3 Milroy Disease

When Maja was born, the first thing her parents noticed was how swollen her legs were. Her edematous limbs were suggestive of primary lymphedema and lymphoscintigraphy confirmed Milroy disease, or congenital hereditary lymphedema. In this disease, hypoplasia of lymphatic vessels leads to accumulation of lymphatic fluid in the subcutaneous tissue under the dermis. Hypertrophy of soft tissue, most pronounced in extremities, results. Maja was referred to Dr. Ricci, a vascular specialist.

Dr. Ricci explained to Maja's parents that there is no cure for this disease, but regular treatment is important to reduce swelling and prevent infection. Untreated lymphedema has many potential complications including lymphorrhea, lymphangitis, cellulitis, and rarely lymphangiosarcoma or intestinal lymphangiectasia. Complete decongestive therapy (CDT), which includes maneuvers to enhance lymphatic drainage, compression bandaging, exercise, and skin care, coordinated by a lymphedema specialist, has been shown to be most effective. Maja's parents are committed to vigilance in managing their daughter's care, but as patient compliance is critical in a successful outcome, Maja will have to take over her own care coordination as she gets older.

Lymph/o is the combining form meaning lymph. Lymph is a watery, clear fluid that flows through lymphatic vessels. It is the fluid collected from between cells and contains protein, fat, salt, and white blood cells. List and define the words in this case study that contain the combining form lymph/o, breaking the terms down into their component parts.

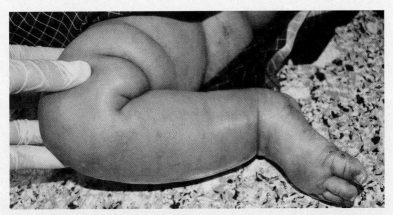

CASE FIGURE: Lymphedema with the possible complication of cellulitis

© Zay Nyi Nyi/Shutterstock

1. What does it mean for a disease to be congenital and hereditary?

2. Complete the table below for the following terms in the case:

Term	Word Parts	Meaning
edematous	*edemat/o; -ous*	*pertaining to swellings*
hypoplasia		
subcutaneous		
hypertrophy		
vascular		
cellulitis		

⌕ *STANDARD CASE STUDY*

5.4 Cooley's Anemia

Spiros Neizan, a 6-month-old infant of Mediterranean origin, is referred to a hematologist for severe anemia. His parents report feeding problems, frequent diarrhea, irritability, and recurrent bouts of fever. Upon physical exam, the hematologist notes pallor, jaundice, and hepatosplenomegaly. A complete blood count shows reduced hemoglobin levels and a low mean corpuscular volume. Peripheral blood smear analysis shows erythroblasts and red blood cells of abnormal morphology. Cells are microcytic, hypochromic, anisocytic, and poikilocytic. The hematologist suspects thalassemia. Hemoglobin electrophoresis and molecular genetic analysis confirm β-thalassemia major, the most severe form of this genetic disease, also known as Cooley's anemia. Thalassemia translates to a blood condition of the sea and is more prevalent in people of Mediterranean descent.

Management of this disease will be lifelong for Spiros. He will need regular transfusions of packed red blood cells to maintain normal levels of hemoglobin. Spiros will also need iron chelation to remove excess iron and prevent iron overload, a major complication of regular transfusion. An overabundance of iron can damage the heart, liver, and endocrine system. Cooley's anemia is inherited as an autosomal recessive disorder; both parents must have a defective gene for a child to be affected. Spiros' parents will receive genetic counseling before making the decision to have another child and Spiros will receive genetic counseling when he is old enough to consider having children himself.

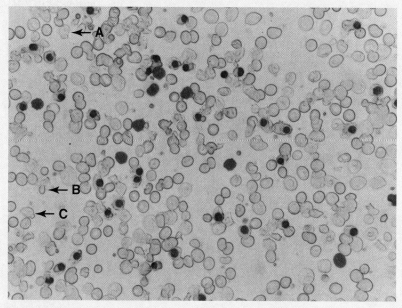

CASE FIGURE: Peripheral blood smear showing (A) hypochromic, (B) anisocytic, and (C) poikilocytic red blood cells

© Schira/Shutterstock

1. Give a short definition for the medical terms *anemia*, *pallor*, and *jaundice*.

    Anemia:

    Pallor:

    Jaundice:

2. Define the word parts for *hepatosplenomegaly*.

    Hepatosplenomegaly: Hepat/o _____, splen/o _____, -megaly _____.

3. Complete the table below for results related to the peripheral blood smear:

Term	Word Parts	Meaning
erythroblasts	*erythr/o; -blasts*	*immature cell of red (immature red blood cells)*
morphology (abnormal)		
microcytic		
hypochromic		
anisocytic		
poikilocytic		

4. Mean corpuscular volume refers to the average size of a single red blood cell. Which term in the table above would indicate a low mean corpuscular volume?

5. Define the word parts and meaning for *hemoglobin electrophoresis*.

Hemoglobin electrophoresis: Hem/o _____, globin/o _____,

electr/o _____, -phoresis _____,

meaning _____.

6. Due to the complex nature of Cooley's anemia, Spiros will need coordinated care throughout his life. The suffix –logist means one who studies. Build medical terms for the following using the suffix –logist for medical personnel who may be involved in Spiros' care.

One who studies blood: _____,

treats issues related to _____.

One who studies the heart: _____,

treats issues related to _____

One who studies the stomach and intestines: _____,

treats issues related to _____.

One who studies glands that secrete within: _____,

treats issues related to _____.

One who studies the mind: _____,

treats issues related to _____.

🔍 *STANDARD CASE STUDY*

5.5 Anaphylactic Shock

An 8-year-old girl presents in the emergency department (ED) with angioedema, pruritus, dyspnea, urticaria, and rhinitis. The patient was stung by a wasp about an hour ago in her classroom. The sting became progressively more inflamed and she began wheezing with presyncope. Anaphylaxis was suspected despite a lack of previous medical history of allergic, or hypersensitivity, reactions. Anaphylaxis is a severe acute immune response that results in increased vascular permeability, driving fluids from systemic circulation into body tissues, resulting in hypovolemia and hypotension. Epinephrine was administered to promote vasoconstriction and bronchodilation to counteract hypotension, laryngeal edema, and shock. She was transferred to critical care and placed on intravenous (IV) therapy and administered antihistamines and glucocorticoids. She was monitored until her full recovery the following day. It was recommended that she carry an autoinjectable epinephrine device (EpiPen) as a precaution, should she be stung again.

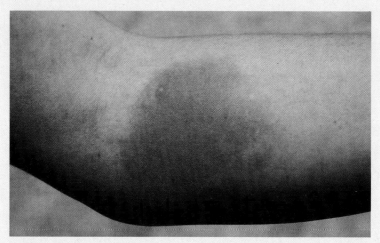

CASE FIGURE: Angioedema and urticaria
© Siegi/Shutterstock

1. Complete the table below for this patient's significant symptoms.

Term	Word Parts	Meaning
angioedema	*angi/o; -edema*	*swelling vessels (swelling of the skin)*
pruritus		
urticaria	NA	
dyspnea		
rhinitis		
rhinorrhea		
presyncope	*pre-; syncop/o*	
hypovolemia		
hypotension		

2. The prefix *ana-* means up and *phylaxia* means protection. The term anaphylaxis was coined in 1902 by Richet and Portier, researchers who studied the severe reaction in laboratory animals. Why are the terms *ana-* and *phylaxia* a good fit for the reaction?

3. Epinephrine was administered to promote vasoconstriction and bronchodilation. Define the word parts and meaning for the terms *vasoconstriction* and *bronchodilation*.

   Vasoconstriction: Vas/o _____, constrict/o _____, -ion _____,

   means _____

   Bronchodilation: Bronch/o _____, dilat/o _____, -ion _____,

   means _____.

🔍 ADVANCED CASE STUDY

5.6 Immune Thrombocytopenia

Yasmine, a 19-year-old college student, had a nosebleed that wouldn't stop. "It's been bleeding for hours," her friend Ruben said to her. "I think it's time for a trip to the ER."

Once at the ER, nasal packing was performed to manage Yasmine's rhinorrhagia. When questioned about other bleeding episodes, Yasmine revealed a history of prolonged epistaxes, menorrhagia, and gingiva that bled easily when brushing her teeth. Notable findings upon physical exam included petechiae on her lower limbs and purpura on the oral mucosa. Yasmine also relayed that she bruised easily, and the bruises were slow to heal. The ER physician ordered blood tests and the results revealed the following:

Test	Result	Reference Range
White blood cell count	10,000/mm^3	4,800–10,800/mm^3
Red blood cell count	4.8 x 10^6/mm^3	4.2–5.4 x 10^6/mm^3
Hemoglobin	13.0 g/dL	12.0–16.0 g/dL
Hematocrit	42%	37–47%
Platelets	4,000/mm^3	150,000–400,000/mm^3

Based on Yasmine's symptoms, laboratory results, and a consultation with a hematologist, she was diagnosed with immune thrombocytopenia and was prescribed corticosteroids as an initial therapeutic agent. Depending on Yasmine's response, other drug treatments may be discussed at a later date. If her condition persists despite pharmaceutical intervention or if relapse is frequent, the option of splenectomy will be considered. Yasmine is advised to avoid contact sports and to use caution with over-the-counter medications such as ibuprofen and aspirin.

(continues)

⌕ ADVANCED CASE STUDY   (continued)

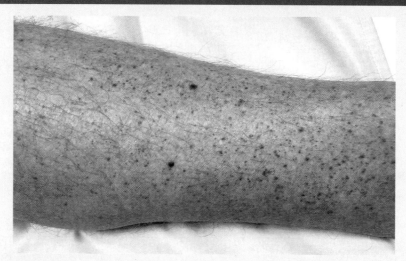

CASE FIGURE: Multiple petechiae on leg

© TisforThan/Shutterstock

1. Yasmine was diagnosed with thrombocytopenia. Define the word parts and meaning for *thrombocytopenia*:

   Thrombocytopenia: Thromb/o _____, cyt/o _____, -penia _____,

   means _____.

2. What lab value provided in the table confirms this diagnosis?

3. White blood cell count and red blood cell count appear to be within reference range. The medical term for white

   blood cells is _____. The medical term for red blood cells is _____.

4. Complete the table below for the following terms:

Term	Word Parts	Meaning
hematologist	*hemat/o; -logist*	*specialist of blood*
rhinorrhagia		
menorrhagia		
hemoglobin		
hematocrit		
splenectomy		

5. List and explain other signs in the case that are indicative of a blood clotting disorder.

6. Why is Yasmine told to avoid contact sports and medications such as ibuprofen and aspirin?

🔍 *ADVANCED CASE STUDY*

5.7 Diabetic Ketoacidosis

A 25-year-old male presents in the emergency department (ED) with generalized weakness, nausea, and diffuse abdominal pain. He is a type 1 diabetic who has not been monitoring his blood glucose, or self-administering insulin, for over a week. He reports anorexia, polydipsia, and polyuria. He is hyperpneic, hypovolemic, and lab tests show hyperketonuria, hyperketonemia, hyperglycemia, and acidemia. He also has abnormally low blood sodium and high blood potassium. He is treated for diabetic ketoacidosis (DKA), a hemodynamic disorder that results from insulin deficiency, which hampers cells' ability to access glucose. With reduced access to glucose, the body begins metabolizing fats, which produces acidic circulating ketones, resulting in metabolic acidosis. The patient is treated with intravenous (IV) fluids, insulin, and bicarbonate.

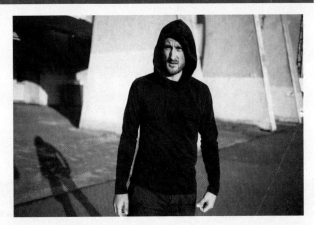

© Svetlana Voroshilova/Moment/Getty Images

1. Complete the table below for this patient's symptoms.

Term	Word Parts	Meaning
anorexia	*an-; -orexia*	*without appetite*
polydipsia		
polyuria		
hyperpneic		
hypovolemic		
hyperketouria		
hyperketonemia		
hyperglycemia		
acidemia		

(continues)

🔍 *ADVANCED CASE STUDY*   *(continued)*

2. The blood test shows low blood sodium and high blood potassium. What are the medical terms for these conditions? Identify their word parts.

3. Type 1 diabetes mellitus is an autoimmune disease. The prefix auto- means self. What is an autoimmune disease?

4. Blood is maintained within a narrow pH range; normal pH of arterial blood is 7.35–7.45. The condition of low blood pH is called *acidemia*, it results from the process of *acidosis*. The condition of high blood pH is called *alkalemia*, it results from the process of *alkalosis*. For the following two statements, fill in the blanks using the italicized terms above.

A person with an arterial blood pH of 7.31 has _____ resulting from _____.

A person with an arterial blood pH of 7.49 has _____ resulting from _____.

🔍 *ADVANCED CASE STUDY*

5.8 The Great Mortality

Recently discovered church documents from the 15th century describe a small Swiss village enduring a wretched winter of death; 30% of the citizens died from a terrifying new illness. The documents thoroughly recorded the symptoms of the stricken.

In one case, a middle-aged male presented to the village apothecary with inguinal lymphadenitis. The patient was described as febrile with "the marks," which were petechial hemorrhages, presumably from disseminated intravascular coagulation (DIC). In DIC, increased coagulation results in the formation of circulating clots and a depletion of available clotting factors leading to hemorrhaging. After two days, the patient exhibited blackened regions in his fingers and toes as thrombi blocked capillaries, reducing perfusion and leading to ischemic necrosis. After several days, the patient's condition further deteriorated, presenting with hematemesis, hemoptysis, hematuria, hematochezia, and ultimately death.

The details of this historical patient record suggest that the patient died of septicemic plague secondary to bubonic plague. Plague is caused by infection by the *Yersinia pestis* bacterium. It is a zoonotic infection that is transmitted to humans from rodents through their fleas. Bubonic plague results from bites from infected fleas. The infection typically spreads through the lymphatic system, causing lymphadenopathy, especially in the inguinal, axillary, and cervical regions. The swollen and rupturing lymph nodes are called buboes, giving bubonic plague its name. If the *Y. pestis* infection moves into systemic circulation, as in this case, it is termed septicemic plague. This type of plague is associated with bacteremia and endotoxemia, which become progressively worse, leading to DIC, driving the thromboembolic and hemorrhaging-associated symptoms described in the present case. Septicemic plague is almost always fatal.

1. A pharmacist is the modern-day apothecary. Define the word parts, and meaning, of *pharmacist*.

Pharmacist: Pharmac/o _____, -ist _____,

means _____.

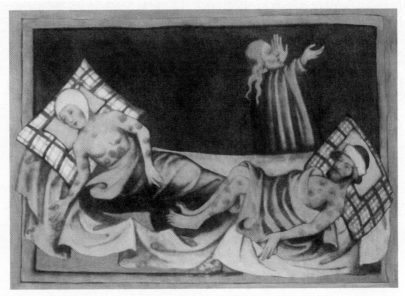

CASE FIGURE: Medieval painting from a German language Bible of 1411

2. Lymphadenitis is a form of adenopathy that can result in visible buboes (painful swellings), characteristic of bubonic plague. Define the following word parts, and meaning, of *inguinal lymphadenitis* and *adenopathy*.

   Inguinal lymphadenitis: Inguin/o _____, -al _____,

   lymph/o _____, aden/o _____, -itis _____,

   means _____.

   Adenopathy: Aden/o _____, -pathy _____,

   means _____.

3. In what body regions are the axillary and cervical lymph nodes?

4. Petechial hemorrhaging may develop as a result of septicemic plague. Explain what is meant by *petechial hemorrhage.*

5. Septicemic plague results from bacteremia and endotoxemia. Indicate and define the component word parts for *bacteremia* and *endotoxemia* and explain their meaning.

(continues)

⌕ *ADVANCED CASE STUDY*   *(continued)*

6. Complete the table below for terms relating to the disseminated intravascular coagulation (DIC) clotting disorder.

Term	Word Parts	Meaning
ischemic	*isch/o; -emic*	*holding back blood (starving tissue of blood supply)*
necrosis		
hematemesis		
hemoptysis		
hematuria		
hematochezia		
thromboembolic		
thrombus		
capillary		

⌕ *ADVANCED CASE STUDY*

5.9 Transfusion Reaction

A 55-year-old female in postoperative recovery became febrile and complained of diffuse abdominal pain. Her urine was a reddish-brown color. She also presented with tachypnea and icteric sclera. It was discovered that during the surgery 12 hours prior, the patient was misidentified before administration of incompatible ABO blood type, which led to a diagnosis of acute hemolytic transfusion reaction (HTR). The donor's ABO blood type was AB, the patient is type O. The patient's antibodies (anti-A and anti-B) were binding to the A and B antigens on the donor's erythrocytes, promoting hemolysis and releasing intracellular potassium and hemoglobin into the blood plasma. Hemolysis was confirmed by visual inspection of centrifuged blood and urine samples; the blood plasma was red, and the centrifuged urine was red and no red blood cells were visible. Laboratory tests revealed hypercreatinemia, hyperkalemia, hyperbilirubinemia, and hyperhemoglobinemia, supporting a diagnosis of HTR. No other test results were significant. The patient was transferred to critical care for close monitoring and supportive care.

Abnormal Test Results:

Test	Result	Reference Range
Serum creatinine	2.5 mg/dL	0.6–1.5 mg/dL
Serum potassium	7.5 mEq/L	3.5–5.0 mEq/L
Serum bilirubin	2.5 mg/dL	<0.4 mg/dL
Serum hemoglobin	5.0 mg/dL	<0.5 mg/dL

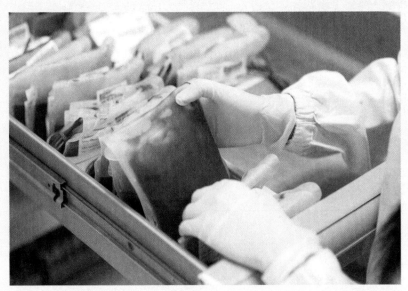

CASE FIGURE: A laboratory technician identifying blood for transfusion

© Komsan Loonprom/Shutterstock

1. Complete the table below for this patient's symptoms and significant test findings.

Term	Word Parts	Meaning
tachypneic	*tachy-; -pnea*	*breathing fast*
icteric sclera		
hypercreatinemia		
hyperkalemia		
hyperbilirubinemia		
hyperhemoglobinemia		

2. The blood type most commonly referred to is the ABO blood grouping. People can have type A, type B, type AB, or type O blood. The type of blood refers to the way that their erythrocytes (red blood cells) are decorated with branching carbohydrate molecules. If a person receives an incompatible blood type, antibodies in their blood serum may cause agglutination and hemolysis of the donor erythrocytes. Define the word parts and meaning for *agglutination*, *hemolysis*, and *erythrocyte*.

Agglutination: Agglutin/o _____, -ation _____,

means _____.

Hemolysis: Hem/o _____, -lysis _____,

means _____.

Erythrocyte: Erythr/o _____, -cyte _____,

means _____.

(continues)

3. Define the word parts and meaning for *hemoglobinuria* and *hematuria*. Then explain why the observations in the case study support hemoglobinuria and do not support hematuria.

Hemoglobinuria: Hem/o _____, globin/o _____,

-emia _____, means _____.

Hematuria: Hemat/o _____, -uria _____,

means _____.

🔍 *ADVANCED CASE STUDY*

5.10 Waldman Disease

A 55-year-old African American female made an appointment with her primary care provider (PCP) to discuss symptoms of generalized abdominal pain, diarrhea, and emesis. She claims that she generally feels tired and she has a 14.6 BMI (5'10" and 140 lbs.), which is underweight. On physical examination, the PCP noted modest lymphedema in the lower extremities. The PCP ordered blood tests and followed up by ordering quantitative serum immunoglobulins (IgG).

Test	Result	Reference Range
Leukocytes	5,500/mm^3	4,800–10,800/mm^3
Lymphocytes	900/mm^3	1,200–3,400/mm^3
Neutrophils (mature)	4,000/mm^3	3,000–5,800/mm^3
Platelets	300 x 10^3/mm^3	150–400 x 10^3/mm^3
Hemoglobin	13 g/dL	12–16 g/dL
Albumin	22 g/L	35–52 g/L
Total protein	40 g/dL	60–84 g/L
IgG	3.5 g/L	7–16 g/L
IgA	1.0 g/L	0.7–3.8 g/L
IgM	0.4 g/L	0.5–2.6 g/L

The tests revealed lymphopenia, hypoalbuminemia, hypoproteinemia, and hypogammaglobulinemia. Subsequent tests measuring components of complement, which are a group of proteins involved in the body's immune defenses, revealed hypocomplementemia. The findings were consistent with an immunodeficiency syndrome secondary to primary intestinal lymphangiectasia (Waldman disease), an exudative enteropathy, which is characterized by a loss of proteins and lymphocytes in the stool. The dilation of the lymphatic vessels associated with the intestinal epithelium leads to oozing of lymphatic materials into the gastrointestinal tract. An enteroscopy, together with a biopsy, confirmed jejunal submucosal lymphangiectasia.

Differential diagnoses, including HIV, were omitted by testing. The PCP prescribed diuretics, and recommended compression socks, to reduce lower limb lymphedema. She referred the patient to a nutritionist to develop a long-term diet strategy, including supplements, to meet the needs of this patient with a protein-losing enteropathy.

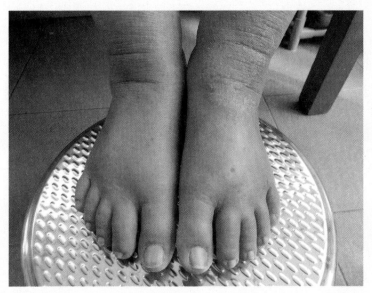

CASE FIGURE: Lymphedema in lower extremities
© AppleDK/Shutterstock

1. Complete the table below for this patient's significant symptoms.

Term	Word Parts	Meaning
diarrhea	*dia-; -rrhea*	complete discharge (watery stool)
emesis		
lymphedema		
lymphopenia		
hypoalbuminemia		
hypoproteinemia		
hypogammaglobulinemia	*hypo-; gammaglobulin (IgG); -emia*	
hypocomplementemia	*hypo-; complement; -emia*	

2. The patient was losing proteins, antibodies, and lymphocytes from the lymphatic system to the gastrointestinal tract due to intestinal lymphangiectasia. Define the word parts, and meaning, for jejunal lymphangiectasia.

Jejunal lymphangiectasia: Jejun/o _____, -al _____,

lymph/o _____, angi/o _____, -ectasis _____,

means _____.

(continues)

⌕ *ADVANCED CASE STUDY*   *(continued)*

3. What is a differential diagnosis?

4. Define the word parts and meaning for *enteroscopy*, *biopsy*, and *enteropathy*.

Enteroscopy: Enter/o _____, -scopy _____,

means _____.

Biopsy: Bi/o _____, -opsy _____,

means _____.

Enteropathy: Enter/o _____, -pathy _____,

means _____.

References

Dennis, D. T., & Mead, P. S. (2006). Plague. *Tropical Infectious Diseases*, 471–481. https://doi.org/10.1016/B978-0-443-06668-9.50047-8

Freeman, A. M., Matto, P. Adenopathy. [Updated 2020 Apr 22]. In: StatPearls [Internet]. Treasure Island (FL): StatPearls Publishing; 2020 Jan-. Available from: https://www.ncbi.nlm.nih.gov/books/NBK513250/

Galanello, R., & Origa, R. (2010). Beta-thalassemia. *Orphanet Journal of Rare Diseases*, *5*(11). doi:10.1186/1750-1172-5-11

Huber, X., Degen, L., Muenst, S., & Trendelenburg, M. (2017). Primary intestinal lymphangiectasia in an elderly female patient: A case report on a rare cause of secondary immunodeficiency. *Medicine*, *96*(31), e7729. https://doi.org/10.1097/MD.0000000000007729

Jimenez-Rodriguez, T. W., Garcia-Neuer, M., Alenazy, L. A., & Castells, M. (2018). Anaphylaxis in the 21st century: phenotypes, endotypes, and biomarkers. *Journal of Asthma and Allergy*, *11*, 121–142. https://doi.org/10.2147/JAA.S159411

Kado, R., & McCune, W. J. (2019). Treatment of primary and secondary immune thrombocytopenia. *Current Opinion in Rheumatology*, *31*(3), 213–222. https://doi.org/10.1097/BOR.0000000000000599

Lynn, J., Knight, A. K., Kamoun, M., & Levinson, A. I. (2004). A 55-year-old man with hypogammaglobulinemia, lymphopenia, and unrelenting cutaneous warts. *The Journal of Allergy and Clinical Immunology*, *114*(2), 409–414. https://doi.org/10.1016/j.jaci.2004.02.033

Mali, S., & Jambure, R. (2012). Anaphylaxis management: Current concepts. *Anesthesia Essays and Researches*, *6*(2), 115–123. https://doi.org/10.4103/0259-1162.108284

Namikawa, A., Shibuya, Y., Ouchi, H., Takahashi, H., & Furuto, Y. (2018). A case of ABO-incompatible blood transfusion treated by plasma exchange therapy and continuous hemodiafiltration. *CEN Case Reports*, *7*(1), 114–120. https://doi.org/10.1007/s13730-018-0307-4

Schamroth, N. R. (2013). An unusual case of Milroy disease. *South African Journal of Child Health*, *7*(3), 118–119. Retrieved January 12, 2020, from http://www.scielo.org.za/scielo.php?script=sci_arttext&pid=S1999-76712013000300010&lng=en&tlng=en

Sicherer, S. H., Simons, F. E. (2017). Epinephrine for first-aid management of anaphylaxis. *Pediatrics*, *139* (3), e20164006. doi: 10.1542/peds.2016-4006

Stedman, T. L. (2005*). Nath's Stedman's medical terminology, 2e*. Philadelphia: Lippincott Williams & Wilkins.

Strobel, E. (2008). Hemolytic transfusion reactions. *Transfusion medicine and hemotherapy: offizielles Organ der Deutschen Gesellschaft fur Transfusionsmedizin und Immunhamatologie*, *35*(5), 346–353. https://doi.org/10.1159/000154811

Teofili, L., Valentini, C.G., Rossi, E., & De Stefano, V. (2019). Indications and use of therapeutic phlebotomy in polycythemia vera: Which role for erythrocytapheresis? *Leukemia*, *33*, 279–281. doi:10.1038/s41375-018-0304-9

Van de Vyver C, Damen J, Haentjens, C. Ballaux, D, & Bouts, B. (2017). An exceptional case of diabetic ketoacidosis. *Case Reports in Emergency Medicine*, *2017*. doi:10.1155/2017/4351620

Venes, D. & Taber, C. W. (2017). *Taber's cyclopedic medical dictionary*. Ed. 23, illustrated in full color/Philadelphia: F.A. Davis.

Young, N. S., Meyers, G., Schrezenmeier, H., Hillmen, P., & Hill, A. (2009). The management of paroxysmal nocturnal hemoglobinuria: Recent advances in diagnosis and treatment and new hope for patients. *Seminars in Hematology*, *46* (1 Suppl 1), S1–S16. doi:10.1053/j.seminhematol.2008.11.004

CHAPTER 6

Respiratory System

The respiratory system is responsible for external respiration, the exchange of oxygen and carbon dioxide between the outside environment and the bloodstream, which occurs in the lungs; and internal respiration, the exchange of oxygen and carbon dioxide between the bloodstream and cells throughout the body. The primary anatomical components of the respiratory system are the nose and nasal cavity, the three divisions of the pharynx, the larynx, the trachea, and the bronchial tubes and lungs. Inhaled air passes sequentially through these structures. The respiratory system includes many supportive structures such as the paranasal sinuses, the tonsils, and the respiratory muscles.

The exterior of the **nose** is muscle and skin, which covers a supporting framework of bone and cartilage. On the underside of the nose are the two **external nares**, also called nostrils, which open into the nasal cavity. The nasal cavity is divided into a right and left half by a wall consisting mostly of cartilage,

called the **nasal septum**. Mucous membranes and hairs line the nasal cavity. These help to trap debris and pathogens and to warm and humidify inspired air. The nasal cavity also has an olfactory region, lined with olfactory receptors, responsible for the sense of smell. The four paired **paranasal sinuses** are air-filled spaces that surround the nasal cavity. They produce mucus and increase resonance of the voice.

The **pharynx** consists of three regions: the **nasopharynx**, the **oropharynx**, and the **laryngopharynx**. The nasopharynx is located in the posterior region of the nasal cavity, connecting inferiorly to the oropharynx. The oropharynx and laryngopharynx are respiratory and digestive pathways and the laryngopharynx opens both to the esophagus and to the larynx. Small masses of lymphatic tissue that play a role in the body's immune response, called **tonsils**, are located in the pharynx. The **larynx** is also called the voicebox and contains the **vocal cords**, which are cartilage and infoldings

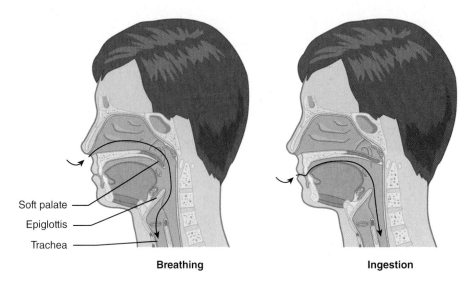

Soft palate
Epiglottis
Trachea

Breathing   **Ingestion**

FIGURE 6.1 The passage of air when breathing and food when eating

of mucous membrane that vibrate to produce voice and sound. The **epiglottis**, a large leaf-shaped flap of cartilage, closes off the larynx during swallowing to ensure that food and liquids do not enter it from the pharynx. The larynx leads to the **trachea**, a tube about 4.5 inches long and an inch wide that is supported by 16–20 C-shaped cartilaginous rings that provide support so that the tracheal wall does not collapse inwardly during inhalation.

In the thoracic cavity, the trachea divides at the **carina**, a projection of the last tracheal cartilage, into the left **primary bronchus** and the right primary bronchus, which enter the lungs. The **bronchi** then branch to smaller secondary and even smaller tertiary bronchi, then to **bronchioles**, which branch repeatedly to end in **terminal bronchioles**. This extensive network of smaller and smaller branching bronchial tubes from the trachea is frequently referred to as the **bronchial tree**. Terminal bronchioles subdivide again to respiratory bronchioles and ultimately terminate in

microscopic air sacs, the alveoli (singular **alveolus**), where gas exchange occurs. In this process, inhaled oxygen diffuses into the bloodstream and waste carbon dioxide diffuses out.

The **lungs** are paired, cone-shaped organs in the **thoracic cavity**. The left lung with two lobes is slightly smaller than the right lung with three lobes. Because the heart and other structures separate the lungs from each other, they reside in two anatomically distinct chambers. This is important clinically because if one lung collapses due to damage, the other may remain expanded. A double layered membrane called the **pleura** covers the lungs. Anatomical features of the lungs include the **apex**, the superior region extending about an inch above the clavicle; the base, which rests on the diaphragm; and the **hilum**, where the primary bronchus, pulmonary arterys and pulmonary vein enter and exit the lung.

The cycle of inhaling and exhaling, or **inspiration** and **expiration**, is **pulmonary ventilation**, also called

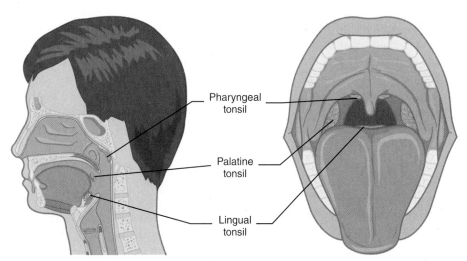

Pharyngeal
tonsil

Palatine
tonsil

Lingual
tonsil

FIGURE 6.2 The major tonsils of the pharynx

Inspiration

Expiration

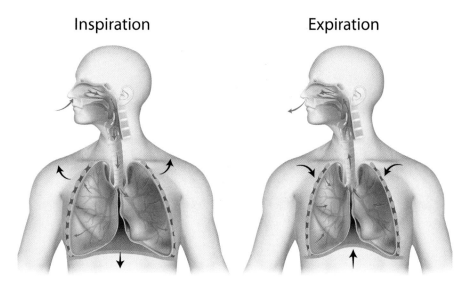

FIGURE 6.3 Pulmonary ventilation

© Alila Medical Media/Shutterstock

breathing. The **diaphragm**, the dome-shaped muscle between the thoracic and abdominal cavity, is the major muscle of pulmonary ventilation. During inhalation, the diaphragm contracts and drops, expanding the chest, and air is pulled in. During exhalation, the diaphragm relaxes and rises, reducing the chest volume, and air is forced out. Normal, also called quiet, breathing is driven by the diaphragm and the **intercostal muscles**. More forceful inspiration and expiration can be achieved by recruiting additional muscles including the **sternocleidomastoid**, **scalene**, and **pectoralis minor muscles**. The respiratory rate, in breaths per minute, is one of the vital signs. A slower or faster respiratory rate than normal can be an indicator of illness.

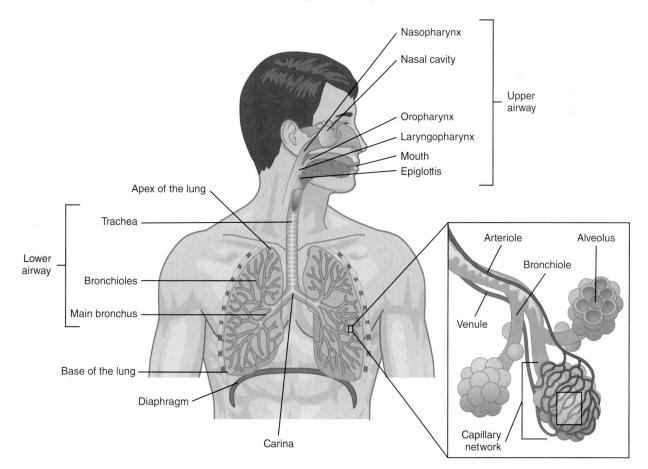

FIGURE 6.4 Major structures of the respiratory system

TABLE 6.1

Key Respiratory System Combining Forms

adenoid/o: adenoids

alveol/o: alveolus, small sac

anthrac/o: coal

asbest/o: asbestos

bronchi/o: bronchus

bronch/o: bronchus

bronchiol/o: bronchiole

capn/o: carbon dioxide

cili/o: cilia

coni/o: dust

chyl/o: chyle (mixture of lymph and fats)

cricothyr/o: ligament between the cricoid, and thyroid, cartilages

eosin/o: rosy

epiglott/o: epiglottis

fibr/o: fiber

laryng/o: larynx

lob/o: lobe

muc/o: mucus

nas/o: nose

odyn/o: pain

ox/i: oxygen

ox/o: oxygen

pharyng/o: pharynx, throat

phon/o: voice, sound

pleur/o: pleura

pneum/o: lung; air

pneumon/o: lung; air

polyp/o: polyp

pulmon/o: lung

rhin/o: nose

segment/o: piece

sept/o: wall

silic/o: glass

sinus/o: sinus

somn/o: sleep

spir/o: breathing

steth/o: chest

thorac/o: chest

thyr/o: thyroid gland; thyroid cartilage

tonsill/o: tonsils

trache/o: trachea

TABLE 6.2

Key Respiratory Suffixes

-capnia: carbon dioxide

-centesis: puncture to withdraw fluid

-ectasis: dilation

-osmia: smelling

-pnea: breathing

-ptysis: spitting

-thorax: pleural cavity, chest

-tubation: putting a tube within

🔍 *STANDARD CASE STUDY*

6.1 Epiglottitis

A 55-year-old female presents to the emergency department (ED) with myalgia, sore throat with lymphadenopathy, fever, odynophagia, dysphasia, and difficult phonation. Differential diagnoses include pharyngitis, laryngitis, and more serious conditions such as epiglottitis, angioedema, caustic ingestion, or foreign-body ingestion. Patient exhibits mild inspiratory stridor without wheezing. Posterior oropharynx is erythematous without exudate. Epiglottitis is suspected and an otorhinolaryngologist is asked to perform nasopharyngolaryngoscopy. Due to the risk of laryngospasm, intubation equipment is in close proximity. An edamatous epiglottis is visible with the classic "thumbprint signal" confirming epiglottitis and management in the intensive care unit is recommended. Soon after ICU admission, hypoxia, tachypnea, and a significant increase in patient respiratory effort necessitated endotracheal intubation. An acute care surgical team was prepared with a tracheostomy tube for emergent cricothyrotomy, which did not become necessary. Dexamethasone and IV antibiotics were administered and decrease of epiglottic swelling was noted the next day. On the second hospital day, the patient was extubated and by the fourth hospital day no epiglottic edema was present. The patient was discharged on hospital day 8 without complication.

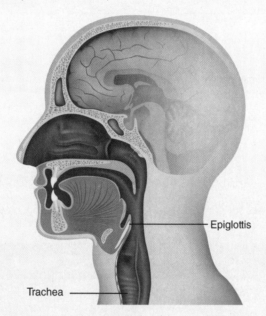

Epiglottis

Trachea

CASE FIGURE: Sagittal section of the upper respiratory system. An epiglottis that is swollen looks like a raised thumb and can readily block the trachea
© Medicalstocks/Shutterstock

1. Complete the table below listing symptoms and differential diagnostics related to epiglottitis:

Term	Word Parts	Meaning
epiglottitis	*epiglott/o; -itis*	*inflammation of the epiglottis*
myalgia		
lymphadenopathy		
odynophagia		
dysphasia		
phonation		

(continues)

🔍 *STANDARD CASE STUDY* (continued)

Term	Word Parts	Meaning
pharyngitis		
angioedema		
hypoxia		
tachypnea		

2. Stridor is a high-pitched sound caused by an obstruction in the pharynx or larynx. What is *inspiratory stridor*?

Inspiratory: In- _____, spir/o _____, -atory _____.

3. Using your knowledge of medical terminology, rewrite the following statement without medical jargon: *Posterior oropharynx is erythematous without exudate.*

4. Complete the table below describing medical specialties and procedures involved in the management of epiglottitis.

Term	Word Parts	Meaning
otorhinolaryngologist	*ot/o; rhin/o; laryng/o; -logist*	*one who studies the ears, nose, and throat*
nasopharyngolaryngoscopy		
endotracheal intubation		
tracheostomy		
cricothyrotomy		
extubation		

5. Indicate the word parts for *laryngospasm* and *edematous*. What is the epiglottis and why do you think an edematous epiglottis necessitates management in the ICU?

🔍 *STANDARD CASE STUDY*

6.2 Mounier-Kuhn Syndrome

David, a 25-year-old teacher, has bronchitis again. Ever since he was a child, he has suffered from recurrent bronchopulmonary infections. Lately, they have increased in frequency, probably due to his exposure to the numerous students who passed through his classroom. His doctor, sensing David's frustration, decides to further investigate the underlying cause of these repeat infections. David is sent for a chest X-ray and the astute radiologist notices a tracheal diameter of 35 mm, significantly larger than the normal range of 15–25 mm for males. Thoracic computed tomography (CT) indicates moderate bronchiectasis. Tracheal and bronchial dilation, along with frequent occurrences of lower respiratory infection, are diagnostic of the rare disease, Mounier-Kuhn syndrome. Treatment for this syndrome is symptomatic with antibiotics for recurrent infections and possible chest physiotherapy and mucolytics to improve mucociliary clearance. Complications can include tracheomalacia in which case a tracheobronchial stent, sometimes coupled with tracheobronchoplasty, can be considered.

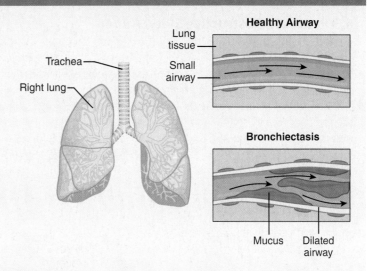

CASE FIGURE: Airways in a healthy lung and in one with bronchiectasis

1. Define the component word parts for *bronchiectasis*.

   Bronchiectasis: Bronchi/o _____, -ectasis _____.

2. Build a term for narrowing of the bronchial tubes, the opposite of what is seen in Mounier-Kuhn syndrome.

3. Trachea is the medical term for the windpipe. List the terms in the case with this root, indicate their word parts, and define the terms.

4. Build a term meaning enlarged trachea and bronchi. This term is a secondary name for Mounier-Kuhn syndrome.

5. Refer to a medical dictionary and define mucociliary clearance. What role do mucolytics play in this?

⌕ *STANDARD CASE STUDY*

6.3 Pediatric Obstructive Sleep Apnea

A mother brings her 8-year-old son to the pediatrician for evaluation of his nighttime snoring, daytime somnolence, and irritability. The mother reports several witnessed episodes of apnea during the night. The child exhibits hyponasal speech and physical exam of the oropharynx reveals adenotonsillar hypertrophy. The pediatrician suspects obstructive sleep apnea and recommends an overnight, attended, polysomnography consisting of electroencephalography, nasal and oral airflow sensors, pulse oximetry, and capnography. An apnea-hypopnea index will be calculated, indicating the total number of apneas and hypopneas per hour of sleep. The child will be seen by a specialist to review the polysomnogram results and to discuss adenotonsillectomy for his marked lymphadenoid hyperplasia.

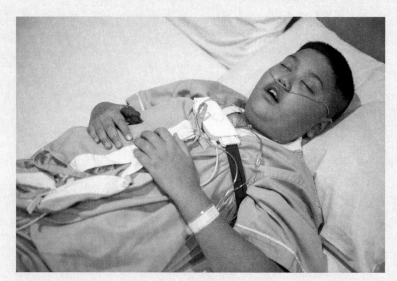

CASE FIGURE: A boy undergoing polysomnography

© Pisit Rapitpunt/Shutterstock

1. Define the component word parts for *apnea* and *hypopnea*.

    Apnea: A- _____, -pnea _____.

    Hypopnea: Hypo- _____, -pnea _____.

2. Use the suffix -pnea to make the terms meaning the following.

Meaning	Term
breathing that is difficult	
breathing that is normal	
breathing that is excessive	
breathing slow	
breathing fast	
breathing straight (describes breathing that is easier when sitting straight)	

3. Complete the table below for procedural terms related to the case.

Term	Word Parts	Meaning
electroencephalography	*electr/o; encephal/o; -grahy*	*recording the electricity of the brain*
polysomnograhy		
oximetry		
capnography		
adenotonsillectomy		

4. The word in the case indicating the boy is sleepy during the day is _____.

5. The word in the case indicating too little air is getting through the boy's nose when he speaks is _____

_____.

6. There are two different terms in the case indicating the boy has enlarged tonsils. List the two terms, indicate their word parts, and define the terms.

7. Define the component word parts for the following areas of specialty and circle the most appropriate follow-up specialist for the boy.

Oncologist: Onc/o _____, -logist _____.

Dermatopathologist: Dermat/o _____, path/o _____,

-logist _____.

Mycologist: Myc/o _____, -logist _____.

Answer: Otorhinolaryngologist: Ot/o _____, rhin/o _____,

laryng/o _____, -logist _____.

Pulmonologist: Pulmon/o _____, -logist _____.

🔍 *STANDARD CASE STUDY*

6.4 Bronchogenic Carcinoma

A 72-year-old male presents to his primary care physician with a yearlong history of chronic bronchitis, dyspnea, hemoptysis, pleurodynia, and anorexia. Patient social history includes heavy drinking, and smoking a pack of cigarettes, each day. Patient medical history includes pulmonary Langerhans cell histiocytosis (LCH), which is characterized by accumulations of Langerhans cells in the lung. Patient physical exam shows wheezing during auscultation. The physician orders chest X-rays, which identify three abnormal lesions (>2x2 cm) in the superior and middle lobes of the right lung. Computed tomography (CT) reveals additional small lesions in the superior lobe of the right lung. Prior sputum cytology is negative for bronchogenic carcinoma, but in light of the current symptoms and large lesions, a transbronchial biopsy is collected by bronchoscope and analyzed by a pathologist who confirmed small lung cell carcinoma (SCLC). The patient is diagnosed with bronchogenic carcinoma, likely secondary to pulmonary LCH. Discussion with the patient led to possible courses of action; he is told that chemotherapy and radiation treatment are likely, and surgical removal of lesions may be considered using wedge resection, segmentectomy, lobectomy, or pneumonectomy. The patient is referred to an oncologist.

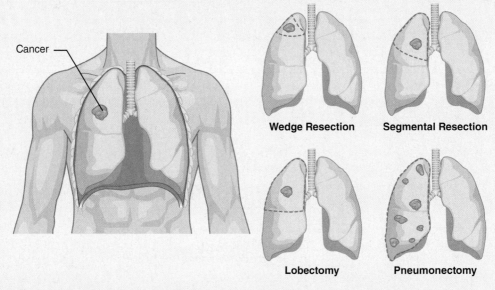

CASE FIGURE: Lung cancer surgery. Dotted blue line indicates region of the lung removed

1. Complete the table below for the terms associated with the patient's symptoms:

Term	Word Parts	Meaning
chronic	*chron/o; -ic*	*pertaining to time (longtime)*
bronchitis		
dyspnea		
hemoptysis		
pleurodynia		
anorexia		

2. Langerhans cells reside in tissues throughout the body and function as part of the immune system. In pulmonary Langerhans cell histiocytosis, these cells accumulate in lung tissue. Define the word parts for pulmonary and histiocytosis and then put this together to explain what is meant by pulmonary Langerhans cell histiocytosis.

   Pulmonary: Pulmon/o _____, -ary _____.

   Histiocytosis: Histi/o _____, -cytosis _____.

3. Auscultation means listening to sounds within the body by stethoscope. Define the component word parts for *stethoscope*.

   Stethoscope: Steth/o _____, -scope _____.

4. Sputum refers to mucus that has been coughed up and spit out. Define the word parts and meaning for *cytology* and then provide the meaning for *sputum cytology*.

   Cytology: Cyt/o _____, -logy _____,

   sputum cytology means _____.

5. Define the following word parts, and meaning, of *bronchogenic carcinoma*.

   Bronchogenic carcinoma: Bronch/o _____, -genic _____,

   carcin/o _____, -oma _____,

   means _____.

6. Complete the table below for the terms associated with the patient's assessment, diagnosis, and treatment:

Term	Word Parts	Meaning
transbronchial	*trans-; bronchi/o; -al*	*pertaining to across the bronchus*
biopsy		
bronchoscope		
pathologist		
oncologist		
segmentectomy		
lobectomy		
pneumonectomy		

⌕ *STANDARD CASE STUDY*

6.5 Eosinophilic Granulomatosis with Polyangiitis

A 45-year-old female presented to the emergency department (ED) with moderate acute asthma exacerbation (AAE). Symptoms included dyspnea, anosmia, speaking in short phrases, and diaphoretic and pale skin. The patient's partner was present, and he explained that she had recently been short of breath and had developed paresis and paresthesia in her hands and feet. Physical examination was significant for tachycardia (120 beats/min), a sonorous wheeze (rhonchi) with auscultation, and nasal polyps. Spirometry showed airway obstruction characteristic of asthma, which she had been treating for 6 years with inhaled corticosteroids and bronchodilators. However, her partner said that her asthma is not well controlled. Blood was drawn for testing and chest X-rays were ordered.

The chest X-rays revealed lesions in the lung tissue. A differential blood cell count showed eosinophilia. A muscle and nerve biopsy were ordered. The muscle biopsy revealed vasculitis and tissue eosinophilia, and the nerve biopsy revealed chronic axonopathy with patchy demyelination. With these results, the criteria are met for a diagnosis of eosinophilic granulomatosis with polyangiitis (EGP), also called Churg Strauss syndrome, a disorder characterized by eosinophilia, asthma, and vasculitis. The patient was prescribed prednisone to reduce inflammation and a follow-up appointment was scheduled.

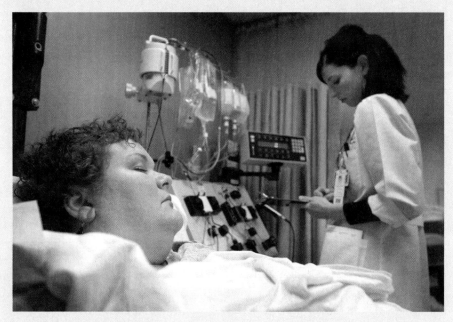

CASE FIGURE: A woman being treated in the emergency department following exacerbation of her asthma

© Darren Durlach/The Boston Globe/Getty Images

1. Complete the table below for the terms associated with the patient's symptoms:

Term	Word Parts	Meaning
dyspnea	*dys-; -pnea*	*breathing that is difficult*
anosmia		
diaphoretic		
paresis		
paresthesia		
tachycardia		

2. The physical examination revealed a sonorous wheeze (rhonchi) with auscultation and nasal polyps. Using a medical dictionary or other resource describe what rhonchi and nasal polyps are.

3. Auscultation means listening to sounds within the body by stethoscope. Spirometry is a procedure for measuring lung capacity. Define the component word parts for *stethoscope* and *spirometry*.

    Stethoscope: Steth/o _____, -scope _____.

    Spirometry: Spir/o _____, -metry _____.

4. The patient has been treating her asthma with inhaled corticosteroids and bronchodilators. Using a medical dictionary, or other resource, briefly explain what these drugs do in the lungs.

    Corticosteroids:

    Bronchodilator:

5. Complete the table below for the terms associated with the patient's diagnosis of eosinophilic granulomatosis with polyangiitis:

Term	Word Parts	Meaning
eosinophilic	*eosin/o; -phil; -ic*	*pertaining to being attracted to red (eosinophils attract a rosy red stain)*
granulomatosis		
polyangiitis		
vasculitis		
eosinophilia		
biopsy		
axonopathy		
demyelination		

✎ *ADVANCED CASE STUDY*

6.6 Pneumoconiosis

Current Complaint: A 50-year-old male presents with chronic cough of several months' duration, dyspnea, anorexia, and weight loss. Cough is worse in the morning and is accompanied by whitish sputum production. Prompting this visit is increasing windedness with even minor exertion and recent hemoptysis.

Past History: Patient has been previously diagnosed with bronchitis and prescribed antibiotics, but symptoms have not abated.

Signs and Symptoms: Inspiratory bilateral rales and expiratory rhonchi are heard on auscultation. Patient is afebrile and no bacteria or atypical cells are present in bronchoalveolar lavage fluid. Arterial blood gasses are within normal range and do not indicate hypoxemia or hypercapnia. Pulmonary function tests using spirometry indicate restrictive ventilatory impairment with decreased total lung capacity. Thoracic radiography reveals numerous small opacities. Transbronchial pulmonary biopsy with video-assisted thoracoscopy indicates peribronchiolar fibrosis with metallic particles found in affected lung tissue.

Diagnosis: Pneumoconiosis. Occupational history reveals a 30-year employment as a dental technician grinding crowns, bridges, and dentures. Findings are consistent with fibrosis induced by silica dust and other particles generated during grinding of dental prostheses. Patient did not routinely wear personal protective equipment.

Treatment: Care will be focused on preventing disease progression. If patient chooses to continue in his current occupation, personal protection equipment should be worn to mitigate additional dust exposure. A pulmonary rehabilitation program is recommended to increase exercise tolerance. Patient will have regular follow-up with a pulmonologist to manage symptoms and monitor lung function.

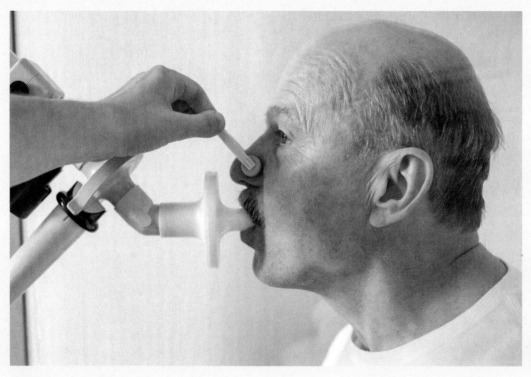

CASE FIGURE: Spirometry to test lung function
© Koldunov/Shutterstock

1. Define the word parts for *pneumoconiosis*.

    Pneumoconiosis: Pneum/o _____, coni/o _____,

    -osis _____.

2. There are several types of pneumoconiosis. Define the word parts for the following and circle the most likely type of pneumoconiosis that applies to the patient in the case study.

   Answer: Silicosis: Silic/o _____, -osis _____.

   Anthracosis: Anthrac/o _____, -osis _____.

   Asbestosis: Asbest/o _____, -osis _____.

3. Complete the table below listing symptoms related to pneumoconiosis:

Term	Word Parts	Meaning
dyspnea	*dys-; -pnea*	*breathing that is difficult*
anorexia		
hemoptysis		
bronchitis		
hypoxemia		
hypercapnia		
peribronchiolar fibrosis		

4. Use a medical dictionary to define the following terms, which cannot be broken down into word parts:

   Sputum:

   Rales:

   Rhonchi:

   Define the word parts that make up the signs *inspiratory bilateral rales* and *expiratory rhonchi*, and provide a meaning for the signs.

   Inspiratory bilateral rales: In- _____, spir/o _____,

               -atory _____, bi- _____,

               later/o _____, -al _____,

               rales: _____,

               means _____.

   Expiratory rhonchi: Ex- _____, spir/o _____,

             -atory _____, rhonchi _____,

            means _____.

(continues)

⚲ ADVANCED CASE STUDY   (continued)

5. Complete the table below listing diagnostic terms related to pneumoconiosis:

Term	Word Parts	Meaning
bronchoalveolar lavage	*bronch/o; alveol/o; -ar lavage*	*wash pertaining to the alveoli and bronchi*
spirometry		
PA thoracic radiography		
transbronchial pulmonary biopsy		
thoracoscopy		
pulmonologist		

6. Auscultation means listening to sounds within the body by stethoscope. Define the component word parts for *stethoscope*.

   Stethoscope: Steth/o _____, -scope _____.

⚲ ADVANCED CASE STUDY

6.7 Chronic Rhinosinusitis

Consultation for Surgery

Subjective: The subject is seen today for recurrent rhinosinusitis. On questioning, she recounts frequent sinus infections over the past 10 years. Past treatments have included antibiotic therapy, nasal lavage with saline, and topical intranasal steroids. She reports both increasing frequency and duration of sinus infections usually with facial pain and pressure, accompanied by hyposmia and mucopurulent rhinorrhea. Patient has seasonal allergies and asthma but is otherwise healthy.

Objective: Examination of the head and neck region does not indicate lymphadenopathy. Ears and mouth are normal with some postnasal discharge in the back of the throat. No polyps are seen with examination of the nasal cavity; however, a significant deviation of the nasal septum to the left side is evident.

Assessment: Chronic pansinusitis without polyposis.

Plan: Sinus computed tomography has been ordered. Multiple possible surgical interventions were discussed including endoscopic sinusotomy, sphenoidotomy, ethmoidectomy, or balloon ostial dilation. The addition of nasal septoplasty to facilitate breathing was also recommended. The patient was instructed to return in 2 weeks, once the results of the CT were available, to further discuss surgical approaches and to have any lingering questions answered.

1. Recurrent means occurring often. Define the component word parts for *rhinosinusitis* and explain what is meant by recurrent rhinosinusitis.

   Rhinosinusitis: Rhin/o _____, sinus/o _____,

   -itis _____.

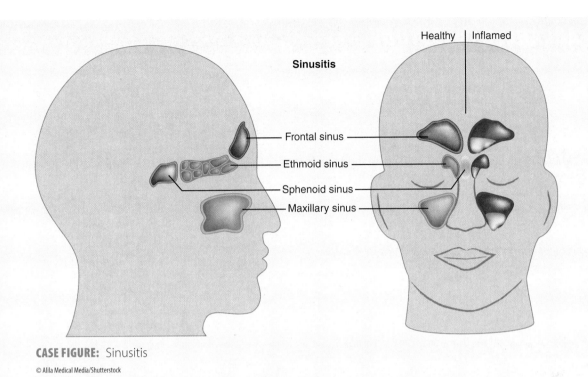

Sinusitis

Healthy | Inflamed

Frontal sinus

Ethmoid sinus

Sphenoid sinus

Maxillary sinus

CASE FIGURE: Sinusitis

© Alila Medical Media/Shutterstock

2. Complete the table below of terms related to the case.

Term	Word Parts	Meaning
hyposmia	*hypo-; -osmia*	*state of insufficient smell*
mucopurulent	*muc/o; purulent*	
rhinorrhea		
lymphadenopathy		
pansinusitis		
polyposis		

3. The patient has tried several treatments. Use the terminology in the case to complete the following:

medications to treat bacterial infections: _____.

rinsing the nose with salt: _____.

an anti-inflammatory used superficially in the nose: _____.

4. Where are the sinuses, what is their purpose, and what is endoscopic sinusotomy?

(continues)

5. Where is the sphenoid bone and what is sphenoidotomy?

6. Where is the ethmoid bone and what is ethmoidectomy?

7. What do you think balloon ostial dilation is?

8. What is the nasal septum and what is septoplasty?

🔍 *ADVANCED CASE STUDY*

6.8 Pneumothorax

A female baby, born premature at 31 weeks of gestation, arrives at the neonatal intensive care unit (NICU) with symptoms of respiratory distress syndrome (RDS). She presents with tachypnea, cyanosis, and hypoxia. The baby is intubated, administered surfactant, and placed on mechanical ventilation. Despite the interventions, her pulmonary status does not improve; and labs show significant findings of acidosis and hypercapnia. An air leak, or air outside of the normal airways, is suspected. A chest X-ray is ordered and shows bilateral pneumothoraces with no evidence of pneumopericardium, pneumomediastinum, anteromedial pneumothorax, or pneumatocele. Chest tubes are inserted; after a gradual improvement in pulmonary status, she is extubated and placed on nasal constant pulmonary airway pressure (NCPAP).

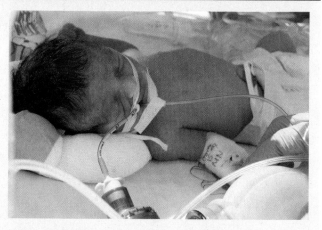

CASE FIGURE: Baby in incubator with ventilation
© Guvendemir/iStock/Getty Images Plus/Getty Images

1. The child in this case was born at 31 weeks of gestation. Refer to a medical dictionary or other resource and indicate what length of time is for normal human gestation (pregnancy).

2. The NICU is an intensive care unit specializing in the care of neonates. Neonates are generally defined as what age group?

3. Define the following word parts, and meaning, of the following RDS symptoms: *tachypnea*, *cyanosis*, *hypoxia*, *acidosis*, and *hypercapnia*.

   Tachypnea: Tachy- _____, -pnea _____,

        means _____.

   Cyanosis: Cyan/o _____, -osis _____,

        means _____.

   Hypoxia: Hypo- _____, ox/o _____, -ia _____,

        means _____.

   Acidosis: Acid- _____, -osis _____,

        means _____.

   Hypercapnia: Hyper- _____, capn/o _____, -ia _____,

        means _____.

4. To intubate is to insert a breathing tube into the trachea to ventilate the lungs. What does extubate mean?

5. Refer to a medical dictionary and define surfactant.

6. The case refers to several air leaks that affect different regions of the chest. Where would you find air in each of the following conditions listed below? You may need to refer to a medical dictionary or other resource.

   Bilateral pneumothorax:

   Pneumopericardium:

   Pneumomediastinum:

   Anteromedial pneumothorax:

   Pneumatocele:

7. What is nasal constant pulmonary airway pressure (NCPAP)?

🔍 *ADVANCED CASE STUDY*

6.9 Cystic Fibrosis

Beatrice is a 45-year-old Caucasian female with cystic fibrosis (CF), a genetic disorder that leads to the production of a thick mucus in multiple organs that can lead to obstruction, inflammation, and infection. In the respiratory system, impaired mucociliary clearance leads to dyspnea, bronchitis, sinusitis, and chronic infection. Her disease had been managed with attention to diet and antibiotics.

Beatrice was in end-stage CF, the buildup of mucus had led to bronchiectasis and the development of cysts and fibrosis in the lungs. She underwent a single lung transplant with a contralateral pneumonectomy, which was performed with single lumen endotracheal intubation and cardiopulmonary bypass (CPB). During recovery, she developed a bronchopleural fistula, pneumonia, and infection of the pneumonectomy space, and she died 4 days later.

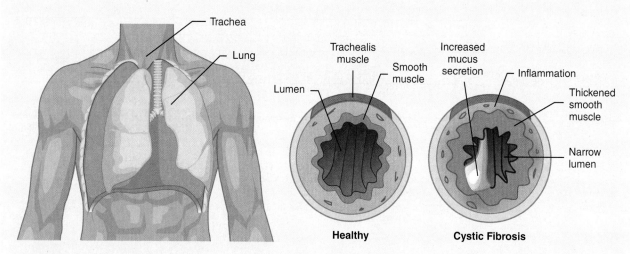

CASE FIGURE: Comparison of a healthy airway to one with mucus buildup from cystic fibrosis

1. Complete the table below for the terms associated with the patient's symptoms:

Term	Word Parts	Meaning
mucociliary	*muc/o; cili/o; -ary*	*pertaining to mucus and cilia (mucus in relation to ciliated respiratory epithelia)*
dyspnea		
bronchitis		
pneumonia		
sinusitis		

2. A lifetime of mucus buildup and inflammation in the patient's lungs had led to bronchiectasis and fibrosis. Define the word parts, and meaning, for *bronchiectasis* and *fibrosis*.

Bronchiectasis: Bronchi/o _____, -ectasis _____,

       means _____.

Fibrosis: Fibr/o _____, -osis _____,

       means _____.

3. Define the word parts, and meaning, for *contralateral pneumonectomy*.

    Contralateral pneumonectomy: Contra- _____, later/o _____,

    -al _____, pneumon/o _____,

    -ectomy _____,

    means _____

4. Define the word parts, and meaning, for *antibiotic*.

    Antibiotic: Anti- _____, bi/o _____, -tic _____,

    means _____

5. Refer to a medical dictionary, or other resource, and describe endotracheal intubation and cardiopulmonary bypass.

6. A fistula is an abnormal connection between two body parts. What two parts are connected with a bronchopleural fistula?

🔍 ADVANCED CASE STUDY

6.10 Lymphangioleiomyomatosis

A 22-year-old female was brought into the emergency department (ED) after collapsing during training with the reserve officers' training corps (ROTC). Prior to collapsing, she experienced dyspnea and minor hemoptysis. In the ED, she reports pain on the left side of her chest. Her physical exam and medical history are unremarkable, except for reduced breath sound on the left. A chest X-ray revealed left-sided pneumothorax and chylothorax. A computed tomography (CT) scan was ordered, which revealed bilateral diffuse ovoid thin-walled cysts (<3 cm) in the lungs and angiomyolipomas in the kidneys. A tube thoracostomy was performed to treat the pneumothorax, but it did not fully resolve. Video-assisted thoracic surgery (VATS) was used to perform a wedge resection of the apex of the left lung to allow for lung expansion and pleurodesis to fuse the visceral and parietal pleura. A biopsy of lung tissue was collected. Thoracentesis and ligation of the thoracic lymphatic duct was performed to treat the chylothorax. The pneumothorax and chylothorax resolved. The biopsy showed characteristics of lymphangioleiomyomatosis, a disorder that results in the abnormal proliferation of smooth muscle in lymphatics, vessels, and airways, leading to abdominal lymphatic tumors, kidney angiomyolipomas, and lung disease, which can cause spontaneous pneumothorax. The patient was started on bronchodilator medication as an initial treatment strategy.

(continues)

ADVANCED CASE STUDY

(continued)

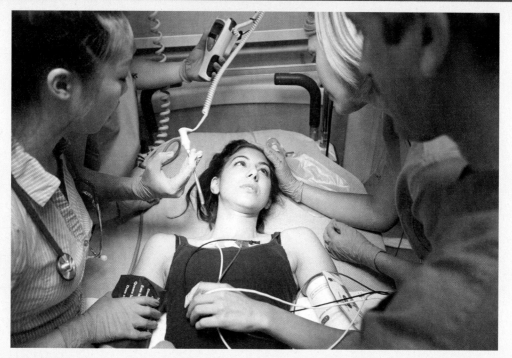

CASE FIGURE: A woman in the emergency department after collapsing during training

© Monkey Business Images/Shutterstock

1. Complete the table below for the terms associated with the patient's symptoms:

Term	Word Parts	Meaning
dyspnea	*dys-; -pnea*	*breathing that is difficult*
hemoptysis		
pneumothorax		
chylothorax		

2. Were the diffuse ovoid thin-walled cysts found in the left lung, right lung, or both lungs?

3. A wedge of tissue was removed from the apex of the left lung to provide adequate space for lung expansion. Is the apex of the lung the medial, lateral, superior, or inferior region of the lung?

4. Define the word parts for *angiomyolipoma* and *lymphangioleiomyomatosis*, then using a medical dictionary, or other resource, describe what they are.

Angiomyolipoma: Angi/o _____, my/o _____,

lip/o _____, -oma _____,

means _____

Description:

Lymphangioleiomyomatosis: Lymph/o _____, angi/o _____, lei/o _____,

myomat/o _____, -osis _____

Description:

5. Complete the table below for the terms associated with the patient's procedures:

Term	Word Parts	Meaning
thoracostomy	*thorac/o; -ostomy*	*surgically create an opening in the chest*
biopsy		
pleurodesis		
thoracocentesis		
ligation		

References

Ali, M. Ghori, U. K., & Musani, A. I. (2019). Orphan lung diseases. *Medical Clinics of North America, 103*(3), 503–515. doi:10.1016/j.mcna.2018.12.009

Bradley, H., & Lucarelli, M. R. (2005). Bronchogenic carcinoma in a 32-year-old with a history of pulmonary Langerhans cell histiocytosis. *Chest, 128*(4 Suppl), 475S.

Capdevila, O. S., Kheirandish-Gozal, L., Dayyat, E., & Gozal, D. (2008). Pediatric obstructive sleep apnea: Complications, management, and long-term outcomes. *Proceedings of the American Thoracic Society, 5*(2), 274–282. https://doi.org/10.1513/pats.200708-138MG

Fernandes, G. L., Teixeira, A. A., Antón, A. G., Reis, A. T., de Freitas, A. C., & Basílio, D. B. (2014). Churg-Strauss syndrome: A case report. *Radiologia Brasileira, 47*(4), 259–261. https://doi.org/10.1590/0100-3984.2013.1817

Lindquist, B., Zachariah, S., & Kulkarni, A. (2017). Adult epiglottitis: A case series. *The Permanente Journal, 21*, 16–089. doi:10.7812/TPP/16-089

Okamoto, M., Tominaga, M., Shimizu, S., Yano, C., Masuda, K., Nakamura, M., Zaizen, Y., Nouno, T., Sakamoto, S., Yokoyama, M., Kawayama, T. & Hoshino, T. (2017). A case of dental technicians' pneumoconiosis. *Internal Medicine, 56*(24), 3323–3326. doi:10.2169/internalmedicine.8860-17

Prasad, S., Fong, E., & Ooi, E. H. (2017). Systematic review of patient-reported outcomes after revision endoscopic sinus surgery. *American Journal of Rhinology & Allergy, 31*(4), 248–255. https://doi.org/10.2500/ajra.2017.31.4446

Razak, A., Mohanty, P. K., & Venkatesh, H. A. (2014). Anteromedial pneumothorax in a neonate: 'The diagnostic dilemma' and the importance of clinical signs. *BMJ Case Reports*. https://doi.org/10.1136/bcr-2013-202487

Reed, B. D., Arya, S., Dufendach, K. R., & Leino, D. (2018). Case 2: Refractory respiratory failure and pneumothorax in a full-term newborn. *NeoReviews, 19*(2) e109–e111. doi:10.1542/neo.19-2-e109

Rhee, J. A., Adial, A., Gumpeni, R., & Iftikhar, A. (2019). Lymphangioleiomyomatosis: A case report and review of literature. *Cureus, 11*(1), e3938. https://doi.org/10.7759/cureus.3938

Riojas, R. A., Bahr, B. A., Thomas, D. B., Perciballi, J., & Noyes, L. (2012). A case report of lymphangioleiomyomatosis presenting as spontaneous pneumothorax. *Military Medicine, 177*(4), 477–480. https://doi.org/10.7205/milmed-d-11-00333

Sakai, M., Hiyama, T., Kuno, H., Mori, K., Saida, T., Ishiguro, T., Takahashi, H., Koyama, K. & Minami, M. (2020). Thoracic abnormal air collections in patients in the intensive care unit: Radiograph findings correlated with CT. *Insights into Imaging, 11*(35), 35. https://doi.org/10.1186/s13244-020-0838-z

Shetty, M., Janapati, R., Krishnaprasad, A., & Nageshwara, R. M. (2014). Churg Strauss syndrome — a case report. *Journal of Clinical and Diagnostic Research, 8*(6), MD05–MD06. https://doi.org/10.7860/JCDR/2014/8271.4494

Souilamas, R., Mostafa, A., Guillemain, R., Boussaud, V., Amrein, C., & Chevalier, P. (2008). Single-lung transplantation for cystic fibrosis and metachronus pneumonectomy: Case reports. *Transplantation Proceedings, 40*(10), 3594–3595. https://doi.org/10.1016/j.transproceed.2008.06.106

Stedman, T. L. (2005). Nath's *Stedman's medical terminology, 2e.* Philadelphia: Lippincott Williams & Wilkins.

Venes, D. & Taber, C. W. (2017). *Taber's cyclopedic medical dictionary.* Ed. 23, illustrated in full color/Philadelphia: F.A. Davis.

CHAPTER 7

Digestive System

KEY TERMS

Anus	Emesis	Peristalsis
Ascending colon	Esophagus	Pharynx
Bile	Feces	Salivary gland
Bolus	Gallbladder	Sigmoid colon
Cecum	Jejunum	Small intestine
Chyme	Liver	Stomach
Common bile duct	Mastication	Transverse colon
Descending colon	Oral cavity	
Duodenum	Pancreas	

The digestive system is composed of a continuous muscular tube, approximately 9 meters in length, and is responsible for the breakdown of food, absorption of nutrients into the bloodstream, and elimination of unabsorbed food as solid waste. It is also known as the gastrointestinal, or GI, system. Its main anatomical parts are the oral cavity, pharynx, esophagus, stomach, and small and large intestines. Accessory organs include the salivary glands, liver, gallbladder, and pancreas.

Mechanical and chemical digestion of food begins in the **oral cavity**. Mechanical digestion is the result of **mastication**, chewing with the teeth to grind the food. The enzyme amylase, secreted by the **salivary glands**, begins to chemically break down carbohydrates. The food, now called a **bolus**, is ready to swallow and moves through the **pharynx** and esophagus to the stomach. The **esophagus** secretes mucus to reduce friction and lubricate the bolus to aid its passage. It takes an average of 6 seconds for solid or semisolid food to move from the mouth to the J-shaped **stomach**, which serves as a mixing

chamber and holding reservoir. Once in the stomach, mechanical and chemical digestion continues. Mixing and churning by the smooth muscle of the stomach's wall, and secretion of gastric juice containing hydrochloric acid and enzymes, reduces the partially digested food to a soupy liquid called **chyme**. Little absorption takes place in the stomach; however, some water, ions, and a few drugs are absorbed here. Chyme leaves the stomach through smooth rhythmic contractions called **peristalsis**. The involuntary forcible expulsion of the stomach contents through the mouth is vomiting or **emesis** and generally occurs due to stomach irritation.

Chyme moves from the lower portion of the stomach, the pylorus, through the pyloric sphincter, to the **duodenum**, the first, and shortest portion of the **small intestine**. The major events of digestion and absorption take place in the small intestine, aided by accessory organs, which are the pancreas, the liver, and the gallbladder. The **pancreas** lies horizontally behind the stomach and is connected

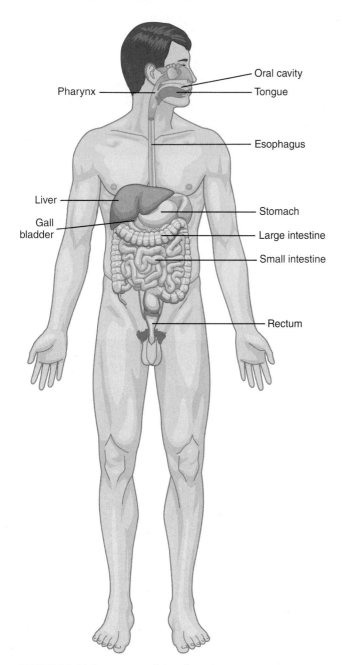

FIGURE 7.1 Major organs of the digestive system

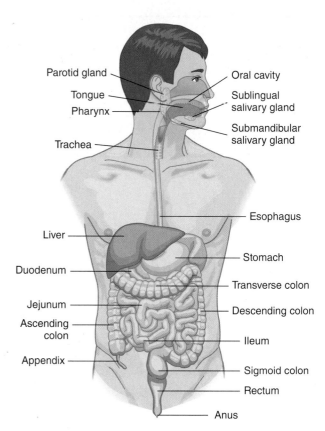

FIGURE 7.2 The abdominal viscera of the digestive system

to the duodenum by two ducts. It produces and secretes about a liter and a half of pancreatic juice every day, containing protein, fat, and carbohydrate-digesting enzymes. The **liver** is the body's largest solid organ and is located in the upper right quadrant of the abdomen, inferior to the diaphragm. The liver has many important metabolic functions, and it makes and secretes **bile**, an alkaline fluid containing bile salts that emulsify, or break down lipids. Bile is released from the liver to the **gallbladder** through several ducts. The bile is stored in the gallbladder and is released when needed, to the duodenum, through the **common bile duct**.

Most digestion and absorption of nutrients into the bloodstream takes place in the small intestine.

Its length of about 3 meters and the circular folds of muscle within it provide significant surface area for this task. The small intestine is made up of the duodenum, the **jejunum**, the middle portion, and the final and longest segment, the **ileum**. Waste products and unabsorbed materials are propelled to the large intestine, which is primarily involved in water reabsorption. Contents move from the **cecum** of the large intestine, to the **ascending colon**, **transverse colon**, **descending colon**, and then the **sigmoid colon**. Once digested material is in the large intestine for 3–10 hours, it becomes solid or semisolid and is then called **feces**. Fecal material moves to the **rectum**, the last 20 cm of the GI tract and is evacuated during defecation through the **anus**, the opening of the rectum to the exterior.

TABLE 7.1
Key Digestive System Combining Forms
abdomin/o: abdomen
alveol/o: small sac; alveolus
amyl/o: starch

Key Digestive System Combining Forms

an/o: anus

appendic/o: appendix

bil/i: bile; gallbladder

bilirubin/o: bilirubin, bile pigment

bucc/o: cheek

calcul/o: little stone

chol/e: bile, gall

cholangi/o: bile duct

cholecyst/o: gallbladder

choledoch/o: common bile duct

cirrh/o: yellow

col/o: colon

colon/o: colon

defec/o: evacuation of feces

diaphar/o: profuse sweating

diverticul/o: pouch

duoden/o: duodenum

enter/o: small intestine

epitheli/o: epithelium

esophag/o: esophagus

faci/o: face

fistul/o: tube, pipe

gastr/o: stomach

hemat/o: blood

hem/o: blood

hepat/o : liver

icter/o: jaundice

ile/o: ileum

jaund/o: yellow

jejun/o: jejunum

lapar/o: abdomen

lith/o: stone

lip/o: fat

maxill/o: maxilla, upper jaw

nas/o: nose

or/o: mouth

ot/o: ear

pancreat/o: pancreas

phag/o: eat, swallow

proct/o: anus, rectum

rect/o: rectum

sarc/o: flesh; connective tissue

sialaden/o: salivary gland

sial/o: saliva

sigmoid/o: sigmoid colon

steat/o: fat

syncop/o: to cut off; faint

TABLE 7.2

Key Digestive System Suffixes

-agogue: bringer of

-ase: enzyme

-chezia: defecation, elimination of waste

-emesis: vomiting

(continues)

TABLE 7.2	(continued)
Key Digestive System Suffixes	
-lithiasis: condition of stones	
-lithotripsy: surgical crushing of stones	
-pepsia: digestion	

-phagia: eating

-phage: to eat

-prandial: meal

-stomia: condition of the mouth

-tresia: opening

🔍 *STANDARD CASE STUDY*

7.1 Eosinophilic Esophagitis

Eating was now a struggle. It used to be one of Lalis' greatest loves, but over the past few years, it was increasingly difficult to swallow food. There were times that it felt like food was getting stuck in her throat or chest, and she would have to strain to push it down. Lalis had tried over the counter heartburn medications, hoping that her problem with food was simply heartburn, but none of these treatments helped. Eating used to be a joy, now it was a source of anxiety. Lalis scheduled an appointment with her primary care physician.

Case Report: A 78-year-old female presents to a referred gastroenterologist with a chief complaint of esophageal dysphagia; episodes are becoming more frequent and severe. Heart rate, blood pressure, and temperature are within normal limits. The patient reports that she has not

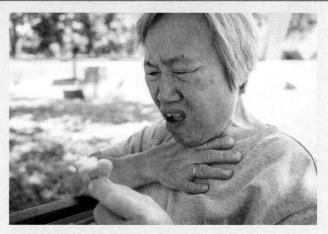

CASE FIGURE: Lalis struggling to swallow
© CGN089/Shutterstock

been feeling nauseous or constipated. She denies hematemesis, hematochezia, or melena. Over-the-counter acid reflux medications have not yielded any apparent benefit. There is no significant family history of gastrointestinal cancer, but both parents had atopic diseases; the mother had eczema and the father had asthma and rhinoconjunctivitis.

An endoscopy was performed, and esophageal biopsies were taken from the distal and proximal esophagus. Endoscopic features include small-caliber esophagus and white vesicles on the mucosal surface. Biopsies reveal significant infiltration of intraepithelial eosinophils [up to 50 eosinophils per high-powered field (HPF)]. Eosinophils are immune cells that are typically associated with parasitic infections and allergic reactions.

Eosinophilic esophagitis (EE or EoE) was diagnosed based on the symptoms, endoscopic features, and presence of eosinophils in the esophageal mucosa. The patient was advised on strategies for identifying possible allergies to foods that may be triggering the EE. The patient was prescribed a topical steroid (fluticasone 125 mcg inhaler, four puffs swallowed three times a day for 6 weeks), and a follow-up appointment was requested.

1. Define the word parts and meaning for *esophageal dysphagia*.

   Esophageal dysphagia: Esophag/o _____, -eal _____,

   dys- _____, phag/o _____, -ia _____,

   means _____

2. Define the word parts for the following symptoms:

   Hematemesis: Hemat/o _____, -emesis _____

   Hematochezia: Hemat/o _____, -chezia

3. The term melena comes from the Greek word *melaina*, which means black. Melena refers to black tarry feces, which contain digested blood. How is melena different than hematochezia?

4. Define the word parts for the following terms relating to the esophageal biopsies:

   Biopsy: Bi/o _____, -opsy _____.

   Distal: Dist/o _____, -al _____.

   Proximal: Proxim/o _____, -al _____.

   Intraepithelial: Intra- _____, epitheli/o _____, -al _____.

5. Define the word parts for *rhinoconjunctivitis*.

   Rhinoconjunctivitis: Rhin/o _____, conjunctiv/o _____, -itis _____.

🔍 STANDARD CASE STUDY

7.2 Bleeding Gastric Ulcer

The patient was a 30-year-old female transported to the ER by her wife following two syncopal episodes. Upon arrival, she was conscious but lethargic, pale, hypotensive, and tachycardic. A patient history revealed ongoing fatigue coupled with epigastric pain and general dyspepsia. The pain increased postprandially. Further questioning revealed ongoing melena and recent hematemesis. Hematochezia was not reported. A bleeding gastric ulcer was suspected and immediate IV fluid replacement was initiated to treat signs of hypovolemia. Once the patient's vital signs were stable, esophagogastroduodenoscopy (EGD) was performed as a diagnostic and therapeutic hemostatic procedure. The presence of a bleeding gastric ulcer was confirmed, and hemostasis was successful. The patient was advised to follow up with a gastroenterologist for further evaluation.

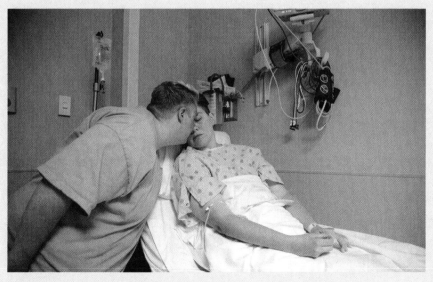

CASE FIGURE: Woman comforting her wife

© Sharon Pruitt/EyeEm/Getty Images

(continues)

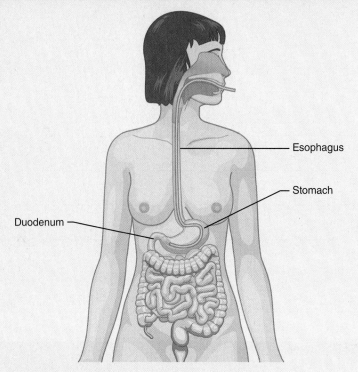

CASE FIGURE: The passage of the viewing instrument during an esophagogastroduodenoscopy

1. Indicate the word parts for *syncopal* and define the term based on those parts.

2. Define the word parts and meaning for the following signs of hypovolemia:

    Hypotensive: Hypo- _____, tens/o _____,

    -ive _____, means _____.

    Tachycardic: Tachy- _____, cardi/o _____, -ic _____,

    means _____.

3. What is hypovolemia?

4. Where would a gastric ulcer be found?

5. Complete the table below for symptoms related to gastric ulcer:

Term	Word Parts	Meaning
epigastric	*epi-; gastr/o; -ic*	*pertaining to above the stomach*
dyspepsia		
postprandial		
melena	N/A	
hematemesis		
hematochezia		

6. Esophagogastroduodenoscopy (EGD) can be both diagnostic and therapeutic. Explain the terms *diagnostic* and *therapeutic*.

7. Indicate the word parts for *esophagogastroduodenoscopy*, define the word parts, and provide the meaning of the term.

8. Define the word parts for *hemostasis* and explain what is meant by this term.

   Hemostasis: Hem/o _____, -stasis _____.

9. The patient is advised to follow up with a gastroenterologist. Indicate the word parts for *gastroenterologist* and determine the specialty of this physician based on those parts.

🔍 STANDARD CASE STUDY

7.3 Sialadenitis

Current Complaint: A 50-year-old man presents to Urgent Care with recurrent parotidomegaly, tenderness of the right parotid gland, and swelling in the right cheek and neck region.

Past History: Patient reports three previous episodes of sialadenitis over the past 2 years. Each episode has resolved with conservative management including sialagogues, warm compresses, and gland massage, which the patient initiated on his own after researching his condition on the Internet.

Signs and Symptoms: Patient reports significant pain during mastication, worse this time than during any previous episode. He also reports xerostomia and hyposialorrhea. During clinical examination, a stony hard mass could be palpated in the region of the right buccal mucosa. Ultrasonography indicates calculus and sialoangiectasis.

Diagnosis: Recurrent sialadenitis with sialolithiasis of the right parotid gland.

Treatments: Attempt to manage conservatively with massage, hydration, sialagogues, anti-inflammatory medications and analgesics. Schedule follow-up appointment with the Department of Oral and Maxillofacial Surgery to discuss other treatment options including sialolithotomy and parotidectomy, if symptoms do not resolve.

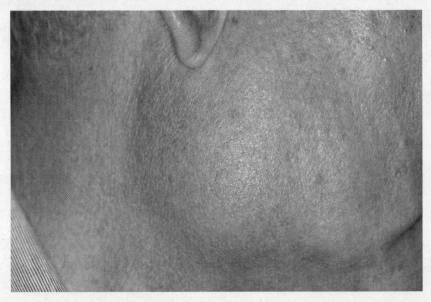

CASE FIGURE: Parotidomegaly

© Karan Bunjean/Shutterstock

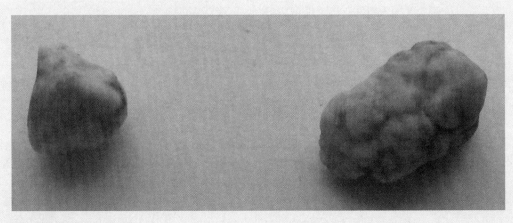

CASE FIGURE: Salivary stones

© ThanikaThaiPhotoStock/Shutterstock

1. Define the word parts for *parotidomegaly* and explain what the condition is.

   Parotidomegaly: Para- _____, ot/o _____, -id _____,

           -megaly _____.

2. The term in the case study that refers to removal of the parotid gland is _____.

3. Sial/o is the combining form meaning saliva. List and define the words in this case study that contain the combining form sial/o, breaking the terms down into their component parts.

4. The patient reports xerostomia (xer/o -stomia), which means _____.

5. Where is the buccal mucosa?

6. Lith/o is the combining form meaning stone. The other term in the case used for stone

   is _____.

7. Salivary stones were detected by ultrasonography. Define the word parts of this procedure and briefly explain the procedure.

   Ultrasonography: Ultra- _____, son/o _____, -graphy _____

8. Which specialist should the patient follow up with? Indicate and define the word parts for this specialist and describe their specialty.

🔍 STANDARD CASE STUDY

7.4 Rectal Prolapse

Surgical Consultation—Doctor's Notes

First Visit

This is my first consultation with Mrs. Clarkson, a 62-year-old accountant suffering from proctoptosis. Initial embarrassment made it hard for her to discuss her symptoms but after gentle questioning, she provided more details. She relayed a long history of frequent constipation and straining to move her bowels. More recently, she has had episodes of fecal incontinence as well as bleeding and pain in the rectal area; assuming she had hemorrhoids, she has been relying on home remedies. The pain and bleeding have not abated and more recently, after defecating, she feels like "something is falling out." Too embarrassed to discuss this initially with a physician, she has been able to "push it back in." I explained to her that she likely has rectal prolapse, which should be repaired surgically because it will continue to worsen over time if untreated. As each episode of prolapse further stretches the anal sphincter, permanent fecal incontinence may result if the prolapse is not addressed. I have scheduled Mrs. Clarkson for several procedures pending further discussion of surgery. Tests scheduled are anorectal manometry, colonoscopy, and defecography.

Follow-Up Visit

This is my second consultation with Mrs. Clarkson. Diagnostic tests previously ordered confirm a significant rectal prolapse and rule out concurrent polyps or cancer of the bowel. At this point, prolapse of other pelvic organs is not present. I discussed two surgical approaches with Mrs. Clarkson, the perineal approach and the abdominal approach. Both perineal rectosigmoidectomy with accompanying levatoroplasty and abdominal rectopexy with possible bowel resection carry risks and benefits. After a lengthy conversation, I scheduled Mrs. Clarkson for a laparoscopic abdominal rectopexy. This intervention typically results in less pain and a shorter hospital stay with a low rate of recurrent prolapse.

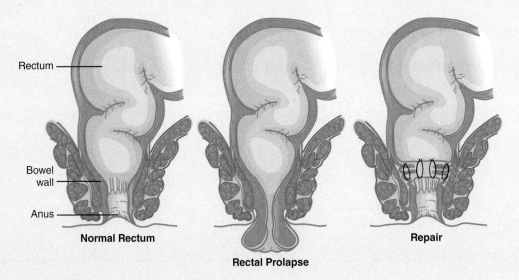

CASE FIGURE: Rectal prolapse and repair

1. Indicate the word parts for *proctoptosis* and provide the meaning of the disorder based on those parts.

2. Why might Mrs. Clarkson believe her symptoms are due to hemorrhoids?

3. Complete the following table for procedures related to proctoptosis.

Term	Word Parts	Meaning
levatoroplasty	*levator/o; -plasty*	*surgical repair of the levator ani muscle (the muscle that draws the anus upward after defecation and supports the pelvic organs)*
colonoscopy		
defecography		
rectosigmoidectomy		
anorectal manometry		
rectopexy		
resection		

4. Contrast an abdominal vs. a perineal procedure by indicating the word parts for each term and defining it.

5. Indicate the word parts for *laparoscopic* and describe a laparoscopic procedure.

🔍 STANDARD CASE STUDY

7.5 Sigmoid Colovesical Fistula

A 60-year-old man presented to the emergency department (ED) with a 3-day history of fecaluria and pneumaturia. Vital signs were within normal range. Physical exam was unremarkable except for mild tenderness in the suprapubic region. Medical history includes hypertension, cystitis, and colonic diverticulosis.

Urine was collected for examination. The urine sample was visibly opaque and microscopic observation revealed high numbers of leukocytes and erythrocytes. A midstream specimen of urine (MSU) test was performed and was positive for nitrate and culture tests were positive for *Escherichia coli*.

A colonoscopy revealed multiple diverticuli in the sigmoid colon. Abdominal computed tomography (CT) images showed air in the bladder and provided some evidence of a fistulous communication between the sigmoid colon and the urinary bladder. A barium enema was performed, passage of dye from the sigmoid colon to the bladder confirmed a colovesical fistula.

A diagnosis of sigmoid colovesical fistula secondary to colonic diverticulosis was made and the patient was transferred to the department of surgery for consultation.

(continues)

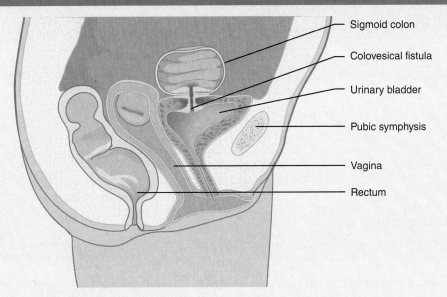

CASE FIGURE: A colovesical fistula

1. Define the word parts for *colovesical fistula*.

   Colovesical fistula: Col/o _____, vesic/o _____, -al _____,

   fistula _____.

2. In general, what does the term *fistula* refer to?

3. What region of the colon is involved in a sigmoid colovesical fistula?

4. Fecaluria or pneumaturia are pathognomic of colovesicular fistula. Define the word parts for *fecaluria* and *pneumaturia*.

   Fecaluria: Fecal _____*feces*_____, -uria _____.

   Pneumaturia: Pneumat/o _____, -uria _____.

5. Define the word parts for the following conditions in the patient's medical history:

   Hypertension: Hyper- _____, -tension _____.

   Cystitis: Cyst/o _____, -itis _____.

   Colonic diverticulosis: Colon/o _____, -ic _____,

   diverticul/o _____, -osis _____.

⌕ ADVANCED CASE STUDY

7.6 Jejunal Atresia

Although baby Amaya was born prematurely, her birth was uneventful. The day following the birth, however, it was clear that something was wrong. She was not nursing well, and her abdomen was swollen. In addition, she was vomiting a yellow green substance. Amaya would have to stay at the hospital and her parents were scared.

Amaya's inability to tolerate feedings, epigastric distension, and bilious vomiting all pointed to a bowel obstruction. Nasogastric intubation was performed to decompress the abdomen and an intravenous (IV) line was inserted to provide nutrients and fluids. A CT scan confirmed jejunal atresia; neither volvulus nor intussusception were detected. Surgical intervention was the only way to correct this congenital defect and Baby Amaya was scheduled for surgery the next day. During the operation the surgeon examined the full length of the small bowel and found a single small area of obstruction. The damaged portion of the bowel was resected, and

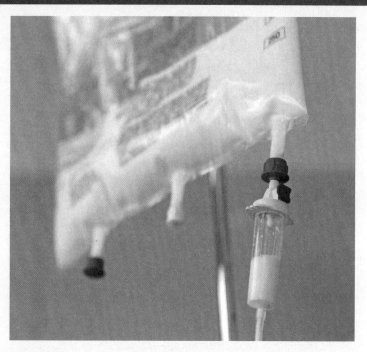

CASE FIGURE: Total parenteral nutrition (TPN) fluid bag

© Martin Carlsson/Shutterstock

anastomosis was performed. Amaya was placed on total parenteral nutrition (TPN) following surgery until she could tolerate oral enteral feeding. Amaya was lucky. Her bowel damage was not extensive, and she has no other coexisting congenital defects. Her prognosis for a complete recovery with a fully functioning digestive tract was very good.

1. Define the word parts for *atresia* and explain what a jejunal atresia is.

    Atresia: A- _____, -tresia _____

2. Amaya's symptoms include epigastric distension and bilious vomiting. Explain these symptoms.

3. Explain the following procedures, using word parts.

    Nasogastric intubation:

    Intravenous:

(continues)

🔍 *ADVANCED CASE STUDY* *(continued)*

4. Volvulus and intussusception are other causes of intestinal blockages. Define these terms.

   Volvulus:

   Intussusception:

5. Resection and anastomosis are common surgical procedures to treat bowel obstructions. Resection is the excision of the damaged area and anastomosis joins the two cut ends to open the structures to each other. The following are surgical procedures opening one structure to another. Define the word parts and meaning for each of the following types of anastomosis and circle the one most likely performed in this case study:

   Gastroenterostomy: Gastr/o _____, enter/o _____,

   -ostomy _____, means _____.

   Duodenocholecystostomy: Duoden/o _____, cholecyst/o _____,

   -ostomy _____, means _____.

   Enteroenterostomy: Enter/o _____, enter/o _____,

   -ostomy _____, means _____.

   Gastroduodenostomy: Gastr/o _____, duoden/o _____,

   -ostomy _____, means _____.

   Arteriovenostomy: Arteri/o _____, ven/o _____,

   -ostomy _____, means _____.

6. Contrast total parenteral nutrition with oral enteral nutrition.

7. When part of the small intestine is removed, short bowel syndrome can result from extensive intestinal blockage. Considering the function of the small intestine, what do you think the likely consequences are of short bowel syndrome?

⌕ ADVANCED CASE STUDY

7.7 Pancreatitis

Mrs. Kumar is a 50-year-old female who presented to the emergency department (ED) after being woken from a sound sleep by severe pain in the left upper quadrant of the abdomen. The pain was more severe when in a supine position. She grimaced as she described the pain as steady and radiating throughout her abdomen and to her back. She appeared acutely ill. She was diaphoretic and tachypneic with a pulse of 140 bpm (normal is 60–100 bpm). Her abdomen was clearly distended upon physical exam and she was jaundiced. Blood work indicated elevated amylase and lipase levels, and hyperbilirubinemia. A CT scan confirmed a diagnosis of pancreatitis, with gallstones as the suspected underlying cause. Mrs. Kumar was admitted to the hospital and placed on IV fluids and provided analgesics for pain relief. After a 48-hr period of NPO for bowel rest, endoscopic retrograde cholangiopancreatography (ERCP) was performed which confirmed cholodocholithiasis as the underlying cause of the pancreatitis. The stones were removed during this procedure using standard basket extraction techniques. Cholecystectomy was recommended to prevent recurrent cholelithiasis and was performed laparoscopically the following morning. By the evening, Mrs. Kumar was able to eat and drink and to ambulate unaided. She was discharged to go home with post-operative instructions and a scheduled follow-up visit with gastroenterology the following week.

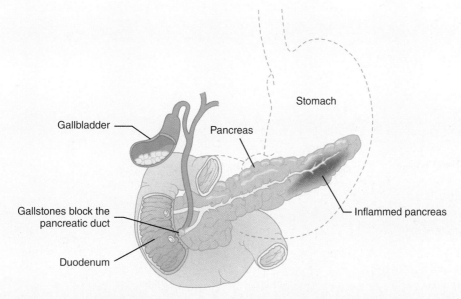

CASE FIGURE: Acute pancreatitis is an inflammation of the pancreas. Gallstones block the flow of pancreatic juices into the duodenum. Digestive enzymes become active in the pancreas, where they destroy healthy tissue

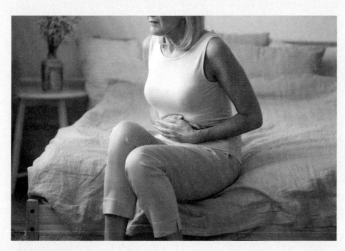

CASE FIGURE: Woman with severe abdominal pain

© Fizkes/Shutterstock

(continues)

🔍 *ADVANCED CASE STUDY*   *(continued)*

1. What organs are located in the left upper quadrant of the abdomen?

2. What is the supine position? What is the opposite of supine?

3. Complete the following table for signs and symptoms related to the patient's diagnosis:

Term	Word Parts	Meaning
pancreatitis	*pancreat/o; -itis*	*inflammation of the pancreas*
diaphoretic		
tachypneic		
jaundice		
amylase (elevated)		
lipase (elevated)		
hyperbilirubinemia		

4. Explain how elevated amylase and lipase, and hyperbilirubinemia, relate to the patient's diagnosis of pancreatitis caused by gallstones.

5. The abbreviation NPO comes from the Latin phrase *nil per os*. What does NPO mean?

6. The following terms all contain the root *chol/e*, which means gall (another word for bile). Define the word parts for each term, and the meaning of the term:

   Cholodocholithiasis: Cholodoch/o _____, -lithiasis _____,

   means _____,

Cholecystectomy: Cholecyst/o _____, -ectomy _____,

means _____

Cholelithiasis: Chol/e _____, -lithiasis _____,

means _____

7. Endoscopic retrograde cholangiopancreatography (ERCP) is a common procedure to investigate pancreatic and biliary disease. Define the word parts for this procedure then explain how the procedure is used. Use a medical dictionary or other valid resource, if needed, to help.

Endoscopic: Endo- _____, -scopic _____

Retrograde: Retro- _____, -grade _____

Cholangiopancreatography: Cholangi/o _____, pancreat/o _____,

-graphy _____

8. If gallstones are large, they must be broken up, so they are small enough to pass through the bile ducts. Construct a medical term for surgical crushing of gallstones in the common bile duct and define each word part.

9. What are the word parts for *laparoscopic*? What is a laparoscopic procedure?

10. Mrs. Kumar is instructed to follow up with the gastroenterology department the following week. Define the word parts for *gastroenterology*.

Gastroenterology: Gastr/o _____, enter/o _____, -logy _____

⌕ ADVANCED CASE STUDY

7.8 Zollinger-Ellison Syndrome

A 35-year-old male presented with severe epigastralgia and a 6-month history of chronic diarrhea and steatorrhea. The patient lost 25 kg (55 lb) in this time period and appeared cachectic. Stool culture and tests for ova and parasites and *Clostridium difficile* were negative. Endoscopic evaluation and computed tomography (CT) scan identified ulcers and a 3 cm mass in the duodenum. Serum gastrin level was significantly elevated at 11,100 pg/mL (normal < 100 pg/mL). Basal acid output test revealed gastric acid hypersecretion of 20 mEq/h and established the diagnosis of Zollinger-Ellison syndrome.

(continues)

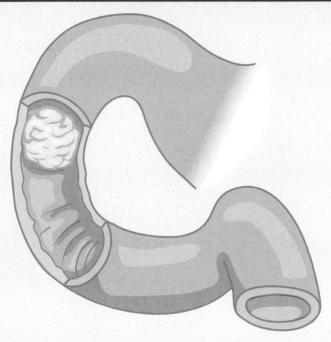

CASE FIGURE: Duodenal mass

1. Define the following word parts to the following conditions:

Epigastralgia: Epi- _____, gastr/o _____, -algia _____.

Diarrhea: Dia- _____, -rrhea _____.

Steatorrhea: Steat/o _____, -rrhea _____.

2. What does cachectic mean?

3. The patient has hypergastrinemia, or a condition of elevated levels of the hormone gastrin in the blood.

Where is the hormone gastrin produced?

What is the primary function of the hormone gastrin?

4. Define the word parts for the following terms and then circle the term you would use to describe the mass that was identified with the CT scan.

Duodenal sarcoma: Duoden/o _____, -al _____,

sarc/o _____, -oma _____.

Pancreatic gastrinoma: Pancreat/o _____, -ic _____,

gastrin _____ *pertaining to stomach* _____, -oma _____.

Duodenal gastrinoma: Duoden/o _____, -al _____,

gastrin _____ *pertaining to stomach* _____,

-oma _____.

Duodenal lipoma: Duoden/o _____, -al _____,

lip/o _____, -oma _____.

🔍 ADVANCED CASE STUDY

7.9 Ulcerative Colitis

A 45-year-old male presented to urgent care with a chief complaint of passing watery diarrhea over 15 times each day and through the night. The patient reported that the diarrhea had become progressively worse over three months, and the introduction of blood to the diarrhea for 2 days motivated the urgent care visit. The patient had lost 20 lb (9.1 kg) since the initial symptoms had started, and he complained of feeling fatigued. He had been diagnosed with ulcerative colitis three years prior, and at that time, responded well to steroid therapy and had remained in remission since.

The patient was afebrile and anicteric. Heart rate and blood pressure were within normal rates. Laboratory values were unremarkable, stool and urine cultures were negative, and no ova or intestinal parasites were present. Mild tenderness was elicited in the hypogastric and left iliac regions.

A gastroscopy showed that the mucosa of the esophagus and stomach were intact and normal, but a colonoscopy revealed severe ulceration and inflammation involving the rectum and the sigmoid colon; the ascending, transverse, and descending colon were spared. The affected intestinal mucosa was erythematous and edematous. Biopsies were collected for histological analysis; biopsies were friable and granular. Histology revealed neutrophil infiltration of the intestinal epithelium and epithelial architectural distortion suggestive of chronicity.

A likely diagnosis of ulcerative colitis was made based on patient history, presenting symptoms, and pathohistology.

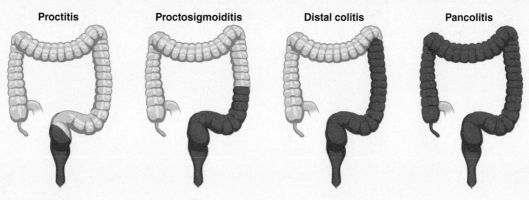

CASE FIGURE: Types of ulcerative colitis

(continues)

🔍 *ADVANCED CASE STUDY*   *(continued)*

1. Define the word parts for the different region-specific types of ulcerative colitis:

    Ulcerative proctitis: proct/o _____, -itis _____.

    Ulcerative proctosigmoiditis: proct/o _____, sigmoid/o _____,

    -itis _____.

    Ulcerative distal colitis: dist/o _____, -al _____,

    col/o _____, -itis _____.

    Ulcerative pancolitis: pan- _____, col/o _____, -itis _____.

2. Based on the results of the endoscopy procedures, what type of region-specific ulcerative colitis do you think the patient has?

3. Define the word parts for the following medical terms relating to the patient examination:

    Anicteric: An- _____, icter/o _____,

    -ic _____.

    Erythematous: Erythr/o _____, hemat/o _____,

    -ous _____.

    Edematous: Edemat/o _____, -ous _____.

4. Give a short definition for the medical terms *febrile*, *friable*, and *chronicity*.

    Febrile:

    Friable:

    Chronicity:

🔍 *ADVANCED CASE STUDY*

7.10 Hepatic Alveolar Echinococcosis

Current Complaint: A 45-year-old male presented to urgent care with a 2-month history of right hypochondriac pain. The patient complained of fatigue, dyspepsia, emesis, and reported that he has lost 10 kg (22 lb), from 80 to 70 kg, since the abdominal pain began.

Past History: The patient's past medical history was unremarkable. At the time of presentation, he was a United States resident, emigrating from Egypt 10 years prior. In Egypt, he grew up and lived in a rural farming community.

Signs and Symptoms: Vital signs were within normal range. Patient had mild hepatomegaly and icteric sclera.

Relevant Laboratory Values

Measured Value	Value	Normal Range
Hemoglobin	14.5 g/dL	14.0–18.0 g/dL
Hematocrit	41%	42–52%
Erythrocytes (RBCs)	4.4×10^6 cells/μL	$4.7–6.1 \times 10^6$ cells/μL
Leukocytes (WBCs)	15,200 cells/μL	4,800–10,800 cells/μL
Eosinophils	3,010 cells/μL	<700 cells/μL
Bilirubin (serum, total)	3.1 mg/dL	<0.4 mg/dL
ALK (serum) (alkaline phosphatase)	220 U/L	36–92 U/L
ALT (serum) (alanine aminotransferase)	60 U/L	1–21 U/L
AST (serum) (aspartate aminotransferase)	78 U/L	7–27 U/L

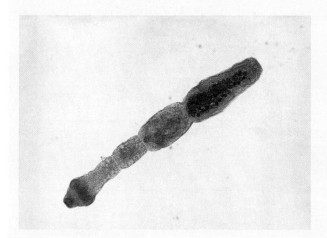

CASE FIGURE: Adult *Echinococcus multilocularis* tapeworm

Courtesy of Dr. Healy/Centers for Disease Control and Prevention

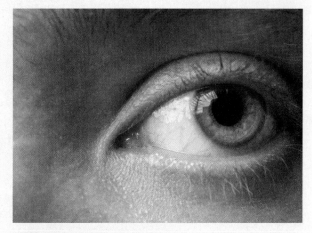

CASE FIGURE: Jaundiced eyes

© DaniiD/Shutterstock

(continues)

$\mathcal{P}$ ADVANCED CASE STUDY

(continued)

An initial sonogram and computed tomography (CT) image revealed two lesions in the right hepatic lobe. The lesions were between 8 and 10 cm in diameter, had an alveolar-like pattern, and were surrounded by dense connective tissue. The lesions had heterogenous contents, including irregular peripheral calcifications and central necrosis.

Patient history: Hematological and serum biochemical profiles, and sonography and CT scan suggested that the legions were hydatid cysts containing the larval stage of the fox tapeworm, *Echinococcus multilocularis*. *E. multilocularis*-specific serum antibodies were detected by serotests.

Diagnosis: Hepatic alveolar echinococcosis caused by *E. multilocularis*.

Treatment: Cysts were surgically removed. Chemotherapy (albendazole) 24 hr before, and for 30 days after, intervention.

1. The patient describes pain in the right hypochondriac region; define the word parts for *hypochondriac* and then describe how the word parts relate to this region.

   Hypochondriac: Hypo- _____, chondr/o _____,

   -iac _____.

   Describe how the word parts relate to this region.

2. What organs are found within the right hypochondriac region?

3. A physical examination of the patient revealed mild hepatomegaly. Define the word parts for *hepatomegaly*.

   Hepatomegaly: Hepat/o _____, -megaly _____.

4. Three cell types were reported in the relevant laboratory values. Define the word parts of the three types of cells, provide their meaning, and circle the type(s) that are/is not within normal range in this patient.

   Erythrocyte: Erythr/o _____, -cyte _____,

   means _____.

   Leukocyte: Leuk/o _____, -cyte _____,

   means _____.

   Eosinophil: Eosin/o _____, -phil _____,

   means _____.

5. What pathological conditions increase the abundance of eosinophils?

6. Define the word parts for the following medical terms included in the results of the medical imaging:

    Alveolar: Alveol/o _____, -ar _____

    Heterogeneous: Hetero- _____, -genous _____

    Peripheral: Peripher/o _____, -al _____

    Necrosis: Necr/o _____, -osis _____

7. How might the biology of *E. multilocularis* be associated with icteric sclera? Consider the definition of icteric sclera and some of the abnormal laboratory values to formulate your response.

References

Aamar, A., Madhani, K., Virk, H., & Butt, Z. (2016). Zollinger-Ellison Syndrome: A rare case of chronic diarrhea. *Gastroenterology Research*, 9(6), 103–104. https://doi.org/10.14740/gr734w

Cañamares-Orbís, P., & Chan, F. (2019). Endoscopic management of nonvariceal upper gastrointestinal bleeding. *Best Practice & Research Clinical Gastroenterology*, 42–43, 101608. https://doi.org/10.1016/j.bpg.2019.04.001

Geramizadeh, B., Nikeghbalian, S., & Malekhosseini, S. A. (2012). Alveolar echinococcosis of the liver: Report of three cases from different geographic areas of Iran. *Hepatitis Monthly*, 12(9), e6143. doi:10.5812/hepatmon.6143

Kim, N. I., Jo, Y., Ahn, S. B., Son, B. K., Kim, S. H., Park, Y. S., Kim, S. H., & Ju, J. E. (2010). A case of eosinophilic esophagitis with food hypersensitivity. *Journal of Neurogastroenterology and Motility*, 16(3), 315–318. https://doi.org/10.5056/jnm.2010.16.3.315

Lee, L., Akhtar, M. M., Gardezisanjliajk, A., & Macfaul, G. (2013). Ulcerative colitis: A case of steroid refractory disease. *BMJ Case Reports*, 2013, bcr2013009784. https://doi.org/10.1136/bcr-2013-009784

Pachisia, S., Mandal, G., Sahu, S., & Ghosh, S. (2019). Submandibular sialolithiasis: A series of three case reports with review of literature. *Clinics and Practice*, 9(1), 32–37. https://doi.org/10.4081/cp.2019.1119

Qu, B., Guo, L., Sheng, G., Yu, F., Chen, G., Wang, Y., Shi, Y., Zhan, H., Yang, Y., & Du, X. (2017). Management of advanced hepatic alveolar echinococcosis: Report of 42 cases. *The American Journal of Tropical Medicine and Hygiene*, 96(3), 680–685. doi:10.4269/ajtmh.16-0557

Rickert, A., & Kienle, P. (2015). Laparoscopic surgery for rectal prolapse and pelvic floor disorders. *World Journal of Gastrointestinal Endoscopy*, 7(12), 1045–1054. https://doi.org/10.4253/wjge.v7.i12.1045

Stedman, T. L. (2005). Nath's *Stedman's medical terminology, 2e*. Philadelphia: Lippincott Williams & Wilkins.

Șurlin, V., Săftoiu, A., & Dumitrescu, D. (2014). Imaging tests for accurate diagnosis of acute biliary pancreatitis. *World Journal of Gastroenterology*, 20(44), 16544–16549. https://doi.org/10.3748/wjg.v20.i44.16544

Venes, D., & Taber, C. W. (2017). *Taber's cyclopedic medical dictionary*. Ed. 23, illustrated in full color/Philadelphia: F.A. Davis.

Verma, A., Rattan, K. N., & Yadav, R. (2016). Neonatal intestinal obstruction: A 15 year experience in a tertiary care hospital. *Journal of Clinical and Diagnostic Research*, 10(2), SC10–SC13. https://doi.org/10.7860/JCDR/2016/17204.7268

Yang, H. Y., Sun, W. Y., Lee, T. G., & Lee, S. J. (2011). A case of colovesical fistula induced by sigmoid diverticulitis. *Journal of the Korean Society of Coloproctology*, 27(2), 94–98. https://doi.org/10.3393/jksc.2011.27.2.94

CHAPTER 8

Urinary System

Calyx	Nephron	Renal pyramid
Glomerular filtration rate (GFR)	Purpura	Ureter
Glomerulus	Renal capsule	Urethra
Hilum	Renal cortex	Urgency
Incontinence	Renal medulla	Urinalysis
Kidney	Renal papilla	Urinary bladder
Micturition	Renal pelvis	Urine

The most important role of the urinary system is to filter blood, conserving needed substances, and removing excess materials and nitrogenous wastes. These wastes, if left to accumulate, would quickly become toxic. By balancing the blood composition, the body can maintain water balance, blood pressure, optimal electrolyte levels, and pH.

The urinary system consists of a pair of kidneys and ureters, the urinary bladder, and the urethra. The **kidneys** are reddish in color and kidney-bean-shaped and are located behind the abdominal cavity (retroperitoneal). The right kidney is a little lower than the left because it is displaced by the liver, which lies just superior to it. The **ureters** are muscular tubes that extend about 25 to 30 cm down from the kidneys to the **urinary bladder**. **Urine** is produced by the kidneys, descends through the ureters, and is stored in the bladder until the urge to void is felt. For a typical adult, this occurs when approximately 250 mL of urine fills the bladder although capacity of the bladder averages between 700 and 800 mL. The bladder is spherical when distended with urine but collapses when empty. Urine exits the bladder through the internal urethral sphincter, which is involuntary, into the **urethra** and is released through the urinary meatus by voluntary relaxation of the external urethral sphincter. In females, the urethra is just 2.5 to 5 cm long compared with a length of 20 cm in males. The discharge of urine is termed **micturition**, urination, or voiding. Lack of voluntary control over this process is called **incontinence**.

The major work of the urinary system is done by the kidneys. Each kidney is surrounded by a layer of dense connective tissue called the **renal capsule**, which helps maintain its shape. Adipose tissue surrounds the renal capsule to help anchor the kidney in place and protect it from trauma. Internally, the kidney consists of two distinct regions, the outer **renal cortex** and the inner **renal medulla**. The renal cortex receives most of the kidney's blood supply. The renal medulla consists of cone-shaped **renal pyramids** with the apex, or pointed end, of each pyramid projecting toward the **hilum**, a deep fissure through which the ureter emerges, along with the renal artery and the renal vein. This apex is called a **renal papilla**. **Nephrons**, the functional units of the kidneys, traverse the renal cortex to the renal medulla. Each kidney has about a million microscopic nephrons, which is where urine formation takes place. This process occurs in three stages: filtration, reabsorption, and secretion.

Glomerular filtration, the first step of urine production, occurs in the renal cortex, within the microscopic ball-shaped collections of capillaries of the nephrons, the glomeruli (singular **glomerulus**). Here water and most solutes from systemic blood move from glomerular capillaries to the glomerular capsule. The filtrate then moves to the renal tubule of the nephron where about 99% of the filtered water and many useful solutes such as small proteins, sodium and chloride ions, and glucose are reabsorbed into the blood. This is the second step of urine formation. During secretion, the final step of urine formation, wastes, drugs, and excess ions, are secreted from blood into the filtrate in the renal tubules. The filtrate moves to the collecting ducts of the nephron, to the renal papillae, then to the cup-like minor calyces (singular **calyx**) then major calyces. The liquid, now defined as urine, collects into the single, large cavity called the **renal pelvis**, which drains into the ureters and urinary bladder.

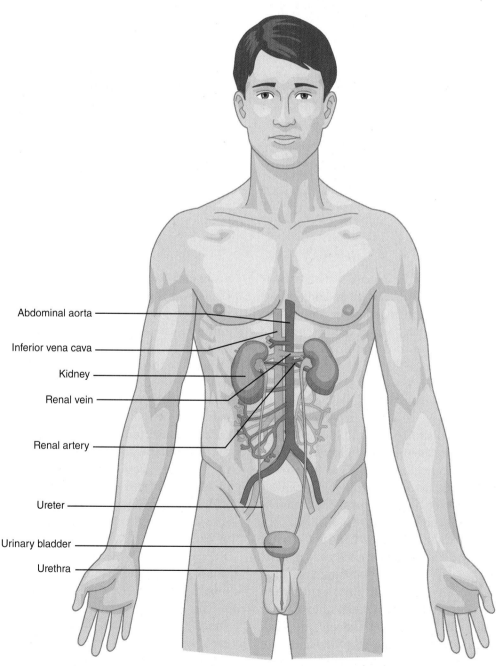

Abdominal aorta

Inferior vena cava

Kidney

Renal vein

Renal artery

Ureter

Urinary bladder

Urethra

FIGURE 8.1 Organs of the urinary system

Kidney

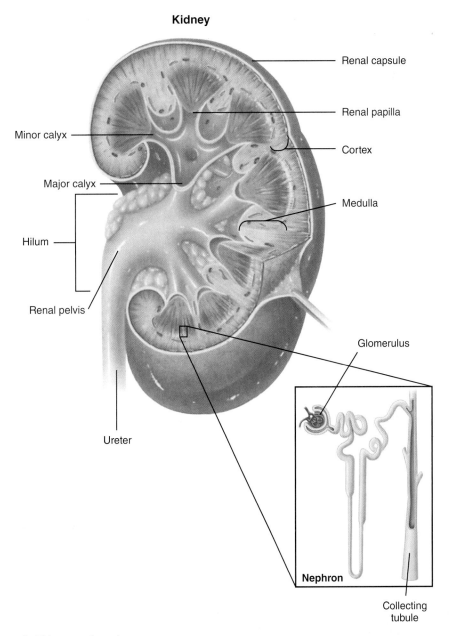

FIGURE 8.2 Anatomy of a kidney and nephron

Glomerular filtration rate (GFR) is an important measure of health. If GFR is too low, too much filtrate will be reabsorbed into the blood and waste products will not be adequately excreted. If GFR is too high, the filtrate will pass too quickly through the kidney tubules and needed substances will be lost in the urine rather than reabsorbed into the blood. A **urinalysis** evaluates the chemical, physical, and microscopic properties of urine and is another important indicator of health. Normal urine is yellow to amber, transparent, and has an average pH of 6. Urine varying from these characteristics or urine with abnormal constituents such as glucose, proteins, red blood cells, or bacteria can be an indicator of disease.

TABLE 8.1
Key Urinary System Prefixes
poly-: many, much
Key urinary system combining forms:
azot/o: nitrogenous waste
bacteri/o: bacteria
capillar/o: capillary

(continues)

TABLE 8.1	(continued)
Key Urinary System Prefixes	
contine/o: hold back, restrain, keep in	
cyst/o: urinary bladder	
dips/o: thirst	
fasci/o: fascia	
globin/o: protein	
glomerul/o: glomerulus	
glycos/o: sugar	
hydr/o: water	
ket/o: ketone	
keton/o: ketone	
laps/o: slip, slide	
lith/o: stone	
nephr/o: kidney	
noct/i: night	
olig/o: scanty	

peritone/o: peritoneum

pyel/o: renal pelvis

py/o: pus

ren/o: kidney

ureter/o: ureter

urethr/o: urethra

urin/o: urine

ur/o: urine

vascul/o: vessels

vesic/o: urinary bladder

TABLE 8.2
Key Urinary System Suffixes
-emia: blood condition
-lithiasis: condition of stones
-uria: urine condition

🔍 STANDARD CASE STUDY

8.1 Floating Kidney

Esha, a 30-year-old extremely thin female, came to the clinic complaining of right unilateral costovertebral pain. The pain increased in severity when she was erect and was relieved when she was in the supine position. Prior imaging including ultrasonography and an abdominal computed tomography (CT) scan, revealed no abnormalities. When questioned, she also described periodic oliguria and slight hematuria. The consulting urologist suspected the rare disorder of nephroptosis and requested dynamic, rather than static, imaging. Intravenous urography, both in the supine and erect position, revealed a craniocaudal migration of the length of 2.5 vertebral bodies of the right kidney. This unusual condition can be associated with the absence of perirenal fat and fascial support of the kidney. Laparoscopic nephropexy is the recommended surgical intervention for symptomatic nephroptosis. After undergoing this procedure, Esha is expected to have complete resolution of her symptoms.

1. Where is Esha's pain? What position improves her symptoms and what position makes them worse?

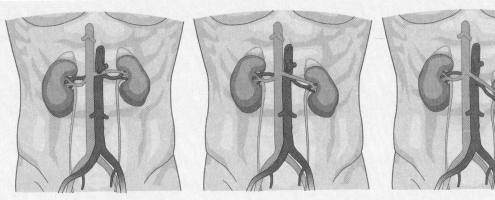

Healthy Kidneys   **Nephroptosis**

CASE FIGURE: Nephroptosis of kidney

2. Esha complains of periodic oliguria. Define the word parts and meaning of this term.

Oliguria: Olig/o _____, -uria _____, means _____.

Esha does not complain of anuria or polyuria, other terms used to refer to urine quantity. Define the word parts and meaning of these terms.

Anuria: An- _____, -uria _____, means _____.

Polyuria: Poly- _____, -uria _____, means _____.

3. Esha complains of slight hematuria, referring to an abnormal substance in the urine. Using a medical dictionary or other resource, complete the following table for hematuria and other terms indicating abnormal substances present in urine. The presence of abnormal substances in the urine can point toward a disease or illness; for each term, indicate what this might be.

Term with Word Parts	Meaning	What It Might Indicate
hemat/o; -uria		
glycos/o; -uria		
keton/o; -uria		
py/o; -uria		
protein; -uria		
bacteri/o; -uria		

4. Dynamic means pertaining to movement while static means pertaining to standing still. Explain Esha's diagnosis of nephroptosis. Be sure to define relevant terms in the case. Why was dynamic imaging necessary for this diagnosis?

(continues)

🔍 STANDARD CASE STUDY   (continued)

5. Complete the table for the procedural terms in the case.

Term	Word Parts	Meaning
ultrasonography	*ultra-; son/o; -graphy*	*process of recording beyond sound*
abdominal computed tomography	*abdomin/o; -al; computed (calculated); tom/o; -graphy*	
intravenous urography		
laparoscopic nephropexy		

🔍 STANDARD CASE STUDY

8.2 Staghorn Renal Calculus

Current Complaint: A 35-year-old male, later transferred to the hospital, presents to Urgent Care with fever, gross hematuria, dysuria, urgency, frequency, and right flank pain.

Relevant Past Illnesses: The patient's record indicates a history of recurrent polymicrobial urinary tract infections and nephrolithiasis.

Signs and Symptoms: The patient appears unwell and is febrile with a temperature of 38.6 °C (normal 37.0 °C). Other vital signs are within normal range. Urine is cloudy with an alkaline pH and blood is present. Intravenous pyelogram of the right kidney shows hydronephrosis and a stone roughly 4.8 cm in size.

Diagnosis: Staghorn calculus (kidney stone) of the right kidney, filling much of the renal pelvis and branching into several of the calyces.

Follow Up and Treatment: Lasix renogram is recommended to assess the level of renal disease. If renal function is significantly compromised, nephrectomy may be recommended. Assuming that kidney damage is not substantial, treatment modalities for staghorn calculus should be evaluated. Extra corporeal shockwave lithotripsy (ECSWL) is ruled out given the size of the stone. Percutaneous nephrolithotomy (PCNL) using ureteroscopy-assisted retrograde nephrostomy (UARN) is recommended due to the large and obstructive nature of the stone.

1. Define the word parts and meaning of *dysuria* and *hematuria*.

    Dysuria: Dys-_____, -uria _____

    Hematuria: Hemat/o _____, -uria _____

2. Define the terms urgency and frequency in the context of urinary system pathology. Use a medical dictionary if necessary.

3. Describe the patient's relevant past illnesses in simple terms.

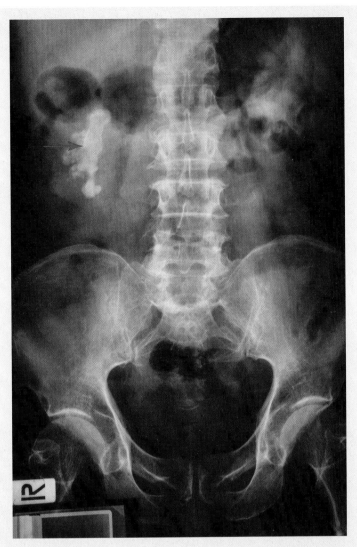

CASE FIGURE: Staghorn renal calculus (arrow). Note how the stone fills the renal pelvis and extends to the calyces

© Puwadol Jaturawutthichai/Shutterstock

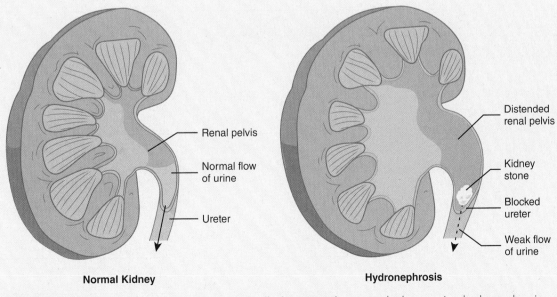

Renal pelvis

Normal flow
of urine

Ureter

Distended
renal pelvis

Kidney
stone

Blocked
ureter

Weak flow
of urine

Normal Kidney

Hydronephrosis

CASE FIGURE: Urine is blocked from passing through the ureter due to a calculus, causing hydronephrosis

(continues)

4. Define the word parts for *hydronephrosis* and explain its occurrence.

Hydronephrosis: Hydro- _____, nephr/o _____,

-osis _____.

5. Define the word parts and meaning of the procedural terms in the case.

Intravenous pyelogram: Intra- _____, ven/o _____

-ous _____ pyel/o _____,

-gram _____.

Lasix is a diuretic that stimulates urine flow

Lasix Renogram: Ren/o _____, -gram _____,

means _____.

Nephrectomy: Nephr/o _____, -ectomy _____,

means _____.

Extracorporeal shock-wave
lithotripsy: Extra- _____, corpor/o _____,

-eal _____, lith/o _____,

-tripsy _____

means _____.

Percutaneous
nephrolithotomy: Per- _____, cutane/o _____

-ous _____, nephr/o _____,

lith/o _____, -otomy _____,

means _____.

Ureteroscopy-assisted retrograde
nephrostomy: Ureter/o _____ ,

-scopy _____ , retro- _____ ,

-grade _____ , nephr/o _____ ,

-ostomy _____ ,

means _____ .

6. What is the renal pelvis and what are calyces? From where do you think the name staghorn calculus comes?

🔍 *STANDARD CASE STUDY*

8.3 Cystocele

A 30-year-old female sees her primary care provider with complaints of nocturia, increased frequency and urgency of urination, urinary incontinence, and persistent urinary tract infections. The symptoms began shortly after having her third child; all children were vaginal deliveries without complications. Cystoscopy, X-ray cystourethrography, and magnetic resonance imaging (MRI) revealed cystocele, also called bladder prolapse, a hernia of the posterior side of the bladder that pushes into the anterior side of the vagina. The patient was successfully treated using laparoscopy to anchor (fix) the bladder from the sacral promontory with an intervesicouterine prosthesis.

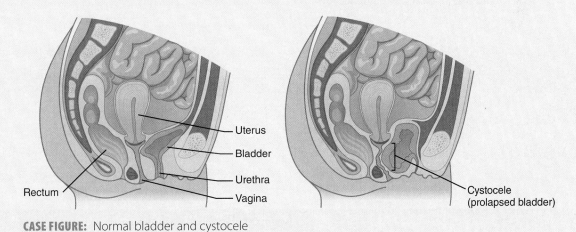

CASE FIGURE: Normal bladder and cystocele

1. The patient in this case was experiencing nocturia. Define the following word parts, and meaning, for the following pathologies: *anuria, nocturia, oliguria, polyuria*.

Anuria: An- _____ , -uria _____ ,

means _____ .

(continues)

🔍 STANDARD CASE STUDY   *(continued)*

Nocturia: Noct/i _____, -uria _____,

means _____.

Oliguria: Olig/o _____, -uria _____,

means _____.

Polyuria: Poly- _____, -uria _____,

means _____.

2. Define the following word parts, and meaning, for the imaging techniques, *cystoscopy* and *cystourethrography*, used in this case.

Cystoscopy: Cyst/o _____, -oscopy _____,

means _____.

Cystourethrography: Cyst/o _____, urethr/o _____,

-graphy _____,

means _____.

3. Complete the table below for the terms related to the diagnosis and treatment:

Term	Word Parts	Meaning
cystocele	*cyst/o; -cele*	*urinary bladder protrusion*
prolapse	*pro- ; laps/o*	
laparoscopic		
sacral		
intervesicouterine		

🔍 STANDARD CASE STUDY

8.4 Bladder Cancer

Urological Surgical Consultation

Mr. Arthur Melun, a 58-year-old male, is here today to discuss his upcoming cystectomy. Mr. Melun, a lifelong smoker, was diagnosed 2 years ago with non-muscle invasive bladder cancer (NMIBC). Initial staging following cystoscopy and transurethral resection of the bladder tumor (TURBT) revealed stage I urothelial cancer. The cancer had grown through the bladder lining but had not reached the muscle layer. Following cystoscopic resection to remove all visible cancer, Mr. Melun was given postoperative intravesical chemotherapy, and several weeks later, intravesical immunotherapy. Mr. Melun has been on maintenance therapy and monitored with regular cystoscopy. His recent cystoscope exam revealed recurrence of his bladder cancer and cystectomy was recommended, necessitating urinary diversion, with many different reconstructive options to consider. Both noncontinent and continent diversions are discussed. Noncontinent diversion includes urostomy, which uses part of the intestine to direct urine to an opening in the abdomen; two examples use an ileal or colonic conduit. These are noncontinent because the urine continuously collects in an ostomy bag. Continent diversions include orthotopic neobladder or continent cutaneous diversion such as appendicovesicostomy. Continent diversions maintain a functional urethral sphincter, or require self-catheterization, both of which achieve urinary continence. Many factors must be weighed when considering continent vs. noncontinent options, such as patient age, overall state of health, motivation to care for oneself, manual dexterity, and risk of complications associated with each procedure.

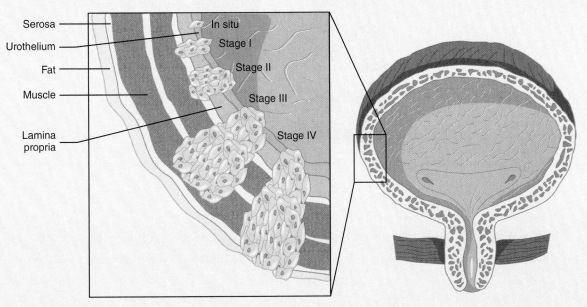

CASE FIGURE: Stages of bladder cancer. Stage I has invaded the urothelial cells that line the bladder but has not invaded the muscle wall

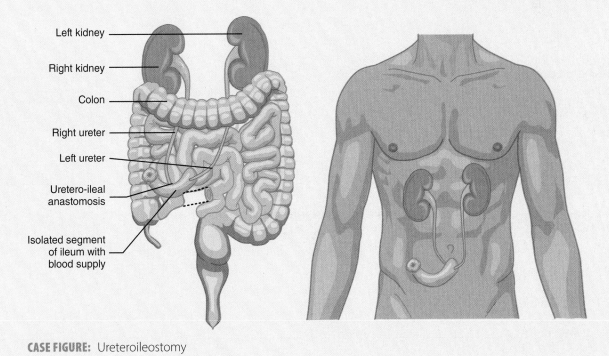

CASE FIGURE: Ureteroileostomy

(continues)

STANDARD CASE STUDY

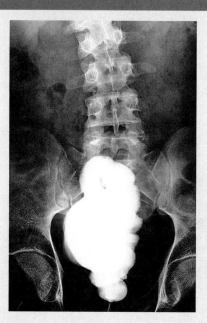

CASE FIGURE: An orthotopic neobladder formed from ileal tissue

© BSIP/Universal Images Group/Getty Images

1. Complete the table for the procedural terms in the case.

Term	Word Parts	Meaning
cystectomy	*cyst/o; -ectomy*	*surgical removal of the bladder*
cystoscopy		
transurethral resection (of the bladder tumor)		
cystoscopic resection		
urostomy		
appendicovesicostomy		

2. Define the word parts for *intravesical*.

    Intravesical: Intra- _____, vesic/o _____, -al _____

    Explain what is meant by intravesical chemotherapy and intravesical immunotherapy.

3. Define the word parts for *diversion*.

    Diversion: Di- _____, vers/o _____, -ion _____,

    means _____.

Continence from the combining form contine/o, to hold back, is defined as the voluntary release of urine. Contrast what is meant by continent urinary diversion vs. noncontinent urinary diversion.

4. A catheter is a tube. Some continent diversions require self-catheterization. Explain.

5. Define the following word parts and then explain what is meant by an orthotopic neobladder.

    orth/o _____

    topic/o _____

    neo- _____

6. What term in the case refers to a channel made with a piece of small intestine through which urine can be diverted?

7. This procedure is also called a ureteroileostomy, which uses part of the ileum to connect the ureters to a stoma on the surface of the abdomen. Define the word parts for *ureteroileostomy* and explain the procedure.

    Ureteroileostomy: Ureter/o _____, ile/o _____,

    -ostomy _____, means _____.

8. What term in the case refers to a similar channel but made with a piece of the large intestine?

🔍 *STANDARD CASE STUDY*

8.5 Acute Kidney Injury

Mr. DeSmet is happy to be going home from the hospital today following a bout with severe gastroenteritis. He had been admitted after suffering for 4 days with profuse watery diarrhea, low-grade fever, vomiting, and abdominal pain. Stool and blood cultures were positive for the bacterium *Salmonella enteritidis*. He was severely dehydrated, hypotensive, and azotemia indicated prerenal acute kidney injury (AKI). Mr. DeSmet had always considered himself a healthy 65-year-old and it had been scary for him that he hadn't responded to initial treatment with antibiotics and intravenous saline hydration. His diarrhea continued and progressive oliguria, decreased glomerular filtration rate (GFR), and worsening uremia all indicated increasingly compromised kidney function. A shift in antibiotic regimen and use of vasopressors had gradually improved his renal function and hemodialysis was averted. Ten days after his hospital admission, Mr. DeSmet was discharged with normal renal function and negative stool and blood cultures.

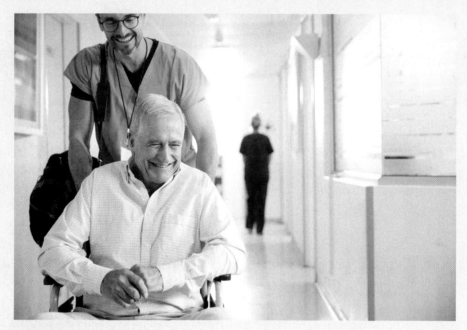

CASE FIGURE: Patient being discharged from the hospital

© Monkey Business Images/Shutterstock

1. Kidney injury can be acute or chronic (chron/o; -ic, meaning pertaining to time). Using a medical dictionary if necessary, differentiate these terms.

2. There are three types of acute kidney injury: prerenal, intrarenal (also called intrinsic), and postrenal. Define these terms using word parts and try to determine what is meant by these terms. Hint: The terms refer to the causative location of the injury.

3. Complete the table for the signs and symptoms in the case.

Term	Word Parts	Meaning
gastroenteritis	*gastr/o; enter/o; -itis*	*inflammation of the stomach and intestine*
hypotensive		
diarrhea		
dehydration (dehydrated)		
azotemia		
oliguria		
uremia		

4. Saline is a salt solution designed to correct electrolyte imbalances. Define the word parts for *intravenous hydration*.

Intravenous hydration: Intra- _____, ven/o _____,

-ous _____, hydr/o _____, -ation _____

Intravenous saline hydration means _____.

5. Vasopressor (vas/o; pressor) literally means a condition of pressing down on a vein. Vasopressors constrict blood vessels. How could these drugs help restore Mr. DeSmet's kidney function?

6. Build a term for a kidney specialist, the type of practitioner with whom Mr. DeSmit would be advised to follow up.

kidney _____, one who studies _____,

a physician who specializes in the kidney is a _____.

ADVANCED CASE STUDY

8.6 Polycystic Kidney Disease

A 55-year-old Japanese female presents to her primary care physician with complaints of persistent headaches, diplopia, flank (lumbar) pain, and macroscopic hematuria. The patient reports a previous medical history of passing several calculi in the previous 5 years. Her family history includes two uncles with nephrolithiasis and one undergoing hemodialysis. A physical assessment is significant for hypertension. Urinalysis confirms hematuria and proteinuria. The patient's estimated glomerular filtration rate (eGFR) is below normal as determined by a creatinine clearance test. Computed tomography (CT) scans reveal six bilateral hypoechoic lesions and calcifications consistent with renal cysts and nephrolithiasis. The patient meets the criteria for a diagnosis of polycystic kidney disease with nephrolithiasis and is referred to a nephrologist for further consultation and treatment.

(continues)

Polycystic Kidney Disease

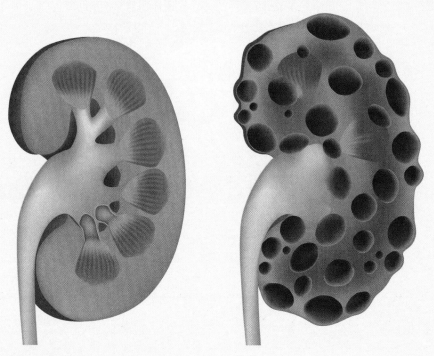

CASE FIGURE: Normal kidney and polycystic kidney disease

© Alila Sao Mai/Shutterstock

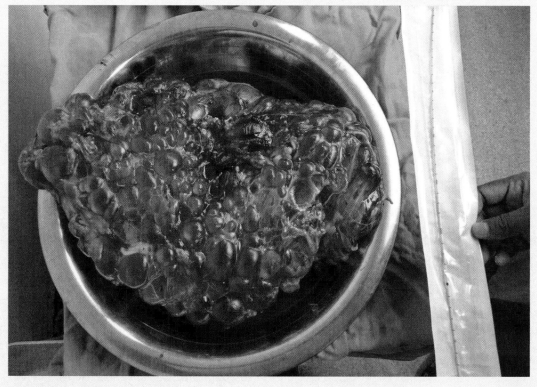

CASE FIGURE: Removed polycystic kidney

© Rare Shot/Barcroft Media/Getty Images

1. Complete the table below for the terms related to this patient's signs and symptoms:

Term	Word Parts	Meaning
macroscopic	*macro-; -scopic*	*pertaining to visually examining something large (visible without a microscope)*
diplopia		
hematuria		
hypertension		
proteinuria		

2. A calculus (plural calculi) translates from Latin to English as stone, or pebble. What does a calculus refer to when discussing the urinary system?

3. The patient's family history includes nephrolithiasis and one uncle undergoing hemodialysis. Define the word parts and meaning for *nephrolithiasis* and *hemodialysis*.

    Nephrolithiasis: Nephr/o _____, -lithiasis _____,

    means _____.

    Hemodialysis: Hem/o _____, dia- _____,

    -lysis _____, means _____

4. A creatinine clearance test is used to estimate the patient's glomerular filtration rate; the rate at which the kidneys are filtering blood. Using a medical dictionary, or other resource, briefly describe a creatinine clearance test.

5. The ultrasound reveals bilateral hypoechoic lesions (damage) consistent with renal cysts. Define the word parts for *bilateral* and *hypoechoic* and then describe how that is consistent with renal cysts (abnormal open pouches in the kidney).

    Bilateral: Bi- _____, later/_____ -al _____.

    Hypoechoic: Hypo- _____, echo-_____ -ic _____.

    Description:

6. Define the following word parts for *nephrologist*:

    Nephrologist: Nephr/o _____, -logist _____

🔍 *ADVANCED CASE STUDY*

8.7 Out with the Old

A 65-year-old Japanese female with end-stage renal disease (ESRD) resulting from polycystic kidney disease (PKD) talks with her nephrologist and a transplant surgeon about preparing for renal transplantation. The patient was diagnosed with PKD 10 years prior. For 3 years, the patient has been undergoing hemodialysis (HD), which entails three visits a week to a center that has a machine that can perform the role of her kidneys, which is to filter her blood. Over the last 10 years, her PKD has advanced. Her large polycystic kidneys have led to rectus abdominis diastasis, urogynecological symptoms including urinary incontinence, and insufficient space in the abdominal cavity for a renal transplant. To increase space, a pretransplant synchronous bilateral retroperitoneoscopic nephrectomy is recommended, as well as repair of rectus abdominis diastasis. She will use peritoneal dialysis (PD) from the time of nephrectomy to renal transplant. PD is a form of dialysis wherein a sterile solute-rich solution, dialysate, is introduced into the peritoneal cavity. Fluid and wastes are filtered from the blood across the peritoneum into the dialysate, which is subsequently drained. PD is performed each day at home. It offers more freedom and less restrictions than hemodialysis. The nephrectomy is scheduled to take place in several weeks, and scheduling a transplant with a new kidney will depend on donated kidney availability.

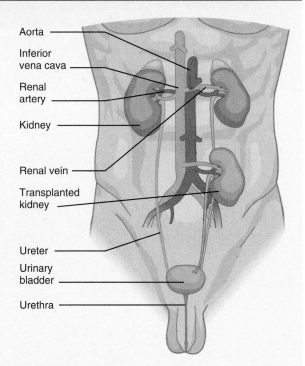

CASE FIGURE: Kidney transplantation

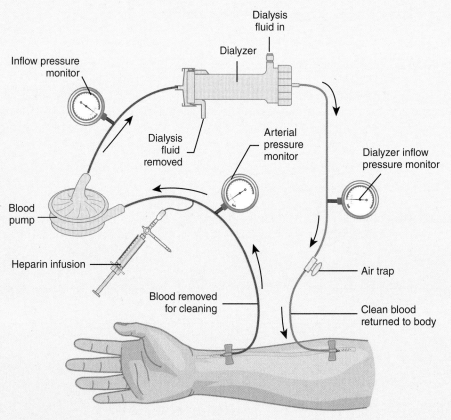

CASE FIGURE: Hemodialysis

Dialysate bag

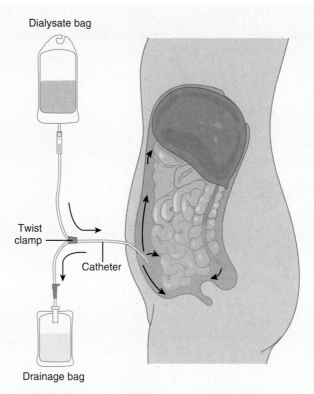

Twist
clamp

Catheter

Drainage bag

CASE FIGURE: Peritoneal dialysis

1. The patient's kidneys have increased in size as the number, and size, of cysts have increased. This has led to diastasis of a set of abdominal muscles, the rectus abdominis muscles, and other urogynecological symptoms. Define the word parts, and meaning, for *diastasis*, *urogynecological*, and *incontinence*, and then describe *rectus abdominis diastasis*, *urogynecological*, and *urinary incontinence*.

Diastasis: Dia- _____, -stasis _____, means _____.

Rectus abdominis diastasis description:

Urogynecological: Ur/o _____, gynec/o _____,

-logical _____, means _____.

Urogynecological symptom description:

Incontinence: In- _____, contine/o _____,

-ence _____, means _____.

Urinary incontinence description:

(continues)

2. A tissue graft is the transplanting of living tissue from one location to another. Define the prefixes for the following types of tissue grafts and use a medical dictionary, or other resource, to briefly describe the type of tissue graft. Circle the type of tissue graft that is planned for this patient.

Allograft: All/o _____, description _____.

Autograft: Auto- _____, description _____.

Isograft: Iso- _____, description _____.

Xenograft: Xeno- _____, description _____.

3. The patient will undergo a bilateral retroperitoneoscopic nephrectomy. Define the word parts, and meaning, for *bilateral*, *retroperitoneoscopic*, and *nephrectomy*.

Bilateral: Bi- _____, later/o _____-al _____,

means _____.

Retroperitoneoscopic: Retro- _____, peritone/o_____,

-scopic _____, means _____.

Nephrectomy: Nephr/o_____, -ectomy _____,

means _____.

4. What is a similarity and a difference between hemodialysis (HD) and peritoneal dialysis (PD)?

🔎 *ADVANCED CASE STUDY*

8.8 Cryoglobulinemic Glomerulonephritis

A 45-year-old woman presents to her primary care physician complaining of diarrhea, arthralgia, and presyncope symptoms, which had become increasingly severe over a period of 6 weeks. Physical exam revealed that the patient was febrile (100.5 °F/38.1 °C), tachycardic (105 beats/min), with bilateral lower limb nonpruritic purpura and pedal edema. The patient had a past medical history of hepatitis C virus (HCV) and is taking medication to treat hypercholesterolemia and hypertension. Lab tests show proteinuria, hypoalbuminemia, uremia, and creatinemia, all suggestive of nephrotic syndrome, which results from vasculitis and damaged glomerular capillaries. This damage allows the abnormal passage of protein into the urine. Blood and urine cultures were sterile and viral tests were negative except for the presence of HCV antibodies. HCV RNA was not present. A serum assay was positive for cryoglobulins, antibodies that precipitate at low temperature and may be produced in some people after some types of infections, including HCV. Kidney biopsy showed endocapillary hypercellularity and leukocytoclastic vasculitis with capillary cryoglobulin granular deposits. The patient was referred to a nephrologist for treatment of renal insufficiency and cryoglobulinemic glomerulonephritis secondary to HCV infection.

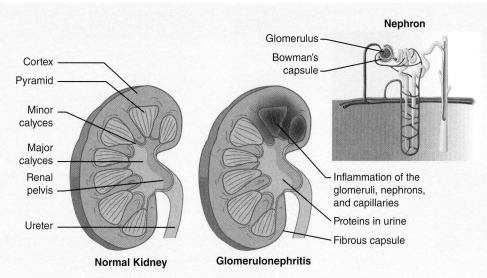

CASE FIGURE: Comparison of a normal kidney with one affected by glomerulonephritis

1. Complete the table below for the terms related to this patient's signs and symptoms:

Term	Word Parts	Meaning
diarrhea	*dia-; -rrhea*	*complete discharge (discharge of watery stool)*
arthralgia		
tachycardic		
hypercholesterolemia		
hypertension		
proteinuria		
hypoalbuminemia		
uremia		
creatinemia	*creatine; -emia*	
vasculitis		

2. The patient has nonpruritic purpura on her lower limbs. What is meant by *nonpruritic purpura*? Use a medical dictionary, or other resource, to complete this answer.

(continues)

3. The patient had symptoms of *presyncope*. What is meant by the term *presyncope*? Use a medical dictionary, or other resource, to complete this answer.

4. The patient had become febrile. What is meant by the term *febrile*?

5. Define the following word parts, and meaning, of *cryoglobulinemia* and *glomerulonephritis*.

   Cryoglobulinemia: Cry/o _____, globin/o _____,

   -emia _____, means _____.

   Glomerulonephritis: Glomerul/o _____, nephr/o _____,

   -itis _____, means _____.

6. Complete the table below for the terms related to the kidney biopsy:

Term	Word Parts	Meaning
biopsy	*bi/o; -opsy*	*view of life*
endocapillary		
hypercellularity	*hyper-; cellular (pertaining to cells); -ity*	
leukocytoclastic		
capillary		
granular		

7. Define the following word parts for *nephrologist*:

   Nephrologist: Nephr/o _____, -logist _____.

8. The suffix *-itis* means inflammation, the term hepatitis in the name of the hepatitis C virus refers to inflammation of a specific organ. What organ is inflamed with hepatitis?

🔍 *ADVANCED CASE STUDY*

8.9 Diabetic Nephropathy

Conrad is a 65-year-old African American male with a 25-year history of diabetes mellitus (DM) and hypertension, a 5-year history of albuminuria, and 1 year ago, he was diagnosed with nonproliferative diabetic retinopathy. He had recently started developing bilateral edematous lower appendages. His hypertension was being treated with drugs that affect angiotensin-converting enzyme (ACE), but a physical exam showed that his blood pressure remained high (150/100 mm Hg) and labs revealed that the antihypertensive drugs had not improved the proteinuria as hoped. His nephrologist was concerned that microvascular damage was advancing due to sustained hyperglycemia, which was a result of poorly managed DM. The microvascular damage was impacting capillaries in the patient's retinas and kidney glomeruli. Damaged glomeruli were not retaining proteins during filtration; instead, proteins were lost in the urine. The loss

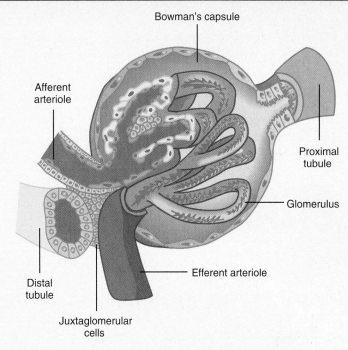

CASE FIGURE: Normal renal corpuscle

of blood proteins reduces the attraction of water to systemic circulation; as a result, water accumulates in tissues, causing swelling, or edema. A kidney biopsy was collected to determine how advanced the diabetic nephropathy had become.

The kidney biopsy showed abnormal podocytes and supporting cells, glomerulosclerosis, afferent and efferent arteriolar nephrosclerosis, and tubular atrophy. The renal and glomerulopathy histology findings are consistent with diabetic nephropathy. The nephrologist and patient will discuss alternative antihypertensive and antihyperglycemic therapies.

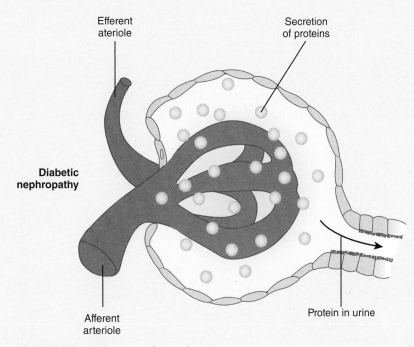

CASE FIGURE: Diabetic nephropathy

(continues)

⌕ *ADVANCED CASE STUDY* *(continued)*

1. Complete the table below for the terms related to this patient's signs and symptoms:

Term	Word Parts	Meaning
hypertension	*hyper-; -tension*	*excessive pressure (high blood pressure)*
albuminuria		
proteinuria		
retinopathy		
bilateral		
edematous		
hyperglycemia		
microvascular		

2. Type 1 diabetes mellitus (DM), once called juvenile diabetes, is an autoimmune disease that reduces the ability of the pancreas to produce insulin, a hormone that normally causes cells of the body to use glucose and reduces the concentration of glucose in the blood. Type 2 DM is a disease that tends to manifest later in life, is often related to lifestyle, and reduces the ability of the cells of the body to respond to insulin, which, like type 1, results in excessive blood glucose. Based on the information in this case, do you think the patient has a 25-year history of type 1 or type 2 DM?

3. Angiotensin converting enzyme (ACE) normally converts a hormone called angiotensin I to angiotensin II, which increases blood pressure through a myriad of mechanisms. Define the word parts angi/o and tens/o and indicate if the patient in this case has probably been prescribed drugs that increase, or inhibit, ACE activity.

   Angi/o _____, tens/o _____.

   Has the patient probably been taking drugs that increase, or inhibit, ACE activity?

4. Complete the table below for the terms related to the results of the biopsy:

Term	Word Parts	Meaning
biopsy	*bi/o; -opsy*	*view of life*
podocytes		

Term	Word Parts	Meaning
glomerulosclerosis		
arteriolar		
nephrosclerosis		
microvascular		
atrophy		
glomerulopathy		
nephropathy		

5. Define the following word parts, and meaning, for *antihypertensive* and *antihyperglycemic*.

Antihypertensive: Anti- _____, hyper- _____,

tens/o _____, -ive _____,

means _____.

Antihyperglycemic: Anti- _____, hyper- _____,

glyc/o _____, -emic _____,

means _____.

🔍 ADVANCED CASE STUDY

8.10 Vesicoureteral Reflux

Hadia, a 6-year-old healthy-appearing little girl came skipping into the urologist's office. She was there for a follow-up visit after last year's surgery.

"How are you feeling?" asks Dr. Morales.

"I feel fine," asserts Hadia. "And I don't get sick anymore," she declares.

Hadia's first diagnosed urinary tract infection (UTI) was when she was 3. Following two more UTIs in close succession, her pediatrician referred her to Dr. Morales who sent her for a test called a voiding cystourethrogram (VCUG). The VCUG confirmed the urologist's suspicion that Hadia had vesicoureteral reflux (VUR), the most common uropathy found in children. VUR is the retrograde flow of urine from the bladder to the kidney, and in Hadia's case, was caused by inadequate closure of the ureterovesical junction. VUR is classified by grade, with grade I as the most moderate and grade V the most severe. Haida's parents were told she had grade III reflux, which resolves spontaneously about 50% of the time. Haida was prescribed low-dose prophylactic antibiotics to prevent UTIs and possible associated pyelonephritis. Initially, this wait-and-see approach seemed like it was working, but after a year, Haida began having breakthrough febrile UTIs. Dr. Morales, concerned about permanent renal damage, recommended robot-assisted ureteroneocystostomy as a corrective surgical approach for the VUR. Haida spent two nights in the hospital following this procedure and follow-up ultrasound and X-ray verified its success.

"Her blood pressure, height, and weight are all within normal range," Dr. Morales told Haida's parents. All of the urinalyses we have done over the past year have been normal, so it appears Haida has had no new UTIs. As she gets older, we will continue to monitor her kidneys by ultrasound to be sure they are growing normally."

(continues)

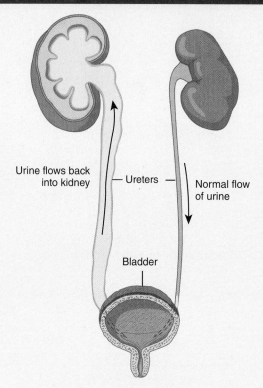

Vesicoureteral Reflux
Urine in the bladder goes back up
to the ureter and the kidneys.
This could cause infections
and kidney damage

CASE FIGURE: Vesicoureteral reflux

1. Define the word parts for *uropathy*.

    Uropathy: Ur/o _____, -pathy _____.

2. Use word parts to explain the test Haida was sent for.

3. Reflux means the flow of fluid in the body in a direction opposite of normal. Explain Haida's diagnosis of vesicoureteral reflux using word parts. What phrase in the case indicates what fluid is flowing opposite of normal for Haida?

4. Indicate and define the word parts for ureterovesical junction and explain how inadequate closure of this junction can lead to reflux.

5. How were antibiotics used prophylactically for Haida?

6. Breakthrough febrile UTIs indicated the lack of effectiveness of this prophylactic approach. Explain, considering the meaning of the terms breakthrough and febrile.

7. Define the word parts for *ureteroneocystostomy*.

Ureteroneocystostomy: Ureter/o _____, neo-_____,

cyst/o _____, -ostomy _____,

means _____.

References

Ciccone, J. M., McCabe, J. C., & Eyre, R. C. (2012). Case report: Successful staged ureteroscopic treatment of a 5 cm Staghorn renal calculus. *Case Reports in Urology*, 873069. https://doi.org/10.1155/2012/873069

Fioretto, P., & Mauer, M. (2007). Histopathology of diabetic nephropathy. *Seminars in Nephrology*, 27(2), 195–207. https://doi.org/10.1016/j.semnephrol.2007.01.012

Fogo, A. B., Lusco, M. A., Najafian, B., & Alpers, C. E. (2016). *AJKD* Atlas of Renal Pathology: Cryoglobulinemic glomerulonephritis. *American Journal of Kidney*, 67(2), E5–E7. https://doi.org/10.1053/j.ajkd.2015.12.007

Kawahara, T., Ito, H., Terao, H., Uemura, H., Kubota, Y., & Matsuzaki, J. (2015). Ureteroscopy-assisted retrograde nephrostomy for a large and obstructive renal pelvic stone: A case report. *Journal of Medical Case Reports*, 9(44). https://doi.org/10.1186/s13256-015-0529-4

Lalvani, A., Newton, P., & Conlon, C. P. (1997). *Salmonella enteritidis* and acute renal failure: Report of five cases and review. *Infectious Diseases in Clinical Practice*, 6(3), 193–195. https://doi.org/10.1097/00019048-199703000-00014

Lee, R. K., Abol-Enein, H., Artibani, W., Bochner, B., Dalbagni, G., Daneshmand, S., Fradet, Y., Hautmann, R. E., Lee, C. T., Lerner, S. P., Pycha, A., Sievert, K. D., Stenzl, A., Thalmann, G., & Shariat, S. F. (2014). Urinary diversion after radical cystectomy for bladder cancer: options, patient selection, and outcomes. *BJU International*, 113(1), 11–23. https://doi.org/10.1111/bju.12121

Lucon, M., Ianhez, L. E., Lucon, A. M., Chambô, J. L., Sabbaga, E., & Srougi, M. (2006). Bilateral nephrectomy of huge polycystic kidneys associated with a rectus abdominis diastasis and umbilical hernia. *Clinics (Sao Paulo, Brazil)*, 61(6), 529–534. https://doi.org/10.1590/s1807-59322006000600007

Sanjeevan, K. V., Bhat, H. S., & Sudhindran, S. (2004). Laparoscopic simultaneous bilateral pretransplant nephrectomy for uncontrolled hypertension. *Transplantation Proceedings*, 36(7), 2011–2012. https://doi.org/10.1016/j.transproceed.2004.06.052

Satish, S., Rajesh, R., George, K., Elango, E. M., & Unni, V. N. (2008). Membranoproliferative glomerulonephritis with essential cryoglobulinemia. *Indian Journal of Nephrology*, 18(2), 80–82. https://doi.org/10.4103/0971-4065.42347

Sidhu, A., Mittal, A., Negroni-Balasquide, X., Constantinescu, A., & Kozakowski, K. (2016). Case report: Cystinuria and polycystic kidney disease. *Pediatrics*, 138(6), e20160674. https://doi.org/10.1542/peds.2016-0674

Slaoui, A., Nah, A., Bargach, S., Slaoui, A., Karmouni, T., El Khader, K., Koutani, A., & Attya A. I. (2018). Two cystoceles that hide different pathophysiological histories: Report of two cases. *Surgery: Case Reports*, 2(2), 37–38.

Srirangam, S. J., Pollard, A. J., Adeyoju, A. A. & O'Reilly, P. H. (2009). Nephroptosis: Seriously misunderstood? *BJU International*, 103, 296–300. doi:10.1111/j.1464-410X.2008.08082.x

Stedman, T. L. (2005). Nath's *Stedman's medical terminology, 2e*. Philadelphia: Lippincott Williams & Wilkins.

Sung, J., & Skoog, S. (2012). Surgical management of vesicoureteral reflux in children. *Pediatric Nephrology*, 27(4), 551–561. https://doi.org/10.1007/s00467-011-1933-7

Tong, L., & Adler, S. G. (2018). Diabetic kidney disease. *Clinical Journal of the American Society of Nephrology*, 13(2), 335–338. https://doi.org/10.2215/CJN.04650417

Venes, D. & Taber, C. W. (2017). *Taber's cyclopedic medical dictionary*. Ed. 23, illustrated in full color/Philadelphia: F.A. Davis.

CHAPTER 9

Reproductive Systems

KEY TERMS

Amnion
Areola
Blastocyst
Bulbourethral gland
Cervix
Chorion
Clitoris
Ejaculation
Ejaculatory duct
Embryo
Epididymis
Fetus
Gamete
Glans penis
Hymen
Labia majora

Labia minora
Lactation
Mammary gland
Mammary papilla
Mons pubis
Oogenesis
Ova
Ovary
Ovulation
Ovum
Penis
Perineum
Placenta
Prepuce
Prostate gland
Scrotum

Semen
Seminal vesicle
Seminiferous tubule
Spermatic cord
Spermatogenesis
Testis
Umbilical cord
Urethra
Urinary meatus
Uterus
Vagina
Vas deferens
Vulva
Zygote

The functions of the reproductive systems are to make, store, and transport **gametes** (i.e., eggs or sperm); produce sex hormones; and in the case of the female, support a developing embryo and fetus before birth and nourish the infant after birth through breastfeeding. Male and female reproductive systems are similar in that they both produce gametes in paired gonads (ovaries or testes), and during development the gonads arise from the same set of cells. A fusion of an egg and sperm, and a combination of the genetic material they carry, is necessary to produce a **zygote**, which is a fertilized egg that can develop into an embryo and then a fetus. The male and female reproductive systems are distinctly different from each other in most other anatomical and physiological contexts.

The male reproductive system external organs are the penis, testes (singular testis), and epididymides (singular epididymis). The **penis** contains erectile tissue encased in skin. The tip of the penis is called the **glans penis** and is covered with a **prepuce**, or foreskin, which can be removed by circumcision. Two **testes**, also called testicles, are suspended outside of the body in a sac called the **scrotum**. This ensures the maintenance of the cooler temperature necessary for **spermatogenesis** (sperm formation), which takes place in the testes. Sperm is formed in the coiled **seminiferous tubules** within each testis and then moves to the epididymides (singular **epididymis**), the large tubes found on the superior and posterior sides of each testis.

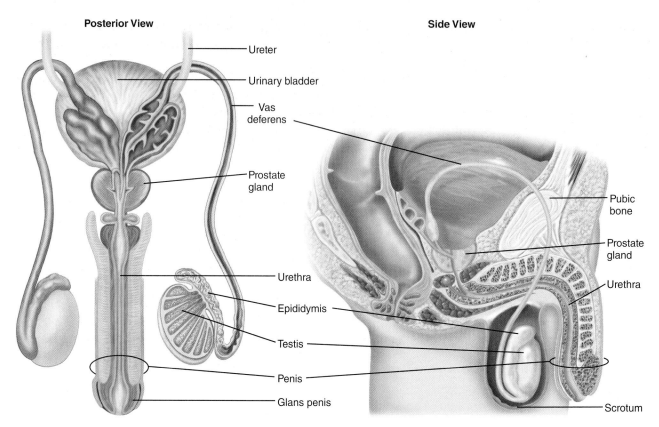

Posterior View

- Ureter
- Urinary bladder
- Vas deferens
- Prostate gland
- Urethra
- Epididymis
- Testis
- Penis
- Glans penis

Side View

- Pubic bone
- Prostate gland
- Urethra
- Scrotum

FIGURE 9.1 The male reproductive system

The male reproductive system internal organs are the vasa deferentia (singular **vas deferens**), seminal vesicles, prostate gland, and bulbourethral glands. During ejaculation, the vasa deferentia (singular **vas deferens**) carry sperm from the epididymis through the **spermatic cords** (which also contains vessels, nerves, and lymphatics), into the pelvic cavity, and then merge with ducts from the seminal vesicle to form the **ejaculatory duct**. The **seminal vesicles** secrete a thick, alkaline, fructose-rich fluid that nourishes the sperm. The basic pH of this seminal fluid helps neutralize the acidic environment of the female reproductive tract that would otherwise kill sperm. Additional liquids that aid in lubrication and the motility of the sperm are secreted by the **prostate gland** and the paired **bulbourethral glands**, also called Cowper's glands. The combination of sperm and fluid from the seminal vesicles, prostate gland, and bulbourethral glands is called **semen**. The semen then moves to the **urethra**, which passes through the penis to the outside of the body. Sperm leaves by **ejaculation** through the **urinary meatus**. In males, the urethra and urinary meatus are shared with both the reproductive and urinary systems as urine also travels through this path.

The external female genitalia are a group of structures collectively referred to as the **vulva**. This region consists of the **labia majora** and **labia minora**, which are protective folds of skin, the **clitoris**, which is a small organ containing sensitive erectile tissue, and the **perineum**, which is the region between the vaginal orifice and the anus. Anterior to the vaginal opening is the **mons pubis**, elevated adipose tissue covered with pubic hair that cushions the pubic symphysis, the cartilaginous joint between the pubic bones. A thin membrane called the **hymen** partially covers the entrance to the vagina and is

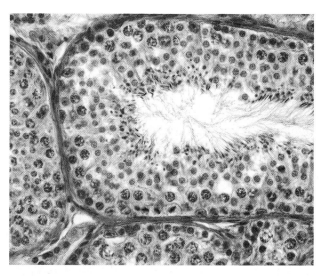

FIGURE 9.2 Cross-section of a seminiferous tubule showing newly formed sperm with tails protruding into the lumen

© Jose Luis Calvo/Shutterstock

broken for the first time during sexual intercourse, physical activity, or tampon use.

The female reproductive system internal organs are a pair of ovaries, paired uterine tubes (also called fallopian tubes or oviducts), the uterus, and the vagina, which extends to the exterior of the body. The **ovaries** are held in place by several ligaments and are the site of **oogenesis** (egg formation). After puberty, **ova** (eggs) mature, and each month one or two follicle(s) containing an **ovum** (singular of ova) ruptures, leaving the ovary in a process called **ovulation**. The ovum passes by fimbriae, finger-like projections, into a uterine tube and is swept along by cilia toward the **uterus**, a muscular organ that is located anterior to the urinary bladder. If sperm are present within about 24 hours of ovulation, fertilization may occur in a region of the oviduct near the ovary called the ampulla. A fertilized ovum is called a zygote. The zygote divides into two cells after about 24 hours, and continues to divide and develop into a blastocyst, which may implant in the endometrium, the inner layer of the uterus. If fertilization does not occur, the ovum will eventually disintegrate and most of the endometrium will be sloughed off during menstruation.

The lower portion of the uterus is the **cervix**. The muscular tube extending from the cervix to the outside of the body is the **vagina**, which allows for the passage of menstrual flow. In addition, the vagina is the repository for male semen, and it serves as the canal through which a baby passes during a vaginal birth.

When pregnancy occurs, the typical gestation period is 38–42 weeks. During that time, a zygote will develop into a mass of cells with a cavity, called a **blastocyst**, then into an **embryo** (2–8 weeks) and a **fetus** (after 8 weeks). The fetus receives nourishment and excretes waste through the

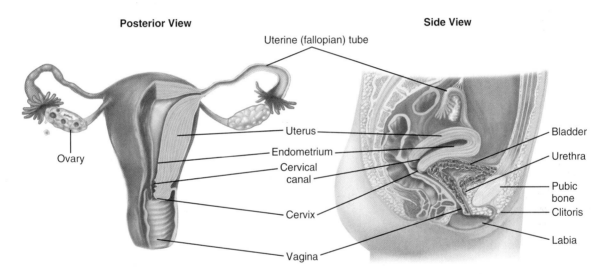

FIGURE 9.3 The female reproductive system

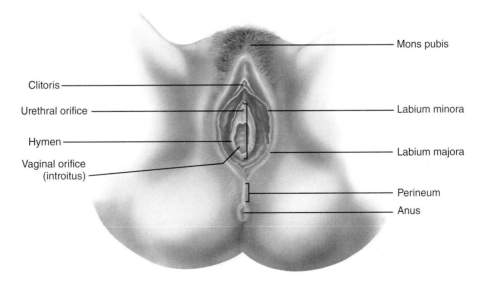

FIGURE 9.4 Female external reproductive anatomy

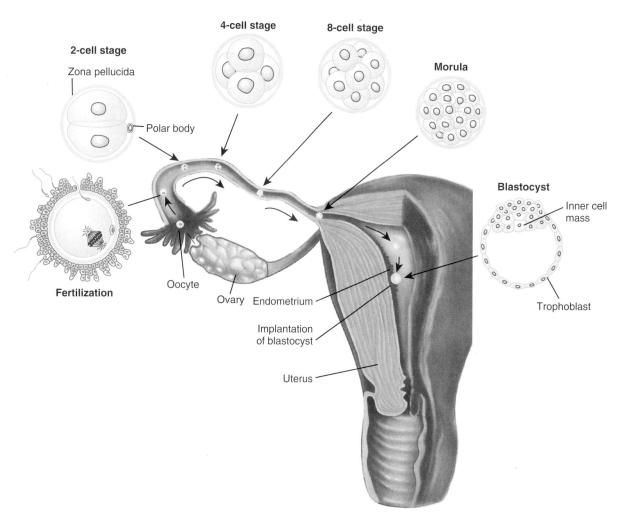

FIGURE 9.5 Fertilization and early development

umbilical cord and **placenta**. The fetus is surrounded by two membranes, the **chorion** and the **amnion**, which contains amniotic fluid. The process of expelling the fetus from the uterus through the vagina is called labor and delivery.

The breasts are accessory organs of the female reproductive system and within them are **mammary glands**, which produce milk to nourish the baby by a process called **lactation**. The nipple of the breast is called the **mammary papilla** and the dark pigmented area surrounding the nipple is the **areola**. The latching on to the nipple by the infant stimulates the release of the hormone oxytocin, which in turn promotes the ejection of milk.

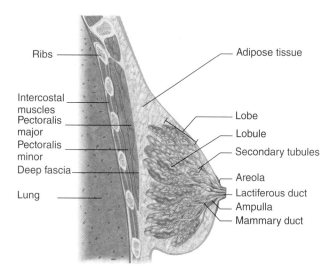

FIGURE 9.6 Breast anatomy

TABLE 9.1
Key Reproductive System Prefixes
asthen-: weakness
multi-: many
nulli-: none
primi-: first

TABLE 9.2

Key Reproduction System Combining Forms

amni/o: amnion

andr/o: male

balan/o: glans penis

cervic/o: cervix

chori/o: chorion

chorion/o: chorion

crypt/o: hidden

epididym/o: epididymis

episi/o: vulva

estr/o: female

fet/o: fetus

glanul/o ; glans penis

gynec/o: woman, female

hyster/o: uterus

lact/o: milk

lapar/o: abdomen

lei/o: smooth

mamm/o: breast

mast/o: breast

meat/o: meatus

men/o: menstruation

metri/o: uterus

metr/o: uterus

my/o: muscle

nat/o: birth

o/o: egg

obstetr/o: pregnancy; childbirth

oophor/o: ovary

ovari/o: ovary

orch/o: testicle, testis

orchi/o: testicle, testis

orchid/o: testicle, testis

ov/o: ovum, egg

ovul/o: egg

pen/o: penis

pelv/o: pelvis

prostat/o: prostate gland

pub/o: pubis

py/o: pus

salping/o: uterine tube, fallopian tube; auditory tube

scrot/o: scrotum

semen/o: semen, seed

spermat/o: sperm cells, semen

sperm/o: sperm cells, semen

terat/o: monster

testicul/o: testes

urethr/o: urethra

vagin/o: vagina

vas/o: vas deferens

vulv/o: vulva

zo/o: animal life

TABLE 9.3	
Key Reproductive System Suffixes	
-arche: beginning	-parous: bearing, bringing forth
-cyesis: state of pregnancy	-partum: childbirth
-genesis: produces, formation	-salpinx: uterine tube
-gravida: pregnancy	-spadia: to tear or cut
-para: to bear, bring forth offspring	-spermia: condition of sperm
	-tocia: labor, childbirth
	-version: act of turning

🔍 STANDARD CASE STUDY

9.1 Prenatal Visit

Thirty-year-old Samiya Benitez, gravida 3 para 1, presents to obstetrics and gynecology following a positive home pregnancy test 2 days ago. Samiya is 5 weeks + 3 days pregnant calculated by her last menstrual period (LMP). Her first pregnancy resulted in an uncomplicated vaginal delivery and her son is now 4-years old. Salpingocyesis caused the loss of her second pregnancy 1 year ago. The ectopic pregnancy was managed by laparoscopic salpingotomy. The contralateral uterine tube was healthy and subsequent hysterosalpingography confirmed the patency of the affected tube. Samiya understands she is at risk for a second ectopic pregnancy and is understandably concerned. The practitioner orders a transvaginal ultrasound, which reveals an intrauterine gestational sac of 40 ± 2 days. This and any subsequent pregnancies will be carefully monitored to reduce risk to Samiya and to the developing fetus.

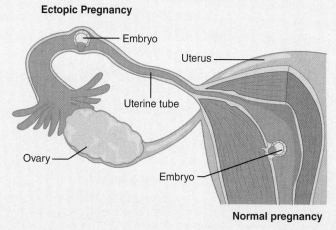

Ectopic Pregnancy

Embryo

Uterus

Uterine tube

Ovary

Embryo

Normal pregnancy

CASE FIGURE: A normal pregnancy implants in the uterus. The most common implantation of an ectopic pregnancy is in a uterine tube

1. Indicate and define the word parts for *prenatal*.

Two other terms with the same meaning are *antepartum* and *antenatal*. Define the word parts for these terms.

Antepartum: Ante-_____, -partum _____

Antenatal: Ante-_____, nat/i _____, -al _____

2. Indicate and define the word parts for obstetrics and gynecology.

3. Samiya is described as gravida 3 para 1. Explain.

   Use the suffixes -gravida and -para to construct terms to mean the following:

   A woman who has been pregnant many times: _____.

   A woman who is pregnant for the first time: _____.

   A woman who has never been pregnant: _____.

   A woman who has given birth to multiple live infants: _____.

   A woman who has given birth to a first live infant: _____.

   A woman who has given birth to no live infants: _____.

4. Define the word parts and meaning of the following procedural terms in the case.

   Laparoscopic salpingotomy: Lapar/o _____, -scopic _____,

   salping/o _____, -otomy _____,

   means _____.

   Hysterosalpingography: Hyster/o _____, salping/o _____,

   -graphy _____,

   means _____.

   Transvaginal ultrasound: Trans- _____, vagin/o _____,

   -al _____, ultra- _____,

   sound, means _____.

5. Indicate and define the word parts for *salpingocyesis* and *ectopic*. Salpingocyesis is one type of ectopic pregnancy. Explain.

   Ectopic pregnancies are extrauterine. Define the word parts for this term.

   Extra- _____, uter/o _____, -ine _____.

(continues)

6. Risk factors for tubal pregnancy include *salpingitis*, *endometriosis*, and *pyosalpinx* from pelvic inflammatory disease. Define the word parts for these risk factors.

Salpingitis: Salping/o _____, -itis _____

Endometriosis: Endo- _____, metri/o _____,

-osis _____

Pyosalpinx: Py/o _____, -salpinx _____

7. The health of the tube contralateral to the affected tube and the patency of the affected tube were likely contributors to the good news Samiya received of an intrauterine gestational sac. Explain, using word parts when appropriate.

🔍 *STANDARD CASE STUDY*

9.2 Uterine Fibroids

Shawna Cox, a 40-year-old African American woman always knew she had uterine fibroids. Dysmenorrhea, metrorrhagia, menorrhagia, and pelvic and back pain had plagued her for years. Both her mother and sister had uterine fibroids and her mother had undergone a total abdominal hysterectomy with bilateral salpingo-oophorectomy after being told a surgical option was the only permanent solution for these benign painful tumors. Shawna's sister's fibroids had shrunk once she entered perimenopause and Shawna hoped hers would as well, but instead they grew larger and her symptoms worsened.

"You know, Shawna," Dr. Mendoza said to her at her appointment, "there are many options now for treating fibroids before major invasive surgery is considered. You are likely beyond the point where watchful waiting or medications to shrink the fibroids are appropriate, but I can outline for you several options for minimally invasive procedures."

"Yes Doctor, I would appreciate that," responded Shawna. "Because I wanted children, I didn't want to consider a hysterectomy earlier, but even though my husband and I don't want more children, I would like to consider something less invasive."

"A few procedures are available that cut off the blood supply to the fibroids," explained Dr. Mendoza. "Uterine artery embolization (UAE), cryomyolysis, and thermocoagulation are a few examples. Depending on the size and location of the fibroids, hysteroscopic or laparoscopic myomectomy are also options." Dr. Mendoza proceeded to describe each procedure for Shawna.

"Wow, that's a lot to take in," said Shawna, a bit overwhelmed. "What should I do next?"

"Let's start with some diagnostic imaging to get more information. I am scheduling you for an ultrasound and a hysteroscopy. I also have a pamphlet to give you explaining the benefits and risks of each procedure we have mentioned today. At your next visit, we can talk in more detail regarding the optimal treatment option for you."

"Thank you so much," replied Shawna. "I am relieved that there are so many options besides the major surgery my mother faced."

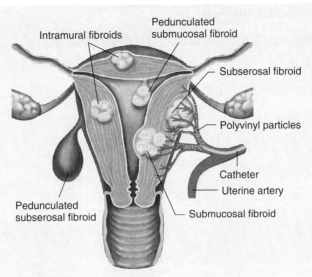

Intramural fibroids

Pedunculated
submucosal fibroid

Subserosal fibroid

Polyvinyl particles

Catheter

Uterine artery

Pedunculated
subserosal fibroid

Submucosal fibroid

CASE FIGURE: Uterine fibroids are benign tumors
that can form in many places within the uterus.
One treatment method is embolization where small
polyvinyl particles are introduced with a catheter
into the arteries that supply blood to the fibroids

1. Uterine fibroids are benign tumors of the smooth muscle of the uterus. Define the word parts for the following
terms and circle the most appropriate synonym for fibroids.

   Lipoma: Lip/o _____, -oma _____

   Myeloma: Myel/o _____, -oma _____

   Neuroblastoma: Neur/o _____, -blast _____,

   -oma _____

   Leiomyoma: Lei/o _____, my/o _____,

   -oma _____

   Condyloma: Condyl/o _____, -oma _____

2. Define the following word parts, and meanings, of Shawna's symptoms.

   Dysmenorrhea: Dys- _____, men/o _____,

   -rrhea _____, means _____

   Metrorrhagia: Metr/o _____, -rrhagia _____,

   means _____.

   Menorrhagia: Men/o _____, -rrhagia _____,

   means _____.

(continues)

🔍 *STANDARD CASE STUDY* *(continued)*

3. Indicate and define the component word parts for *abdominal hysterectomy with bilateral salpingo-oophorectomy* and explain what is meant by this procedure.

4. Complete the table for some of the procedural terms in the case.

Term	Word Parts	Meaning
thermocoagulation	*therm/o; coagul/o; -ation*	*process of clotting with heat*
cryomyolysis		
hysteroscopic myomectomy		
laparoscopic myomectomy		
hysteroscopy		

5. The word embolus means plug. How do you think uterine artery embolization works to treat fibroids?

6. Explain the term perimenopause. Why do you think fibroids often shrink during this time?

🔍 *STANDARD CASE STUDY*

9.3 Scrotal Pain and Swelling

Subjective: Edgar Benton is a 25-year-old male who reports swelling and pain of his scrotum, increasing in severity over the past 2 weeks. He also describes urethral discharge of about the same duration. He was born with undescended testicles, which were repaired surgically when he was 15 months old and he knows this puts him at increased risk for testicular cancer, which is his biggest fear.

Objective: Mr. Benton appears distressed and uncomfortable. Physical exam reveals swelling and erythema of the scrotum with hydrocele. Tenderness along the superior and posterior aspect of the left testis and of the testis itself is apparent on palpation. Some balanorrhea is evident. Exam is not consistent with signs of testicular cancer.

Assessment: Epididymo-orchitis, most likely caused by sexually transmitted chlamydia or gonorrhea.

Plan: Follow-up testing for presence of *Chlamydia trachomatis* or *Neisseria gonorrhoeae*. Antibiotic therapy commencing immediately based on presumptive sexually transmitted infection. Mr. Benton should refrain from sexual intercourse until asymptomatic and should refer sexual contacts to their primary care physician for evaluation. He is also instructed to do regular testicular self-exams due to his increased risk for testicular cancer.

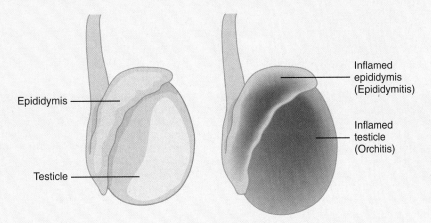

CASE FIGURE: Inflamed testis and epididymis or epididymo-orchitis

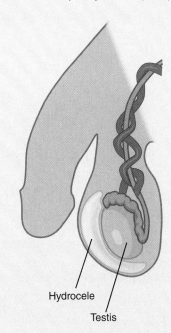

CASE FIGURE: An accumulation of fluid around the testis is known as a hydrocele

1. The medical term for undescended testicles literally translates to condition of hidden testicles. Build this medical term.

   Hidden _____, testicle _____,

   condition of _____, term is _____.

   Undescended testicles are repaired by surgical fixation of the testicle. Build this medical term.

   Testicle _____, surgical fixation _____,

   term is _____.

(continues)

2. Explain the directional terms *superior* and *posterior*.

3. Complete the table for the following terms.

Term	Word Parts	Meaning
urethral	*urethr/o; -al*	*pertaining to the urethra*
testicular		
balanorrhea		
erythema		
hydrocele		
epididymo-orchitis		

4. Provide a brief explanation of the term *palpation*.

🔍 *STANDARD CASE STUDY*

9.4 Hypospadias

Mr. and Mrs. House bring 6-month-old Elvin to the pediatric urologist for a surgical consult. Zola House remembers Elvin's birth well. Her labor was slow to progress and amniotomy was indicated. Elvin was a large baby and episiotomy was necessary to facilitate his birth. Then the doctor told them Elvin was born with the opening of his urethra on the underside of his penis, a congenital defect known as hypospadias. This would require corrective surgery, typically performed between 6 and 18 months of age. Dr. Moya examines Elvin today.

"Elvin has a subcoronal presentation of hypospadias along with chordee," Dr. Moya states. "I am hopeful a single surgery will correct the defect. The operation will have a multi-faceted approach," she further explains. "Orthoplasty, urethroplasty, meatoplasty, glanuloplasty, and scrotoplasty will all be part of the surgery. The prepuce may be used to achieve normal skin coverage. The operation will give Elvin a normal appearance cosmetically and will allow him to void from a standing position."

Elvin's parents are understandably concerned about surgery at such a young age and ask about possible complications.

"There are some potential complications," acknowledges Dr. Moya. "Some of the more serious ones are urethrocutaneous fistula, meatal stenosis, and a chronic form of balanitis. From my experience though the psychosocial consequences later in life if the surgery is not performed outweigh the potential complications. Our operating team is very experienced in this procedure in pediatric patients. It can actually be performed as outpatient surgery and Elvin will be able to go home the same day."

The Houses agree that the surgery is in the best interest of Elvin and ask Dr. Moya to have it scheduled.

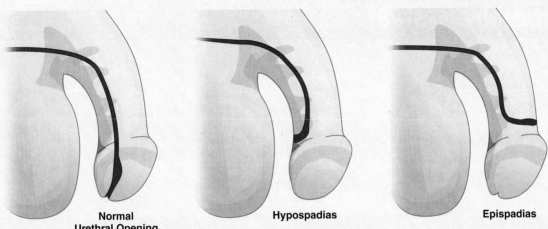

CASE FIGURE: Positions of urethral opening

1. Define the word parts, meaning, and the purpose of *amniotomy* and *episiotomy*.

   Amniotomy: Amni/o _____, -otomy _____,

   means _____.

   Episiotomy: Episi/o _____, -otomy _____,

   means _____.

   Build a term meaning surgical suturing of the vulva, the procedure used to repair an episiotomy.

2. The suffix -spadia means to tear or cut and hypospadias refers to the urethral opening below or on the underside of the penis. Epispadias is also a congenital defect. Provide a brief definition of congenital and explain what epispadias is.

3. Hypospadias can occur in three different regions of the penis: subcoronal, midshaft, and penoscrotal. Explain these using the directional terms distal and proximal.

(continues)

Chordee is a term used to describe ventral bending of the penile shaft. Explain.

4.   Complete the table for the following procedural terms in the case.

Term	Word Parts	Meaning
orthoplasty	*ortho-; -plasty*	*surgical repair of straight (refers to straightening of the penis)*
urethroplasty		
meatoplasty		
glanuloplasty		
scrotoplasty		

5.   What is the common term for prepuce?

6.   A fistula is an abnormal passage from one surface to another. Provide brief explanations for *urethrocutaneous fistula*, *meatal stenosis*, and *balanitis*.

🔍 *STANDARD CASE STUDY*

9.5 Obstructive Azoospermia

Ryan Buono, a 35-year-old male, scheduled a consultation with a reproductive endocrinologist, Dr. Michael Gomez, to determine why, after a year of trying, he and his wife were still unable to conceive. Mr. Buono was currently in good health, but of note in his medical history was a left testis spermatocelectomy. The patient's hormone levels were normal. A semenogram yielded normal semen characteristics except an absence of sperm. Dr. Gomez ordered a scrotal ultrasound, transrectal ultrasound (TRUS), and a testicular biopsy, and scheduled a follow-up appointment to discuss the results.

At the follow-up appointment Dr. Gomez reported to Mr. Buono that spermatogenesis was not the problem; the testis biopsy revealed normal sperm production in the seminiferous tubules. Dr. Gomez thought the best evidence explaining the absence of sperm in the semen came from the ultrasounds. There appeared to be iatrogenic damage from the spermatocelectomy to the left vas deferens and rather severe right epididymal aplasia. He further explained that the vas deferens and epididymis are a part of the seminal tract that transports sperm during ejaculation; interruption of these structures may be causing obstructive azoospermia (OA). OA is defined by an absence of sperm in the semen despite normal spermatogenesis. Dr. Gomez suggested a left vasoepididymostomy to complete a route for sperm produced in the left seminal tract.

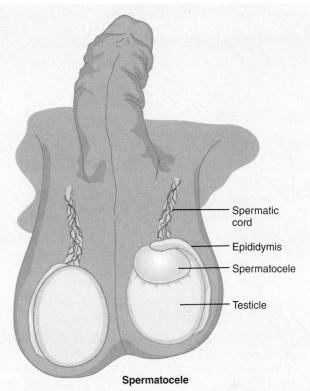

Spermatocele

CASE FIGURE: A spermatocele is a fluid-filled mass that develops in the epididymis

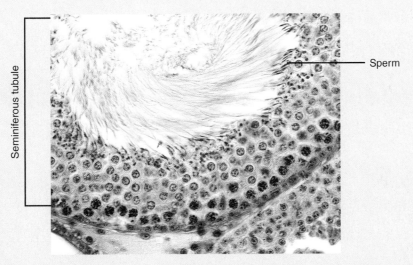

CASE FIGURE: Testis histology showing normal sperm production in the seminiferous tubules

© Jose Luis Calvo/Shutterstock

1. A reproductive endocrinologist is a physician with expertise in reproduction and endocrinology. Define the word parts, and meaning, for *endocrinologist*, then explain what a reproductive endocrinologist specializes in.

   Endocrinologist: Endo- _____, crin/o _____,

   -logist _____, means _____.

2. A semenogram revealed semen azoospermia. What are the word parts, and meaning, for *semenogram*?

   Semenogram: Semen/o _____, -gram _____,

   means _____.

3. Complete the table below for the following terms that describe the abundance and behavior of sperm that can be revealed by a semenogram.

Term	Word Parts	Meaning
aspermia	*a-; -sperm/o; -ia*	condition of no sperm
azoospermia		
hypospermia		
hyperspermia		
oligozoospermia		
asthenozoospermia		
teratozoospermia		
necrozoospermia		
leucocytospermia		

4. Define the following word parts for the three diagnostic procedures that were ordered: *scrotal ultrasound*, *transrectal ultrasound*, and a *testicular biopsy*.

   Scrotal ultrasound: Scrot/o _____, -al _____,

   ultra- _____,

   sound, means _____.

   Transrectal ultrasound: Trans- _____, rect/o _____,

   -al _____, ultra- _____,

   sound, means _____.

   Testicular biopsy: Testicul/o _____, -ar _____,

   bi/o _____, -opsy _____,

   means _____.

5. The diagnostic procedures provided evidence for iatrogenic damage from the spermatocelectomy and epididymal aplasia. What are the word parts, and meaning, for *iatrogenic, spermatocelectomy,* and *epididymal aplasia*?

   Iatrogenic: Iatr/o _____, -genic _____,

   means _____.

Spermatocelectomy: Spermat/o _____, -cele _____,

-ectomy _____, means _____.

Epididymal aplasia: Epididym/o _____, -al _____,

a- _____, -plasia _____,

means _____.

6. Obstructive azoospermia is defined by spermatogenesis with azoospermia. What are the word parts, and meaning, of *spermatogenesis*?

Spermatogenesis: Spermat/o _____, -genesis _____,

means _____.

7. Vasoepididymostomy was recommended. What are the word parts of *vasoepididymostomy*?

Vasoepididymostomy: Vas/o _____, epididym/o _____,

-ostomy _____,

means _____.

🔍 ADVANCED CASE STUDY

9.6 Breastfeeding Challenges

A 28-year-old female presents at 2-months postpartum to her nurse midwife. She complains of fever, general malaise, mastalgia, and decreased lactorrhea. She states that her right breast is swollen and hot to the touch. Upon examination, an erythematous, edematous, wedge-shaped tender region on her right breast is visible. Trauma to the mammary papilla and the areolar region on both breasts is noticeable and the patient confirms her struggle to get her newborn to latch on properly. The nurse midwife diagnoses a breast infection subsequent to milk stasis from a blocked lactiferous duct. Antibiotics are prescribed to treat the acute infection and the patient is referred to a lactation consultant for help with properly positioning her baby. In the meantime, she is instructed to continue breastfeeding, starting on the affected side first. She should be cognizant of fully emptying her breasts of milk, expressing by hand or pump if necessary. Warm compresses and analgesics can be used to relieve pain.

1. Define the following pathologies related to the female reproductive system and then circle your diagnosis for this case study:

Vulvovaginitis: Vulv/o _____, vagin/o _____,

-itis _____.

Metritis: Metr/o _____, -itis _____.

Mastitis: Mast/o _____, -itis _____.

Endocervicitis: Endo- _____, cervic/o _____,

-itis _____.

(continues)

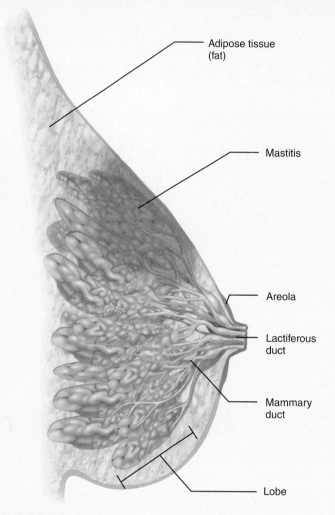

CASE FIGURE: Mastitis

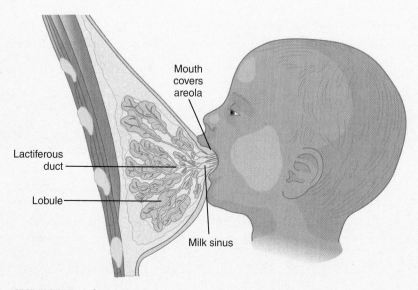

CASE FIGURE: Infant latched on to breast for breast-feeding

2. Define the word parts for *postpartum*.

   Postpartum: Post- _____, -partum _____.

3. Provide a brief definition of malaise.

4. Indicate and define the component word parts for *mastalgia*, *lactorrhea*, *edematous*, and *erythematous*.

5. What is the common word for a mammary papilla and where is the areolar region?

6. Explain what is meant by milk stasis, a blocked lactiferous duct, and how a lactation consultant can help the patient. Use a medical dictionary or other reliable resource for help.

🔍 ADVANCED CASE STUDY

9.7 Zika Virus Infection

We report on a case of a woman who traveled from her home in Boston, MA, USA, to Brasilia, Brazil for a 2-week family visit during a Zika virus outbreak. The woman arrived in Brazil in her 8th week of gestation and arrived home in her 10th week. A week following her return home she became febrile with myalgia, arthralgia, and a pruritic maculopapular rash. The woman tested positive for Zika virus. The woman was informed that intrauterine Zika infections can manifest in arthrogryposis and atonia and a wide range of profound neurodevelopmental defects including microcephaly, anencephaly, hydranencephaly, cerebral atrophy, polymicrogyria, pachygyria, and schizencephaly can develop. Concerned about these outcomes, an amniocentesis was ordered to screen the amniotic fluid for Zika virus, which might indicate fetal infection. Moreover, the patient will undergo biweekly pelvic ultrasonography to monitor fetal neurodevelopment. The patient is informed of prenatal and postnatal neurodevelopmental abnormalities and sequelae associated with Zika infection and referred to a maternal–fetal medicine specialist with expertise in infectious diseases to provide her with guidance including abortifacient options or postnatal treatment and support.

(continues)

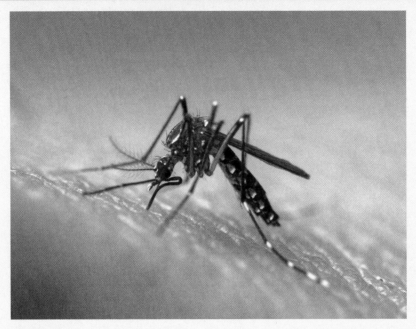

CASE FIGURE: *Aedes aegypti* mosquitoes are the primary vector for Zika virus

© Joao Paulo Burini/Moment/Getty Images

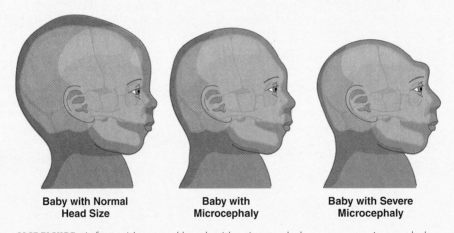

Baby with Normal
Head Size

Baby with
Microcephaly

Baby with Severe
Microcephaly

CASE FIGURE: Infant with normal head, with microcephaly, or severe microcephaly

1. Complete the table below for terms relating to the symptoms that the patient has.

Term	Word Parts	Meaning
febrile	*febri-;-ile*	*pertaining to fever*
myalgia		
arthralgia		
pruritic		
maculopapular		

2. Zika is a mosquito-borne virus spread by a bite from an infected mosquito of the genus *Aedes*, specifically the *Aedes aegypti* species. The woman in this case was probably bitten between gestational weeks 8 and 10, making intrauterine viral infection of the fetus a possibility. Define the word parts for intrauterine and state the gestational range of a full-term pregnancy.

   Intrauterine: Intra- _____, uter/o _____,

           -ine _____.

3. Complete the table below for terms relating to the developmental defects associated with intrauterine Zika virus infection. Refer to other chapters for help with word parts from other body systems.

Term	Word Parts	Meaning
arthrogryposis	*arthr/o; gryposis (abnormal curvature)*	*abnormal curvature of joints*
atonia		
microcephaly		
anencephaly		
hydranencephaly		
cerebral atrophy		
polymicrogyria		
pachygyria		
schizencephaly		

4. Two procedures were ordered, an amniocentesis to screen for the presence of virus and pelvic ultrasonography to monitor neurodevelopment. What are the word parts, and meaning, of *amniocentesis* and *pelvic ultrasonography*?

   Amniocentesis: Amni/o _____, -centesis _____,

           means _____.

   Pelvic ultrasonography: Pelv/o _____, -ic _____,

           ultra- _____, son/o _____, -graphy _____,

           means _____.

5. What do prenatal and postnatal refer to?

6. The patient was provided guidance including abortifacient options or postnatal treatment and support. What does abortifacient mean? Use a medical dictionary or other reliable resource for help.

⌕ *ADVANCED CASE STUDY*

9.8 Prostate Cancer

A 55-year-old male presents to a urologist with a chief complaint of nocturia and increasing severity of obstructive voiding symptoms. His past medical history is significant for benign prostatic hyperplasia (BPH), which he has been treating with medications that should make urination easier, but the urination symptoms have not resolved. The patient's prostate-specific antigen concentration was 45 ng/mL (normal <0.4 ng/mL) suggesting prostate cancer (PCa). Digital rectal examination (DRE) revealed a hard, nodular prostate. A pelvic ultrasound showed hypoechoic lesions, and a biopsy confirmed prostate adenocarcinoma. A bilateral orchiectomy was scheduled to remove the primary source of androgens (primarily male hormones), which should inhibit growth, or shrink, the prostate cancer. The patient will be closely monitored to see if PSA levels decrease. If PSA levels do not decline, a suprapubic radical prostatectomy may be considered.

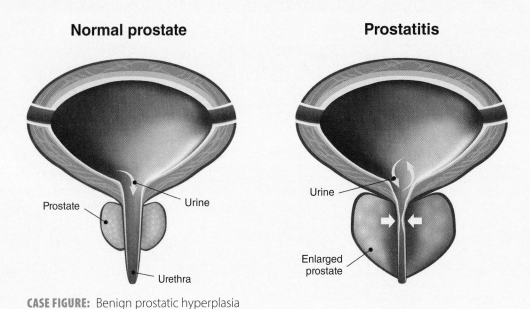

CASE FIGURE: Benign prostatic hyperplasia

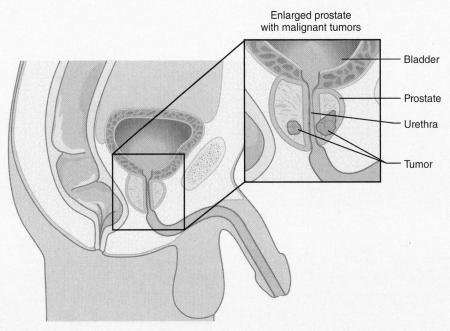

CASE FIGURE: Stages of prostate cancer

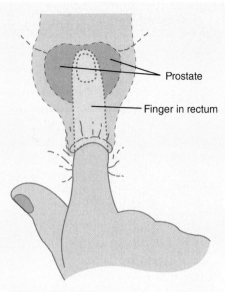

CASE FIGURE: Digital rectal examination

Data from The Prostate Book: Sound Advice on Symptoms and Treatment, Updated Edition by Stephen N. Rous, illustrated by Betty Goodwin. Copyright © 1992, 1988 by Stephen Rous.

1. What are the word parts, and meaning, for *urologist*?

   Urologist: Ur/o _____, -logist _____,

   means _____.

2. The patient's past medical history is significant for benign *prostatic hyperplasia*. Benign refers to a tumor or growth that is not cancerous. What are the word parts, and meaning, for *prostatic hyperplasia*?

   Prostatic hyperplasia: Prostat/o _____, -ic _____,

   hyper- _____, -plasia _____,

   means _____.

3. The diagnostic procedures in this case were measuring prostate-specific antigen (PSA), digital rectal exam (DRE), and pelvic ultrasound. Briefly explain these procedures. Use a medical dictionary or other reliable resource for help.

   Prostate-specific antigen:

   Digital rectal exam:

   Pelvic ultrasound:

   Biopsy:

(continues)

The diagnostic procedures, in particular the hypoechoic lesions and the biopsy, led to a diagnosis of prostate adenocarcinoma. Define the word parts, and meaning, of *hypoechoic* and *adenocarcinoma*.

Hypoechoic: Hypo- _____, echo- _____, -ic _____,

means _____.

Adenocarcinoma: Aden/o _____, carcin/o _____,

-oma _____, means _____.

4. Two therapeutic procedures are considered: a bilateral orchiectomy and a suprapubic radical (complete, or total) prostatectomy. Define the word parts, and meaning, of *bilateral orchiectomy* and *suprapubic prostatectomy*.

Bilateral orchiectomy: Bi- _____, later/o _____,

-al _____, orch/i _____,

-ectomy _____, means _____.

Suprapubic prostatectomy: Supra- _____, pub/o _____,

-ic _____, prostat/o _____,

-ectomy _____, means _____.

9.9 Postmenopausal Endometriosis

A 55-year-old nulliparous woman presented to her gynecologist with malaise and acyclic pelvic pain. The patient's menarche occurred at 14-years-old and her menopause at 50. Her cancer antigen serum markers were negative. Ultrasound revealed a hypoechoic adnexal mass with perilesional and intralesional vascular flow on her right ovarian ligament and endometriosis was suspected. A lesion with a 3-cm diameter was excised through a small inguinal incision. Histopathology confirmed the lesion was endometriosis. The patient was pain free at follow-up with no recurrence at 12 months.

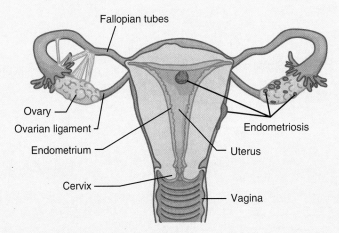

CASE FIGURE: Endometriosis

1. What are the word parts, and meaning, for *gynecologist*?

    Gynecologist: Gynec/o _____, -logist _____,

    means _____.

2. The patient in this case is a nulliparous woman. Define the word parts, and meaning, for the following related terms: *nulliparous, primiparous, multiparous.*

    Nulliparous: Nulli- _____, -parous _____,

    means _____.

    Primiparous: Primi- _____, -parous _____,

    means _____.

    Multiparous: Multi- _____, -parous _____,

    means _____.

3. This case uses terms for the onset, and cessation, of menstrual cycles. Define the word parts, and meaning, for the following related terms: *menarche, perimenopause, menopause.*

    Menarche: Men/o _____, -arche _____,

    means _____.

    Perimenopause: Peri- _____, men/o _____,

    pause _____ *discontinue* _____, means _____.

    Menopause: Men/o _____, pause _____ *discontinue* _____,

    means _____.

    Postmenopause: Post- _____, men/o _____,

    pause _____ *discontinue* _____, means _____.

4. Ultrasound revealed a hypoechoic adnexal mass with perilesional and intralesional vascular flow on her right ovarian ligament. Adnexal refers to the area around the uterus, ovaries, and uterine tubes. A lesion is a damaged area. What is meant when the adnexal mass is described as hypoechoic with perilesional and intralesional vascular flow?

    Hypoechoic:

    Intralesional:

(continues)

⌕ ADVANCED CASE STUDY   (continued)

Perilesional:

Vascular flow:

5. The mass was removed through an incision. In what anatomical region (with the common name) was the incision?

6. Define the word parts, and meaning, for *histopathology* and *endometriosis*.

Histopathology: Hist/o _____, path/o _____,

-logy _____, means _____.

Endometriosis: Endo- _____, metri/o _____,

-osis _____, means _____.

7. Endometriosis is the presence of endometrial tissue outside the uterine endometrial cavity and is often associated with cyclic (monthly) pelvic pain. The condition is rare after menopause. Why do you think this patient had acyclic pain?

⌕ ADVANCED CASE STUDY

9.10 Preeclampsia

A 35-year-old woman, with a monochorionic diamniotic monozygotic twin pregnancy at 28 weeks of gestation, presents to her obstetrician with headache, tachypnea, and abdominal pain. She is afebrile with hypertension (155/120 mm Hg) and edematous face and hands. She has no significant previous medical history. Her family history includes gestational hypertension and preeclampsia, which is defined by the onset of hypertension after 20 weeks of gestation and the development of proteinuria. Preeclampsia can be associated with edema and HELLP syndrome, the constellation of Hemolysis with Elevated Liver enzymes and Low Platelets. The lab work includes significant findings of proteinuria, hematuria, and thrombocytopenia. The diagnosis is preterm preeclampsia; she was scheduled for an emergency caesarean section (C-section).

1. What are the word parts, and meaning, for *obstetrician*?

Obstetrician: Obstetr/o _____, -ician _____,

means _____.

MONOCHORIONIC DIAMNIOTIC TWINS

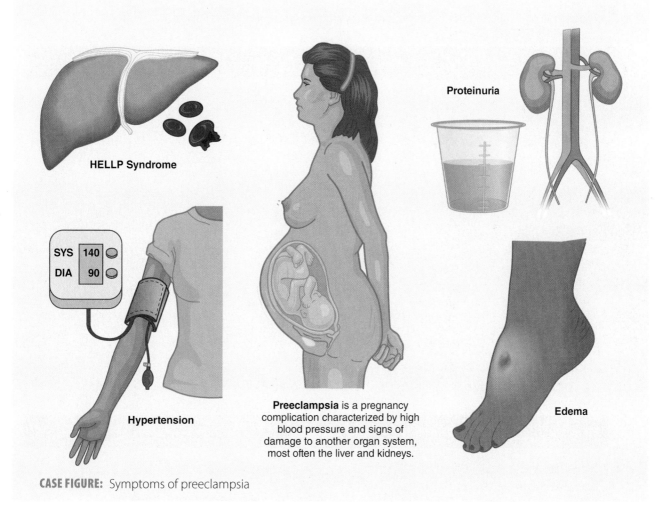

CHORIONIC SAC

AMNIOTIC SAC

FETUS

FETUS

PLACENTA

UMBILICAL CORD

CASE FIGURE: Monochorionic diamniotic twins

© Betty Ray/Shutterstock

HELLP Syndrome

Proteinuria

SYS 140
DIA 90

Hypertension

Preeclampsia is a pregnancy complication characterized by high blood pressure and signs of damage to another organ system, most often the liver and kidneys.

Edema

CASE FIGURE: Symptoms of preeclampsia

(continues)

ADVANCED CASE STUDY

(continued)

2. The patient is pregnant with monochorionic diamniotic monozygotic twins. Define the word parts, and meaning, for *monochorionic*, *diamniotic*, and *monozygotic*. Then put it all together and explain the meaning of *monochorionic diamniotic monozygotic twins*.

Monochorionic: Mono- _____, chorion/o _____,

-ic _____, means _____.

Diamniotic: Di- _____, amni/o _____, -tic _____,

means _____.

Monozygotic: Mono- _____, zygote _____*zygote*_____,

-ic _____, means _____.

Monochorionic diamniotic monozygotic twins:

Complete the table below for terms relating to the signs and symptoms of the patient.

Term	Word Parts	Meaning
afebrile	*a-; febri-;-ile*	*without fever*
tachypnea		
hypertension		
edematous		
proteinuria		
hemolysis		
hemoglobinuria		
thrombocytopenia		

3. Preeclampsia is defined by hypertension after 20 weeks of gestation together with the development of proteinuria. It is different from, but may occur with, HELLP syndrome. Complete the table below for hemolysis and low platelets.

Signs	Word Parts	Meaning
hemolysis		
		abnormal decrease of clotting cells (low platelets)

4. In medicine, what is meant by constellation? Use a medical dictionary or other reliable resource for help.

5. The woman in the case was diagnosed with preterm preeclampsia. What is preterm in gestational weeks? Use a medical dictionary or other reliable resource for help.

References

Baskin, L. S., & Ebbers, M. B. (2006). Hypospadias: Anatomy, etiology, and technique. *Journal of Pediatric Surgery, 41*(3), 463–472. https://doi.org/10.1016/j.jpedsurg.2005.11.059

Berens P. D. (2015). Breast pain: Engorgement, nipple pain, and mastitis. *Clinical Obstetrics and Gynecology, 58*(4), 902–914. https://doi.org/10.1097/GRF.0000000000000153

Deb, P., Chander, Y., & Rai, R. S. (2007). Testicular metastasis from carcinoma of prostate: Report of two cases. *Prostate Cancer and Prostatic Diseases, 10*(2), 202–204. https://doi.org/10.1038/sj.pcan.4500942

Donnez, J., & Dolmans, M. M. (2016). Uterine fibroid management: From the present to the future. *Human Reproduction Update, 22*(6), 665–686. https://doi.org/10.1093/humupd/dmw023

Fujishita, A. Masuzaki, H., Khan, K. N., Kitajima, M., Hiraki, K., & Ishimaru, T. (2004). Laparoscopic salpingotomy for tubal pregnancy: Comparison of linear salpingotomy with and without suturing, *Human Reproduction, 19*(5), 1195–1200. https://doi.org/10.1093/humrep/deh196

Goncé, A., Martínez, M. J., Marbán-Castro, E., Saco, A., Soler, A., Alvarez-Mora, M. I., Peiro, A., Gonzalo, V., Hale, G., Bhatnagar, J., López, M., Zaki, S., Ordi, J., & Bardají, A. (2018). Spontaneous abortion associated with Zika virus infection and persistent viremia. *Emerging Infectious Diseases, 24*(5), 933–935. https://doi.org/10.3201/eid2405.171479

Goodman, H. M., Kredentser, D., & Deligdisch, L. (1989). Postmenopausal endometriosis associated with hormone replacement therapy. A case report. *Journal of Reproductive Medicine, 34*(3), 231–233.

Kovac, J. R., Lehmann, K. J., & Fischer, M. A. (2014). A single-center study examining the outcomes of percutaneous epididymal sperm aspiration in the treatment of obstructive azoospermia. *Urology Annals, 6*(1), 41–45. https://doi.org/10.4103/0974-7796.127026

Langer, R., Bukovsky, I., Herman, A., Sherman, D., Sadovsky, G., & Caspi, E. (1982). Conservative surgery for tubal pregnancy. *Fertility and Sterility, 38*(4), 427–430. https://doi.org/10.1016/s0015-0282(16)46576-3

Parikh, N. I., & Gonzalez, J. (2017). Preeclampsia and hypertension: Courting a long while: Time to make it official. *JAMA Internal Medicine, 177*(7), 917–918. https://doi.org/10.1001/jamainternmed.2017.1422

Rao, D., Chaudhari, N. K., Moore, R. M., & Jim, B. (2016). HELLP syndrome: A diagnostic conundrum with severe complications. *BMJ Case Reports, 2016*, bcr2016216802. https://doi.org/10.1136/bcr-2016-216802

Rupp, T.J. & Leslie S.W. (Updated 2020 May 29). Epididymitis. In: StatPearls. Treasure Island (FL): StatPearls Publishing; 2020 Jan. https://www.ncbi.nlm.nih.gov/books/NBK430814/

Saadeh, F. A., Wahab, N. A., & Gleeson, N. (2014). An unusual presentation of endometriosis. *BMJ Case Reports*, bcr2014204270. https://doi.org/10.1136/bcr-2014-204270

Stedman, T. L. (2005). Nath's *Stedman's medical terminology, 2e.* Philadelphia: Lippincott Williams & Wilkins.

Tsuchihashi, K., Okubo, K., Ichioka, K., Soda, T., Yoshimura, K., Kanematsu, A., Ogawa, O., & Nishiyama, H. (2011). Obstructive azoospermia as an unusual complication associated with herniorrhaphy of an omphalocele: A case report. *Journal of Medical Case Reports, 5*(234). https://doi.org/10.1186/1752-1947-5-234

Venes, D. & Taber, C. W. (2017). *Taber's cyclopedic medical dictionary.* Ed. 23, illustrated in full color/Philadelphia: F. A. Davis.

CHAPTER 10

Endocrine System

KEY TERMS

Adenohypophysis	Glucagon	Parathyroid gland
Adrenal cortex	Gonad	Parathyroid hormone
Adrenal gland	Hormone	Pineal gland
Adrenal medulla	Human growth hormone (hGH)	Pituitary gland
Adrenocorticotropic hormone (ACTH)	Hypophysis	Progesterone
Aldosterone	Hypothalamus	Prolactin (PRL)
Androgens	Infundibulum	Spermatogenesis
Antidiuretic hormone (ADH)	Insulin	Testosterone
Calcitonin	Luteinizing hormone (LH)	Thymosin
Epinephrine	Melatonin	Thymus gland
Estrogen	Neurohypophysis	Thyroid gland
Follicle-stimulating hormone (FSH)	Norepinephrine	Thyroid-stimulating hormone (TSH)
Gamete	Oxytocin	Thyroxine (T_4)
Gland	Pancreas	Tri-iodothyronine (T_3)

The endocrine system coordinates the activities of all of the other body systems. It generally adjusts physiological processes to oppose change and maintain homeostasis. Unlike the nervous system, which has quick and targeted effects, the endocrine system tends to work on longer timelines (e.g., seconds, hours, years) and have broad effects. The endocrine system regulates metabolism, growth, reproduction, behavior, and the transport of chemicals. It functions using **glands**, tissues that are composed of highly specialized cells that synthesize, store, and secrete specific signaling molecules. There are approximately 30 different signaling molecules and these are the **hormones** of the endocrine system.

Hormones can be divided into two broad chemical classes: those that are lipid-soluble and those that are water-soluble. Lipid-soluble hormones include steroid and thyroid hormones, and water-soluble hormones include protein hormones and prostaglandins. In addition to the two types of hormones exerting their effects differently, these two types of hormones must be administered differently to patients needing them. Lipid-soluble hormones may be taken orally since they can cross the intestinal lining and are not destroyed by digestive enzymes. By contrast, water-soluble hormones, such as insulin, must be injected due to their susceptibility to the digestive process.

The major endocrine glands are the hypothalamus, pituitary gland, pineal gland, thyroid gland, parathyroid glands, thymus, pancreas, adrenal glands, and the ovaries and testes. Some organs from other body systems also secrete important endocrine hormones; the kidney and liver are examples. Once endocrine hormones enter the bloodstream, they are dispersed throughout the body and have the ability to affect almost every cell, but only cells that have the matching receptor are ultimately affected. In this way, a hormone can have both broad and specific influence. Once a hormone binds to its target cell, it modifies the function of the cell, generally by altering the activity, or abundance, of specific proteins within the cell.

Hormone-producing cells within each gland are usually dedicated to synthesizing and secreting one predominant hormone. The secretion of this hormone is typically regulated by a negative feedback loop. This type of feedback decreases secretion when the hormone (or its downstream effect) is abundant and increases secretion when the hormone (or its effect) is deficient, thereby keeping the circulating hormone within a narrow, optimal, range. Because the effects of a hormone may be far-reaching and dramatic, inappropriate levels of a hormone may have serious consequences.

Pituitary Gland and Hypothalamus

The **pituitary gland** is also known as the hypophysis. It is a small, 1.0–1.5 cm, pea-shaped structure located underneath the brain and attached to the hypothalamus by a stalk called the **infundibulum**. It has two distinct lobes, the anterior lobe, or the **adenohypophysis** and the posterior lobe, or the **neurohypophysis**. Some of the hormones synthesized by the anterior pituitary include **human growth hormone (hGH)**, which promotes growth of body cells and tissue repair, **thyroid-stimulating hormone (TSH)**, which regulates function of the thyroid glands, **follicle-stimulating hormone (FSH)** and **luteinizing hormone (LH)**, which influence the gonads (i.e., ovaries and testes) and the hormones they secrete, **prolactin (PRL)**, which promotes milk secretion by the mammary glands, and **adrenocorticotropic hormone (ACTH)**, which helps mediate the stress response and secretion of hormones from the adrenal cortex. The release of all of these pituitary hormones is controlled by the **hypothalamus**. The posterior lobe of the pituitary gland stores and releases two hormones that are produced by the hypothalamus, **oxytocin**, which stimulates uterine wall contractions during childbirth and milk ejection from mammary glands, and

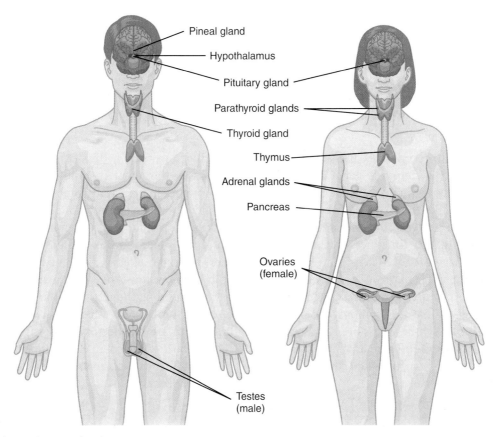

Pineal gland
Hypothalamus
Pituitary gland
Parathyroid glands
Thyroid gland
Thymus
Adrenal glands
Pancreas
Ovaries (female)
Testes (male)

FIGURE 10.1 The endocrine glands

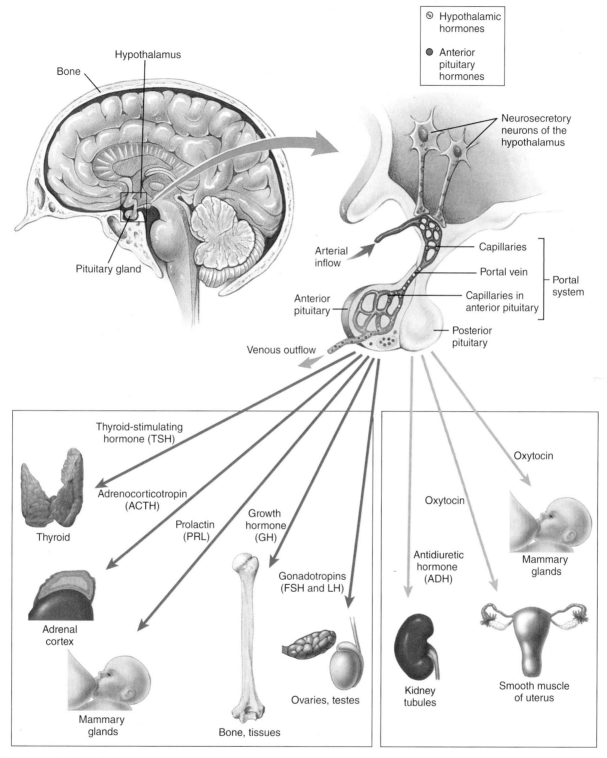

FIGURE 10.2 The hypothalamus and the pituitary glands and the targets of their hormones

antidiuretic hormone (ADH), involved in regulating water balance and blood pressure.

Pineal Gland

The **pineal gland** is a small, pine cone-shaped gland about the size of a grain of rice located near the center of the brain between the cerebral hemispheres. It secretes

the hormone **melatonin**, which plays a role in the regulation of the body's sleep cycle and biological clock.

Thyroid Gland and Parathyroid Glands

The butterfly-shaped **thyroid gland** is located inferior to the larynx. Two hormones produced by this gland, **thyroxine (T$_4$)** and **tri-iodothyronine (T$_3$)**,

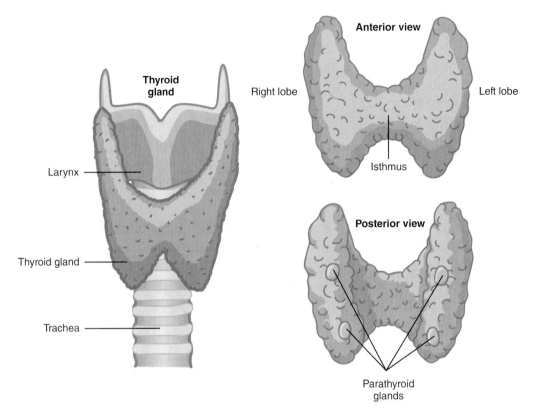

FIGURE 10.3 The thyroid gland and parathyroid glands

increase basal metabolic rate, stimulate protein synthesis, and accelerate body growth. The thyroid gland also secretes **calcitonin**, which is involved in decreasing blood calcium concentration. The four small **parathyroid glands**, with a mass of approximately 40 mg, are embedded in the posterior surface of the thyroid gland. **Parathyroid hormone**, secreted by these glands, is involved in increasing blood calcium concentration.

Thymus Gland

The **thymus gland** is located posterior to the sternum in the mediastinal cavity between the lungs. **Thymosin**, the major hormone it secretes, is involved in the development of T cell lymphocytes, which are an important cell type involved in the immune response.

Pancreas

The **pancreas** is both an endocrine gland and a digestive organ and is located in the upper left abdominal quadrant behind the stomach. As an endocrine gland, it secretes the hormones **insulin**, which decreases blood glucose concentration, and **glucagon**, which has the opposite effect. The endocrine cells of the pancreas, insulin-secreting beta cells and glucagon-secreting alpha cells, are grouped together in the pancreas in structures called islets of Langerhans.

Adrenal Glands

The paired **adrenal glands**, also called the suprarenal glands, lie superior to each kidney. The outer layer of the adrenal glands is called the **adrenal cortex** and this makes up over 80% of each gland. The inner region of the glands is called the

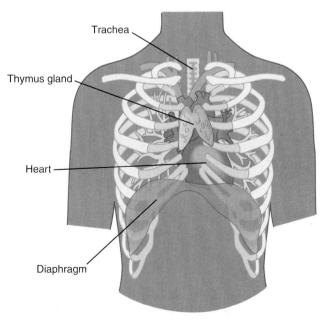

FIGURE 10.4 The thymus gland

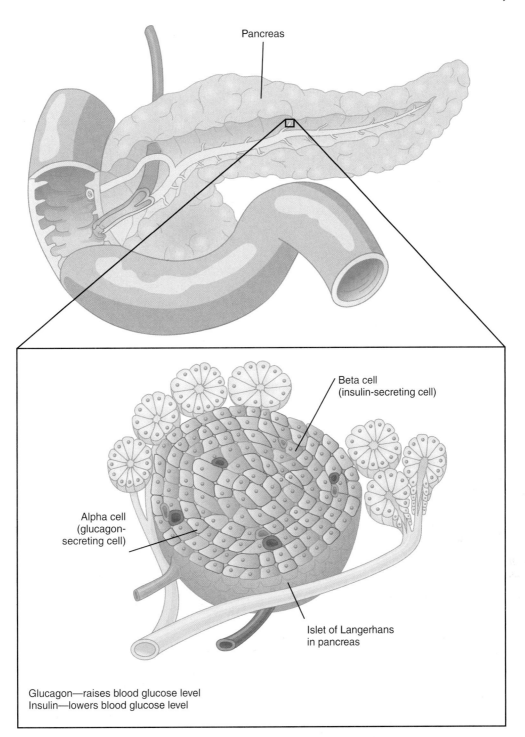

FIGURE 10.5 The pancreas and an islet of Langerhans

adrenal medulla. The main hormones secreted by the adrenal cortex are **aldosterone**, involved in blood pressure regulation, **cortisol**, involved with the body's stress response, and supplemental **androgens**, which regulate development and maintenance of secondary sex characteristics. The adrenal medulla secretes **epinephrine** and **norepinephrine**, which respond to strong emotions during the fight or flight response.

Ovaries and Testes

In addition to their role in **gamete** (i.e., eggs and sperm) production, the **gonads** also secrete hormones. The ovaries produce and secrete **estrogen** and **progesterone**, which regulate the menstrual cycle and help maintain pregnancy. The testes produce and secrete **testosterone**, which regulates **spermatogenesis** and the development of male secondary sex characteristics.

TABLE 10.1

Key Endocrine System Combining Forms

acr/o: extremities

aden/o: gland

adren/o: adrenal glands

adrenal/o: adrenal glands

andr/o: male

calc/o: calcium

cortic/o: outer layer

crin/o: secreting

estr/o: female

gluc/o: sugar

glyc/o: sugar

glycos/o: sugar

gnath/o: jaw

gonad/o: sex glands; gonads

gynec/o: woman

immun/o: immune, protection

iod/o: iodine

hirsut/o: hairy

kal/i: potassium

keton/o: ketones

mast/o: breast

mineral/o: minerals, electrolytes

natr/o: sodium

neur/o: nerve

noct/o: nighttime

orch/o: testes

ovari/o: ovary

pancreat/o: pancreas

parathyroid/o: parathyroid gland

pineal/o: pineal gland

Key Endocrine System Combining Forms

pituit/o: pituitary gland

pituitar/o: pituitary gland

radi/o: radiation

seb/o: oil

somat/o: body

testicul/o: testis

thym/o: thymus gland

thyr/o: thyroid gland

thryoid/o: thyroid gland

toxic/o: poison

trich/o: hair

TABLE 10.2

Key Endocrine System Prefixes

endo-: within

auto-: self

TABLE 10.3

Key Endocrine System Suffixes

-crine: secretion

-dipsia: condition of thirst

-phagia: condition of eating

-pressin: to press down

-statin: to stop

-trophic: pertaining to development

-trophy: development

-tropic: pertaining to stimulating

-tropin: to act on, stimulate

-uria: condition of urine

-volemia: blood volume

Endocrine System **227**

🔍 STANDARD CASE STUDY

10.1 Insulin-Dependent Diabetes Mellitus

"You can't possibly be thirsty again," exclaimed Phillipa to her 9-year-old daughter Medea. "All you have been doing all summer since school ended is eating and drinking. And you are so moody. I just don't understand it! Why don't we go to the pool with your cousins?" suggested Phillipa. "It might put you in a better frame of mind."

"Maybe tomorrow," answered Medea. "I'm tired today. I keep having to get up at night to pee and I can't sleep. I think I'll just lay on my bed and read a book."

Phillipa took a hard look at her usually active and upbeat daughter and realized something wasn't right. Medea didn't look well and in addition, her mother realized she had lost weight. Phillipa called the pediatrician and made an appointment for the following day.

Dr. Angelman listened to Phillipa describe her daughter's symptoms. "The lethargy, weight loss, polyphagia, polydipsia, polyuria, and nocturia you are describing are classic hallmarks of diabetes. Let's do a quick urinalysis and finger-prick glucometer reading on Medea."

The glucometer reading indicated severe hyperglycemia and Medea's urinalysis indicated both glycosuria and ketonuria. Dr. Angelman was alarmed. "You need to take Medea to the hospital now," he told Phillipa.

Once at the hospital, Medea was admitted, and a blood test confirmed type I diabetes mellitus. Medea spent several days in the hospital while her healthcare team worked to bring her blood sugar into normal range. Medea and her parents were educated on what managing her diabetes would mean once she was discharged. Testing her blood sugar regularly, daily insulin injections, and a carefully coordinated diet would all be part of Medea's future.

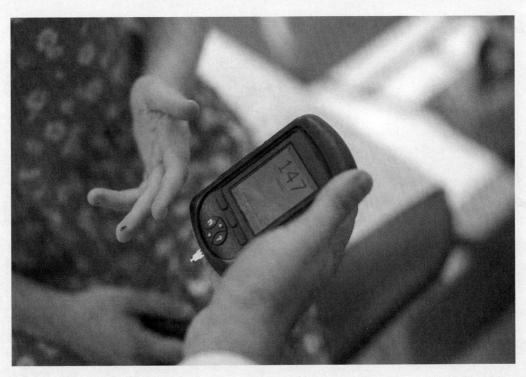

CASE FIGURE: A young girl has her blood sugar tested with a glucometer

© EVOK/M.Poehlman/Evok Images/Getty Images

1. Provide a brief definition of the term lethargy. Use a medical dictionary, if necessary.

(continues)

🔍 STANDARD CASE STUDY   *(continued)*

2. Complete the table below for the signs and symptoms related to diabetes in this case:

Term	Word Parts	Meaning
polyphagia	*poly-; -phagia*	condition of much eating
polydipsia		
polyuria		
nocturia		
hyperglycemia		
glycosuria		
ketonuria		

3. Define the word parts and meaning of *glucometer*.

   Glucometer: Gluc/o _____, -meter _____,

   means _____.

4. It is critical that blood sugar be well managed in diabetes to avoid long-term complications, affecting many body systems. Complete the table for these possible complications. Refer to other chapters for help with word parts from other body systems.

Term	Word Parts	Meaning
retinopathy	*retin/o; -pathy*	*disease of the retina*
macular edema		
polyradiculoneuropathy		
dermopathy		
glomerulosclerosis		
nephropathy		
arteriosclerosis		
tissue necrosis		
microvascular disease		
macrovascular disease		

Term	Word Parts	Meaning
gastroparesis		
periodontitis		
ketoacidosis		

🔍 STANDARD CASE STUDY

10.2 Kallman Syndrome

Endocrinology Consultation Report

Subjective: Noah Free is an 18-year-old male concerned about delayed onset puberty. He has not developed the secondary sex characteristics typical of a male his age, such as growth of body and facial hair, deepening of his voice, and increase in stature. He has no other health concerns but states as an aside that his sense of smell is virtually nonexistent.

Objective: Noah appears physically immature for his chronological age. Signs of hypogonadism are present. Sexual development is inconsistent with age. Physical exam reveals microphallus, testicular atrophy, and slight gynecomastia. Facial, body, and pubic hair are all absent. Height, weight, and muscle mass are below normal range for his age.

Assessment: Failure of onset of puberty coupled with hyposmia or anosmia is consistent with Kallman syndrome, a form of hypogonadotropic hypogonadism.

Plan: Follow-up blood work to determine testosterone and gonadotropin (follicle-stimulating hormone; FH and luteinizing hormone; LH) levels. MRI to evaluate pituitary and assess abnormalities of the olfactory system. Low levels of both testosterone and gonadotropins along with hypoplasia or agenesis of olfactory bulb are indicative of Kallman syndrome. Treatment options are dependent on desire for fertility. Azoospermia is present in the majority of males with Kallman syndrome. Androgen replacement therapy will promote pubertal development but will not restore fertility. Gonadotropin therapy is necessary to promote spermatogenesis and attempt achievement of fertility. Males presenting without cryptorchism have a higher chance of successfully attaining fertility. Without any hormone treatment, the patient has a high risk of developing osteopenia or osteoporosis. Molecular testing for gene mutations associated with Kallman syndrome is suggested to assess risk to family members and potential offspring.

1. Define the word parts of *hypogonadotropic hypogonadism* and then put them together to describe this disorder.

    Hypogonadotropic hypogonadism: Hypo- _____, gonad/o _____,

    -tropic _____, hypo- _____,

    gonad/o _____, -ism _____.

(continues)

Male Hypothalamic-Pituitary-Gonadal Axis

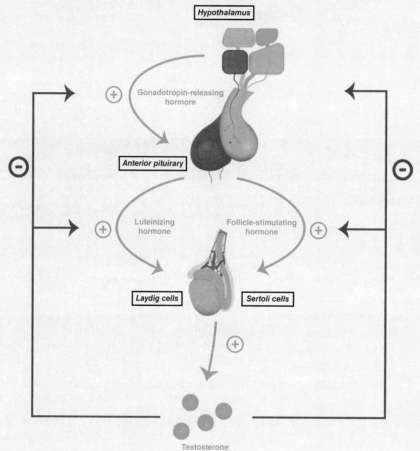

CASE FIGURE: The influence of gonadotropin-releasing hormones and gonadotropins (FSH and LH) on testosterone production and the development of secondary sex characteristics

© Joshya/Shutterstock

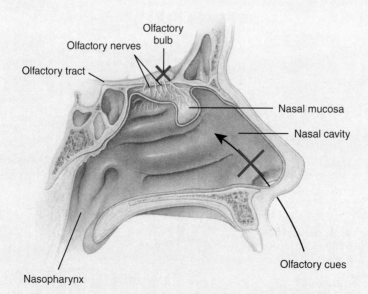

CASE FIGURE: Inability to smell is consistent with Kallman syndrome due to lack of development of the olfactory bulb

2. Complete the table for the following signs of hypogonadism.

Term	Word Parts	Meaning
microphallus	*micro-; phall/o; -us*	*structure of small penis*
testicular atrophy		
gynecomastia		
azoospermia		
cryptorchism		

3. In addition to issues relating to sexual maturity, a hallmark of Kallman syndrome is issues related to smell. List the terms in the case related to smell, indicate the component word parts, and define the terms.

4. Define the word parts for the following therapy-related terms for Kallman syndrome.

   Androgen: Andr/o _____, -gen _____,

   means _____.

   Gonadotropin: Gonad/o _____, -tropin _____,

   means _____.

   Spermatogenesis: Spermat/o _____, -genesis _____,

   means _____.

5. Both male and female hypogonadism are associated with *osteopenia* and *osteoporosis*. Indicate and define the word parts for these terms.

🔍 STANDARD CASE STUDY

10.3 Graves' Disease

A 30-year-old female presents to her primary care physician complaining of anxiety, tremors, heat-intolerance, amenorrhea, diplopia, xerophthalmia, and unexplained weight loss of 6-months' duration. The physician's initial observations of the patient include distinct exophthalmos and a clearly visible goiter. The patient's skin is warm and smooth to the touch. Physical exam reveals tachycardia, diaphoresis, hyperreflexia, and onycholysis. Thyrotoxicosis is suspected and laboratory tests confirm the autoimmune disorder Graves' disease. The patient is advised of treatment options including pharmacologic antithyroid agents, ablative radioiodine, or thyroidectomy. Sustained remission is often achieved with antithyroid drugs and that is the initial recommended therapy. Steroids may be needed to treat the accompanying thyroid ophthalmopathy.

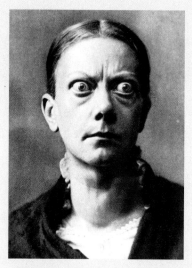

CASE FIGURE: Exophthalmic goiter

© Corbis Historical/Getty Images

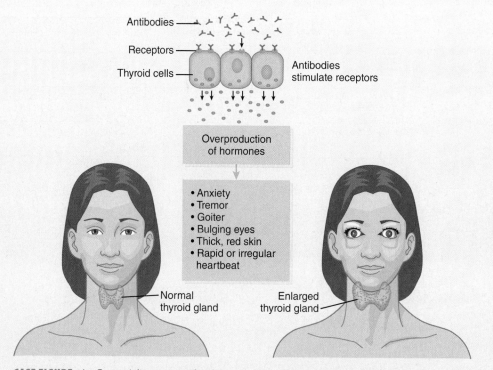

CASE FIGURE: In Graves' disease, antibodies are produced that bind to receptors on the thyroid gland causing it to overproduce thyroid hormone. This leads to many systemic effects

1. Complete the table for the following signs and symptoms of Graves' disease.

Term	Word Parts	Meaning
amenorrhea	*a-; men/o; -rrhea*	*flow without menstruation, lack of menstruation*
diplopia		
xerophthalmia		
exophthalmos		
tachycardia		
diaphoresis		
hyperreflexia		
onycholysis		
ophthalmopathy		

2. A goiter is an enlarged thyroid gland, in this case from hyperthyroidism. Construct a medical term meaning enlarged thyroid gland and define the word parts for *hyperthyroidism*.

   Hyperthyroidism: Hyper- _____ ,

   thyroid/o _____ ,

   -ism _____ .

3. Indicate and define the component word parts for *thyrotoxicosis*, another term for hyperthyroidism.

4. Indicate and define the component word parts for *autoimmune* and provide a brief explanation of autoimmune disease.

5. Provide a brief explanation of pharmacologic antithyroid agents, ablative radioiodine, and thyroidectomy, the possible treatments mentioned in the case for Graves' disease. Use word parts if appropriate and a medical dictionary or other reliable resource if needed.

⌕ *STANDARD CASE STUDY*

10.4 Cushing's Disease

A 35-year-old African American woman presented to the clinic with symptoms of amenorrhea, hirsutism, violaceous striae, facial acne, and weight gain. A physical assessment showed hypertension. Laboratory tests showed high cortisol and adrenocorticotropic (ACTH) levels. Based on high ACTH levels, magnetic resonance imaging (MRI) was performed, which revealed a visible pituitary adenoma. The diagnosis was Cushing's disease, which results from increased production of ACTH from a pituitary tumor, which in turn stimulates increased secretion of cortisol from the adrenal glands. She was scheduled for a consultation with a neurologist, neuroradiologist, neuroendocrinologist, and an otolaryngologist, who collectively recommended a trans-sphenoidal resection of her pituitary adenoma. The patient was monitored for syndrome of inappropriate antidiuretic hormone (SIADH), and diabetes insipidus, which can occur postoperatively, but she remained clear of signs. Her postoperative levels of cortisol were low, so she was placed on hydrocortisone until endogenous cortisol production increased.

The patient returned 6 weeks later, and her cortisol and ACTH levels were within normal range. She had lost 10 lbs., and the hirsutism and facial acne had resolved. She will continue to be monitored for recurrence of pituitary adenoma.

Signs and Symptoms of Cushing's Disease

Adrenal glands

Excess control

CNS irritability
Emotional disturbances

Red and round face

Pituitary tumor

Hypertension

Cardiac hypertrophy

Obesity
(fat deposition
on abdomen
and back of neck)

Purple striae

Osteoporosis

Muscle wasting

Skin ulcers

In females:
- amenorrhea, hirsutism

In males:
- erectile dysfunction

CASE FIGURE: Cushing's syndrome

© Designua/Shutterstock

1. The patient in this case had symptoms including amenorrhea, hirsutism, and a sign of hypertension. Define the following word parts, and meaning, of *amenorrhea, hirsutism,* and *hypertension.*

   Amenorrhea: A- _____, men/o _____,

   -rrhea _____, means _____.

   Hirsutism: Hirsut/o _____, -ism _____,

   means _____.

   Hypertension: Hyper-_____, -tension _____, means _____.

2. One of the symptoms that the patient in this case presented with were violet stretch marks. Review the symptoms in this case and identify which one refers to violet lines.

3. The prefix hyper- means excessive, iso- means equal, and hypo- means insufficient. This case describes two hormones, cortisol and adrenocorticotropic hormone (ACTH). Identify if the levels of cortisol and ACTH would be described as hypersecretion, isosecretion, or hyposecretion of

   Cortisol:

   ACTH:

4. Adrenocorticotropic hormone secreted from the anterior pituitary stimulates cortisol secretion from the cortex of the adrenal gland. Define the following word parts of *adrenocorticotropic hormone.*

   Adrenocorticotropic: Adren/o _____, cortic/o _____,

   -tropic _____, means _____.

5. List the different types of specialists this patient visited and define their component word parts to determine their specialization.

(continues)

STANDARD CASE STUDY *(continued)*

6. The specialists recommended a trans-sphenoidal resection (removal) of the patient's pituitary adenoma. Define the following word parts, and meaning, of *adenoma* and *trans-sphenoidal*.

Adenoma: Aden/o _____, -oma _____,

means _____.

Transsphenoidal: Trans- _____, sphenoid _____ *sphenoid bone* _____,

-al _____, means _____.

STANDARD CASE STUDY

10.5 Done Counting Sheep

Gabby King, an 18-year-old female, visited her primary care physician (PCP) to discuss her persistent insomnia.

Gabby explained, "I haven't had a good night sleep in 6 months. It takes me forever to fall asleep. From what I read, this is called sleep onset latency. I work overnight, third shift, as a certified nurse assistant, which has definitely made sleeping normally almost impossible. I come home from a crazy, busy, night, then I expect to fall asleep after the sun has come up. Not happening."

Her PCP, Dr. Lin Roseman, agreed, "I've been there. It's a common consequence of confusing your body's circadian rhythm… your day and night cycle. It's ruled by your pineal gland, which sits at the back of your brain and looks like a tiny pinecone. It receives cues about light, which it interprets as day, and it increases secretion of a hormone called melatonin when night falls. Melatonin has another name, the darkness hormone, and it makes you sleepy. It is thought to be a pleiotropic molecule, having lots of other effects, like combating inflammation and coagulopathy, and functioning as an antioxidant."

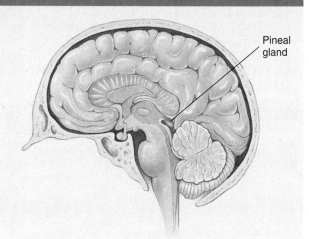

Pineal gland

CASE FIGURE: Midsagittal section of the brain showing the pineal gland

Gabby replied, "I've heard that melatonin secretion can change by looking at screens before bed too. What do you suggest?"

Lin recommended, "First, I'm glad you came to see me to talk about this. Sleep disorders can have significant long-term detrimental effects and have been associated with mental illness, gastrointestinal disorders, obesity, and increased risk of cardiovascular disease. I would suggest that we start simple with over-the-counter melatonin, you can just take exogenous melatonin about 3 hours before you want to start sleeping. There is some evidence that this can help with sleep onset latency and results in longer, more restful sleep. Some risks may include arthritis, and amenorrhea, but only when used at high doses, but these effects seem to be relieved when you stop taking the supplement. The risks are actually quite low, and I think it could help, so let's start with that, and make another appointment to check in through a virtual health visit in about a month."

1. Melatonin is a pleiotropic molecule. Define the word parts, and meaning, for *pleiotropic*, *insomnia*, *coagulopathy*, and *antioxidant*.

Pleiotropic: Plei/o _____, -tropic _____,

means _____.

Insomnia: In- _____, somn/o _____, -ia _____,

means _____.

Coagulopathy: Coagul/o _____, -pathy _____,

means _____

Antioxidant: Anti- _____, oxidant <u>*oxidizer*</u>, means _____.

2. It is recommended that Gabby take exogenous melatonin. Define the following word parts, and meaning, for endogenous and exogenous.

    Endogenous: Endo- _____, gen/o _____, -ous _____

    means _____

    Exogenous: Exo- _____, gen/o _____

    -ous _____, means _____

3. Complete the table below for the following terms related to sleep disorders and melatonin.

Term	Word Parts	Meaning
gastrointestinal	*gastr/o; intestin/o; -al*	*pertaining to stomach and intestines*
cardiovascular		
arthritis		
amenorrhea		

🔍 ADVANCED CASE STUDY

10.6 Acromegaly

Wayne hadn't seen his college roommate Devante in 10 years. They were both in their 30s now, married with children. The first thing Wayne noticed when he saw Devante was the change in his facial features. His forehead was so prominent, his jaw was protruding, and his tongue seemed so big.

"What happened to you?" asked Wayne, a bit shocked.

"I was just diagnosed with acromegaly," answered Devante. "First my hands and feet started growing. I thought I was imagining it, but then my wedding ring didn't fit, and I had to buy shoes a size larger. Then the headaches and the joint pain started. Next thing you know, my skin was getting darker, thicker, oily, and I was getting really hairy. I was always sweating. My doctor threw all sorts of terms at me and sent me to all sorts of specialists: a dermatologist for the hyperpigmentation, seborrhea, pachyderma, and hypertrichosis; an orthopedist for the arthralgia; and an orthodontist for macroglossia and prognathism that led to a widening gap in my front teeth. I was even referred to a psychologist for the headaches and hyperhidrosis. No one could figure out what was wrong with me. Finally, I was referred to an endocrinologist who took one look at me, sent me for some lab tests, and confirmed that I had a tumor on my pituitary gland, specifically a macroadenoma that is causing hypersecretion of growth hormone."

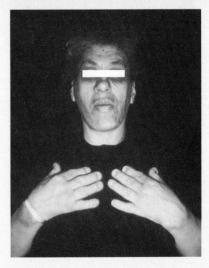

CASE FIGURE: Patient affected with acromegaly

Courtesy of Leonard V. Crowley, MD, Century College

(continues)

ꙩ *ADVANCED CASE STUDY* (continued)

"Oh, wow man, I'm sorry," said Wayne. "Now what?"

"Right now, I'm taking a drug called a somatostatin analogue to shrink the tumor. Then I'll have surgery to remove what's left. I may have reconstructive surgery on my jaw at a later date and my hormone levels will be monitored throughout my life. I'm hopeful that many of my symptoms will resolve following the surgery. Honestly, as bad as it sounds, I am relieved to have a diagnosis and a path forward," Devante affirmed. "Now let's get that burger you came to meet me for!"

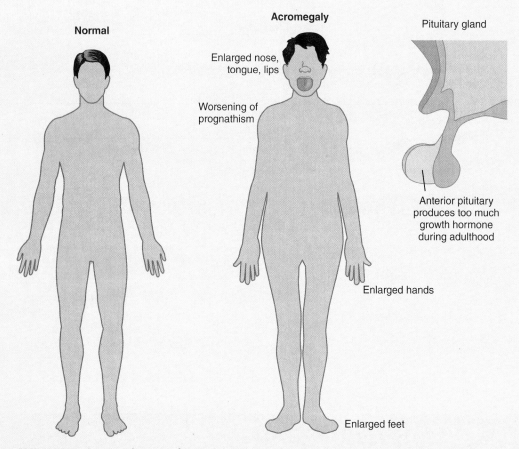

CASE FIGURE: Overproduction of growth hormone in adulthood leads to acromegaly

1. Define the word parts for *acromegaly*.

   Acromegaly: Acr/o _____, -megaly _____

2. List the different types of physicians Devante visited and define their component word parts to determine their specialization.

3. Complete the table for the varied signs and symptoms of acromegaly.

Term	Word Parts	Meaning
seborrhea	*seb/o; -rrhea*	*discharge of oil*
pachyderma		
hypertrichosis		
arthralgia		
prognathism		
macroglossia		
hyperhidrosis		

4. Define the word parts for *macroadenoma*.

   Macroadenoma: Macro- _____, aden/o _____,

   -oma _____

5. The medical term for growth hormone is *somatotropin*. List and define the component word parts of this term.

6. Somatostatin is also known as growth hormone inhibiting hormone. It is released by the hypothalamus and acts on the pituitary to inhibit the release of somatotropin. List and define the component word parts for somatostatin and explain how a somatostatin analogue could counteract the hypersecretion of somatotropin. You may need to use other resources.

7. A common surgical procedure for removal of pituitary adenomas is *endonasal trans-sphenoidal* surgery. Define the word parts and meaning for this procedure.

   Endonasal trans-sphenoidal: Endo- _____, nas/o _____,

   -al _____, trans- _____,

   sphenoid _____*sphenoid bone*_____, -al _____,

   means _____

   _____

⌕ *ADVANCED CASE STUDY*

10.7 Addison's Disease

A 50-year-old Caucasian male presents in the emergency department (ED) with vomiting and diarrhea. He reports symptoms of exhaustion, thirst, and infrequent urination. His medical history is remarkable for mucocutaneous candidiasis and autoimmune polyglandular endocrinopathy. The polyglandular endocrinopathy includes adrenal insufficiency resulting from autoimmune adrenalitis, which is called Addison's disease. A physical assessment reveals hypotension, tachycardia, and skin hyperpigmentation, and blood work suggests acute adrenal crisis based on hyponatremia, hyperkalemia, and hypoglycemia. His signs and symptoms indicate dehydration and hypovolemia. He is transferred to the intensive care unit (ICU) and treated with intravenous (IV) normal saline and dextrose (also called glucose) to correct hypovolemia and hypoglycemia. A series of blood hormone tests show depressed cortisol and aldosterone concentrations and elevated adrenocorticotropic hormone concentration, which suggests an Addisonian crisis. The patient is stabilized, transferred to a step-down unit, and prescribed hydrocortisone as hormone replacement for low cortisol and fludrocortisone to compensate for low aldosterone.

Signs and symptoms of Addison's disease

Adrenal crisis:
- Fever
- Syncope
- Hypoglycemia
- Hyponatremia
- Severe vomiting and diarrhea

Adrenal glands do not produce sufficient steroid hormones

Skin Hyperpigmentation

Gastrointestinal
Nausea
Diarrhea
Vomiting
Constipation
Abdominal pain

Skin Vitiligo

Low blood pressure
Weakness
Weight loss

CASE FIGURE: Addison's disease or chronic adrenal insufficiency

1. The patient's previous medical history included mucocutaneous candidiasis and autoimmune polyglandular endocrinopathy. Define the following word parts for *mucocutaneous candidiasis*, *autoimmune polyglandular endocrinopathy*, *autoimmune adrenalitis*, and provide a simple meaning for the condition. Use a medical dictionary if necessary.

Mucocutaneous candidiasis: Muc/o _____, cutane/o _____,

-ous _____, candid _____*Candida yeast*_____,

-iasis _____.

Mucocutaneous candidiasis means:

Autoimmune polyglandular endocrinopathy: Auto- _____,

immun/o _____, poly- _____,

glandul/o _____, -ar _____.

Autoimmune polyglandular endocrinopathy means:

Autoimmune adrenalitis: Auto- _____, immun/o _____,

adrenal/o _____, -itis _____.

Autoimmune adrenalitis means:

2. Complete the table below for the following terms related to the patient's signs and symptoms:

Term	Word Parts	Meaning
hypotension	*hypo-; -tension*	*insufficient pressure (low blood pressure)*
tachycardia		
hyperpigmentation	*hyper-; pigment; -ation*	
hyponatremia		
hyperkalemia		
hypoglycemia		
dehydration		
hypovolemia		

3. Adrenal insufficiency may be categorized as primary or secondary. Primary adrenal insufficiency results from damage to the adrenal gland so that production of cortisol and aldosterone, the major hormones of the adrenal cortex, are impaired. Secondary adrenal insufficiency results when the adrenal gland does not produce enough cortisol and aldosterone because adrenocorticotropic hormone (ACTH), a pituitary hormone that stimulates the adrenal gland, is reduced. Would you classify this as primary or secondary adrenal insufficiency? Explain your answer.

🔍 *ADVANCED CASE STUDY*   *(continued)*

4. The patient in this case is not producing sufficient cortisol. The patient is prescribed hydrocortisone, which is cortisol when used as a medication. Cortisol has many critical functions. It is a type of glucocorticoid hormone, which can increase glucose availability during times of stress through gluconeogenesis and glycogenolysis. Define the word parts, and meaning, for *gluconeogenesis* and *glycogenolysis*.

Gluconeogenesis: Gluc/o _____, neo- _____,

-genesis _____, means _____.

Glycogenolysis: Glycogen/o _____, -lysis _____,

means _____.

5. The patient in this case is in acute adrenal crisis. Define *acute*, *adrenal*, and *crisis*. Use a medical dictionary or other reliable resource if necessary.

Acute means:

Adrenal means:

Crisis means:

🔍 *ADVANCED CASE STUDY*

10.8 Panhypopituitarism

A 25-year-old male presents to his primary care physician with complaints of underdeveloped secondary (postpubescent) sexual characteristics, including an absence of hair on his face, and in the axillary and pubic regions. The patient claims that he can produce an erection, but not ejaculate. The patient's height was not atypical, but he claimed that he was always much smaller than his peers growing up and features of eunuchoidism persisted into adulthood. There were no symptoms of hypothyroidism or signs of orthostatic hypotension. There was no gynecomastia. Laboratory tests to measure concentrations of key hormones were ordered. Several hormones produced by the adenohypophysis were out of range, and hormones that are produced in other glands (e.g., testes and adrenal glands) were also out of range; testosterone and cortisol were low. Hormones produced by the neurohypophysis (ADH and oxytocin) were within normal range. The results of the adenohypophysis hormones are listed in the table below.

Hormone	Result	Reference Range
Adrenocorticotropic hormone (ACTH)	2.0 ng/L	4.7–48.8 ng/L
Growth hormone (GH)	<0.1 µg/L	0–1 µg/L (men) 0–10 µg/L (women)
Thyroid-stimulating hormone (TSH)	5.0 µU/mL	0.35–5.5 µU/mL
Prolactin (PRL)	16 µg/L	2.1–17.7 µg/L (men) 2.8–29.2 µg/L (nonpregnant women) 9.7–208 µg/L (pregnant women) 1.8–20.3 µg/L (menopausal women)
Follicle-stimulating hormone (FSH)	1.2 mU/mL	1.4–18.1 mU/mL (men) 2.5–10.2 mU/L (women in the follicular phase) 3.4–33.4 mU/mL (women in the ovulatory period) 1.5–9.1 mU/mL (women in the luteal phase) 23–116 mU/mL (menopausal women)
Luteinizing hormone (LH)	0.2 mU/mL	1.5–9.3 mU/mL (men) 1.9–12.5 mU/mL (women in the follicular phase) 8.7–76.3 mU/mL (women in the ovulatory period) 0.5–16.9 mU/mL (women in the luteal phase)

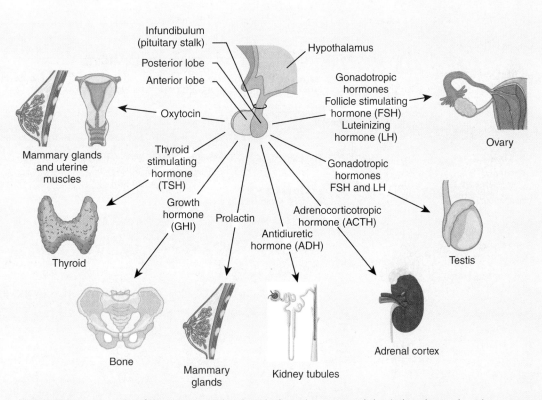

CASE FIGURE: Anatomy of the pituitary gland, including the anterior lobe (adenohypophysis), posterior lobe (neurohypophysis), and the hormones they secrete

(continues)

🔍 ADVANCED CASE STUDY

Magnetic resonance imaging (MRI) was ordered and revealed agenesis of the infundibulum and a hypertrophic adenohypophysis and an ectopic neurohypophysis. The patient was put on hormone replacement therapy to normalize deficiencies. A 3-month follow-up appointment was scheduled to assess development of secondary sexual characteristics.

1. The pituitary has an anterior lobe (adenohypophysis) and a posterior lobe (neurohypophysis). The anterior lobe is made of glandular tissue whereas the posterior lobe is an extension of the hypophysis in the brain. Hypophysis translates to outgrowth in Greek. Define the following word parts, and meaning, of *anterior pituitary*, *adenohypophysis*, *posterior pituitary*, and *neurohypophysis*.

   Anterior pituitary: Anter/o _____, -ior _____,

   pituit/o _____, -ary _____,

   means _____.

   Adenohypophysis: Aden/o _____, hypophysis _____,

   means _____.

   Posterior pituitary: Poster/o _____, -ior _____,

   pituit/o _____, -ary _____,

   means _____.

   Neurohypophysis: Neur/o _____, hypophysis _____,

   means _____.

2. Complete the table below for the following terms that relate to this patient's signs and symptoms.

Term	Word Parts	Meaning
eunuchoidism	*eunuch; -oid; -ism*	*state of resembling a eunuch (persistent prepubertal characteristics)*
hypothyroidism		
orthostatic hypotension		
gynecomastia		

3. List the full name and abbreviation of the hormones that are out of range and indicate if they are below or above range.

4. Adrenocorticotropic hormone, secreted from the adenohypothysis, stimulates cortisol secretion from the cortex of the adrenal gland. Define the following word parts of *adrenocorticotropic hormone.*

   Adrenocorticotropic: Adren/o _____, cortic/o _____,

   -tropic _____, means _____

5. Luteinizing hormone and follicle-stimulating hormone are both a type of gonadotropin. Define the following word parts, and meaning, of *gonadotropin.*

   Gonadotropin: Gonad/o _____, -tropin _____,

   means _____

6. Tropic hormones (suffix -tropic), like adrenocorticotropic hormone and the gonadotropins, act on other glands. What evidence from this case supports this principle?

7. MRI revealed agenesis of the infundibulum and a hypotrophic adenohypophysis and an ectopic neurohypophysis. Define the following word parts, and meaning, of *agenesis*, *hypotrophic*, and *ectopic*. Please be careful because there is a difference between *-trophic* and *-tropic*.

   Agenesis: A- _____, -genesis _____,

   means _____

   Hypotrophic: Hypo- _____, troph/o _____,

   -ic _____, means _____

   Ectopic: Ec- _____, topic/o _____, -ic _____,

   means _____

8. This patient has the signs and symptoms of panhypopituitarism. Define the following word parts, and meaning, of *panhypopituitarism.*

   Panhypopituitarism: Pan- _____, hypo- _____,

   pituitar/o _____, -ism _____,

   means _____

   (Note: pan means all, but this disorder results in insufficiency of many, not necessarily all, adenohypophyseal hormones).

🔍 *ADVANCED CASE STUDY*

10.9 Reninoma

An 8-year-old female, Kyla, is brought to her pediatrician by her mother, Stephanie, who explains that her daughter has been experiencing constant headaches and increased frequency of urination through the day and night. Her family history includes a father with type 2 diabetes and reninoma.

The physician explains to Stephanie, who has some background in biology, that reninoma is a very rare type of tumor that arises from a cell of a renal juxtaglomerular apparatus (JGA). JGAs are cellular complexes that regulate the function of kidney nephrons, the microscopic tubules that are responsible for filtering the blood and producing urine. The tumor is called reninoma because its cells typically secrete renin, an enzyme hormone that is normally synthesized and released by the juxtaglomerular apparatus in response to renal hypotension and hypernatremia, and as a result, is a key regulator of blood volume and pressure. Renin is an upstream player in a broader hormonal system, which also includes angiotensin I, angiotensin II, and aldosterone, called the renin-angiotensin-aldosterone system (RAAS). Circulating renin enzyme activates angiotensinogen, secreted by the liver, by cleaving it into Angiotensin I. Angiotensin I is then converted into angiotensin II by angiotensin converting enzyme (ACE), which is expressed in the lung and kidney vascular epithelia. Angiotensin II has multisystemic effects that decrease blood potassium (through urine excretion) and increase blood sodium (through urine sparing), which draws water into circulation through osmosis increasing blood volume. In the adrenal gland, it stimulates the release of aldosterone, which promotes the excretion of potassium and reabsorption of sodium in the kidney nephrons. In arterioles, it causes vasoconstriction, which increases vascular resistance and blood pressure. In the brain, it causes thirst and the release of antidiuretic hormone (ADH), which together increase fluid intake and retention, increasing blood volume.

The physician thinks that reninoma should be a strong consideration based on Kayla's symptoms and family history. A physical exam shows that Kayla has hypertension. Blood work showing hypernatremia, hypokalemia, and elevation in aldosterone and plasma renin activity confirmed the suspicion that elevated renin was responsible for the hypertension. Elevated aldosterone was also present in her urine. Abdominal ultrasonography does not reveal any abdominal masses but magnetic resonance imaging (MRI) reveals a superficial mass in her right kidney.

The physician explains that if the mass is reninoma and has not metastasized, a surgical resection of the tumor will probably be very effective in relieving Kayla's symptoms, and that this procedure has a history of good outcomes in cases like this. Stephanie is understandably relieved and agrees that scheduling a consultation to discuss laparoscopic transperitoneal resection of the tumor, with a biopsy to confirm reninoma, is the right pathway forward for Kayla.

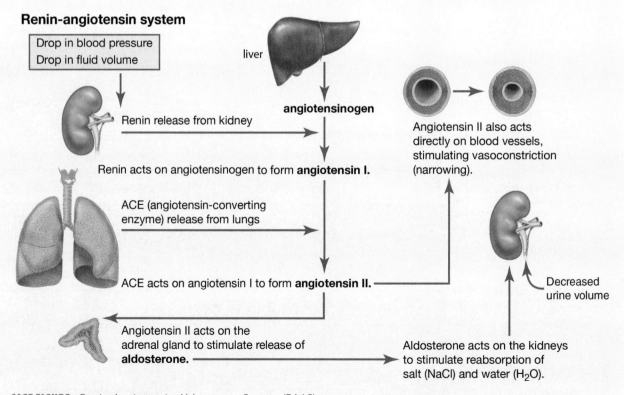

Renin-angiotensin system

Drop in blood pressure
Drop in fluid volume

liver

Renin release from kidney

angiotensinogen

Angiotensin II also acts directly on blood vessels, stimulating vasoconstriction (narrowing).

Renin acts on angiotensinogen to form **angiotensin I.**

ACE (angiotensin-converting enzyme) release from lungs

ACE acts on angiotensin I to form **angiotensin II.**

Decreased urine volume

Angiotensin II acts on the adrenal gland to stimulate release of **aldosterone.**

Aldosterone acts on the kidneys to stimulate reabsorption of salt (NaCl) and water (H_2O).

CASE FIGURE: Renin-Angiotensin-Aldosterone System (RAAS)

1. Kayla has a family history that includes reninoma, a tumor that arises from a renal juxtaglomerular apparatus cell. Define the following word parts, and meaning, of *renal juxtaglomerular*.

   Renal juxtaglomerular: Ren/o _____, -al _____,

   juxta- _____, glomerul/o _____,

   -al _____,

   means _____.

2. Complete the table below for the following terms that relate to this case and renin function:

Term	Word Parts	Meaning
hypotension	*hypo-; -tension*	*insufficient pressure (low blood pressure)*
hypernatremia		
hypokalemia		
hypovolemia		

3. Define the following word parts, and meaning, of *abdominal ultrasonography*.

   Abdominal ultrasonography: Abdomin/o _____, -al _____,

   ultra- _____, son/o _____,

   -graphy _____,

   means _____.

4. Kayla is scheduled to undergo a laparoscopic transperitoneal resection, and biopsy, of the tumor. Define the following word parts, and meaning, of *laparoscopic, transperitoneal*, and *biopsy*.

   Laparoscopic: Lapar/o _____, -scopic _____,

   means _____.

   Transperitoneal: Trans- _____, peritone/o _____,

   -al _____,

   means _____.

   Biopsy: Bi/o _____, -opsy _____,

   means _____.

(continues)

⌕ *ADVANCED CASE STUDY*   *(continued)*

5. List the five key hormones and enzymes involved in RAAS below. With each hormone or enzyme, identify word parts, or variations on word parts, and use them to describe their function.

6. Kayla's condition is leading to hypersecretion of antidiuretic hormone (ADH), which will affect urination frequency and volume. Define the following word parts, and meaning, of *anuria*, *nocturia*, *oliguria*, and *polyuria* and then circle any that Kayla would be predicted to experience.

Anuria: An- _____, -uria _____,

     means _____.

Nocturia: Noct/o _____, -uria _____,

     means _____.

Oliguria: Olig/o _____, -uria _____,

     means _____.

Polyuria: Poly- _____, -uria _____,

     means _____.

⌕ *ADVANCED CASE STUDY*

10.10 Pseudohypoparathyroidism

Ten-year old Anton is brought to the hospital emergency room by his parents after suffering a seizure. Anton is examined immediately, and all vital signs are within normal range, but the emergency room physician notices muscle twitches and carpopedal spasms indicative of tetany. When questioned, Anton describes periodic paresthesia of his hands and feet and perioral numbness. Biochemical testing of blood reveals the following:

Test	Reference Range	Patient Results
Calcium	8.5–10.5 mg/dL	5.04 mg/dL
Glucose	70–100 mg/dL	90 mg/dL
Magnesium	1.5–2.0 mEq/L	1.0 mEq/L

Test	Reference Range	Patient Results
Phosphorus	3.0–4.5 mg/dL	8.04 mg/dL
Parathyroid hormone (PTH)	<25 pg/mL	219 pg/mL

Pseudohypoparathyroidism (PHP) is suspected. Absent the features of osteodystrophy, a hallmark of PHP type 1a, PHP type 1b is most likely. In pseudohypoparathyroidism, the body fails to respond to PTH, in contrast to hypoparathyroidism, when insufficient PTH is made. In type 1b, hormone resistance is localized to the kidneys. Anton's blood results were concerning, and the emergency room physician thought it prudent that he be monitored for cardiac arrhythmias and admitted to the hospital. Once admitted, he was given a calcium-gluconate infusion, which brought his calcium and phosphate levels closer to normal range. After 2 days, calcium-phosphate homeostasis was normalized enough for Anton to be discharged with instructions to his parents that he begin oral calcium supplementation combined with oral calcitriol (the active form of vitamin D) to help promote calcium absorption. Anton's parents were instructed to have him follow up with a pediatric endocrinologist and be tested for other endocrinopathies. Anton would also need to undergo regular biochemical screening to maintain a correctly adjusted therapeutic dose of calcium throughout his life.

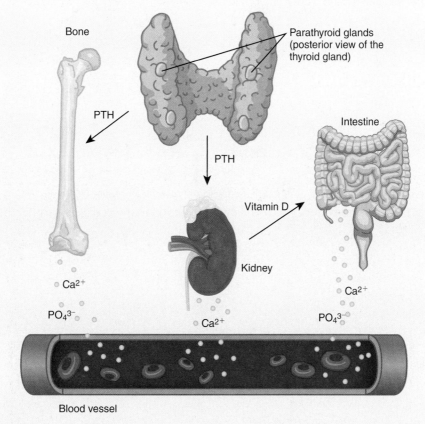

CASE FIGURE: Parathyroid glands and calcium (Ca^{2+}) and phosphate (PO_4^{3-}) metabolism

1. Define the meaning of the prefixes *hypo-*, *hyper-*, and *eu-* and the suffix *-emia*.

Hypo- _____

Hyper- _____

Eu- _____

-emia _____

(continues)

🔍 *ADVANCED CASE STUDY*   *(continued)*

Examine the table of Anton's lab values and circle the correct answer for each of the following:

Anton has (hypocalcemia, eucalcemia, hypercalcemia).

Anton has (hypoglycemia, euglycemia, hyperglycemia).

Anton has (hypomagnesemia, eumagnesemia, hypermagnesemia).

Anton has (hypophosphatemia, euphosphatemia, hyperphosphatemia).

2. Indicate and define the word parts for *pseudohypoparathyroidism*.

3. Using information in the case, contrast hypoparathyroidism to pseudohypoparathyroidism and explain why the levels of PTH are high in the patient's blood.

4. Provide a brief description of the following effects of hypocalcemia: *carpopedal spasms*, *tetany*, *paresthesia*, *perioral numbness*, and *cardiac arrhythmia*. Use word parts if appropriate and a medical dictionary or other reliable resource if necessary.

5. Define the word parts and meaning of the word *homeostasis*.

    Homeostasis: Home/o _____, -stasis _____,

        means _____.

6. Define the word parts and meaning of *osteodystrophy* and connect this term to calcium metabolism.

    Osteodystrophy: Oste/o _____, dys- _____,

        -trophy _____

        means _____.

7. Define the word parts and meaning for *endocrinologist* and *endocrinopathy*.

Endocrinologist: Endo- _____ , crin/o _____ ,

-logist _____ ,

means _____ .

Endocrinopathy: Endo- _____ , crin/o _____ ,

-pathy _____ ,

means _____ .

References

Brent G. A. (2008). Graves' disease. *The New England Journal of Medicine*, *358*(24), 2594–2605. https://doi.org/10.1056/NEJMcp0801880

Carroll, R. W., Katz, M. L., Paul, E., & Jüppner, H. (2017). Case 17-2017—A 14-year-old boy with acute fear of choking while swallowing. *The New England Journal of Medicine*, *376*(23), 2266–2275. https://doi.org/10.1056/NEJMcpc1616019

Chaudhry HS, Singh G. Cushing Syndrome. [Updated 2020 Jul 2]. In: StatPearls [Internet]. Treasure Island (FL): StatPearls Publishing; 2020 Jan-. https://www.ncbi.nlm.nih.gov/books/NBK470218/

Danzig J. (2007). Acromegaly. *BMJ*, *335*(7624), 824–825. https://doi.org/10.1136/bmj.39253.602141.AD

Den Ouden, D. T., Kroon, M., Hoogland, P. H., Geelhoed-Duijvestijn, P. H., & Wit, J. M. (2002). A 43-year-old male with untreated panhypopituitarism due to absence of the pituitary stalk: from dwarf to giant. *The Journal of Clinical Endocrinology & Metabolism, 87*(12), 5430–5434. https://doi.org/10.1210/jc.2002-020672

DiMeglio, L. A., Evans-Molina, C., & Oram, R. A. (2018). Type 1 diabetes. *The Lancet*, *391*(10138), 2449–2462. https://doi.org/10.1016/S0140-6736(18)31320-5

Donghi, V., Mora, S., Zamproni, I., Chiumello, G., & Weber, G. (2009). Pseudohypoparathyroidism, an often delayed diagnosis: A case series. *Cases Journal, 2*(6734). https://doi.org/10.1186/1757-1626-2-6734

Fountain JH, Lappin SL. Physiology, Renin Angiotensin System. [Updated 2019 May 5]. In: StatPearls [Internet]. Treasure Island (FL): StatPearls Publishing; 2020 Jan-. Available from: https://www.ncbi.nlm.nih.gov/books/NBK470410/

Masters, A., Pandi-Perumal, S. R., Seixas, A., Girardin, J. L., & McFarlane, S. I. (2014). Melatonin, the hormone of darkness: From sleep promotion to Ebola treatment. *Brain Disorders & Therapy*, *4*(1), 1000151. https://doi.org/10.4172/2168-975X.1000151

Melmed S. (2020). Pituitary-tumor endocrinopathies. *The New England Journal of Medicine*, *382*(10), 937–950. https://doi.org/10.1056/NEJMra1810772

Munir S, Waseem M. Addison Disease. [Updated 2020 Jul 5]. In: StatPearls [Internet]. Treasure Island (FL): StatPearls Publishing; 2020 Jan-. Available from: https://www.ncbi.nlm.nih.gov/books/NBK441994/

Navarro, P., Halperin, I., Rodríguez, C., González, J. M., Vidal, J., & Vilardell, E. (1994). Congenital panhypopituitarism of late onset. *Journal of Endocrinological Investigation*, *17*(5), 347–350. https://doi.org/10.1007/BF03348997

Stamou, M. I., & Georgopoulos, N. A. (2018). Kallmann syndrome: Phenotype and genotype of hypogonadotropic hypogonadism. *Metabolism*, *86*, 124–134. https://doi.org/10.1016/j.metabol.2017.10.012

Stedman, T. L. (2005). Nath's *Stedman's medical terminology, 2e.* Philadelphia: Lippincott Williams & Wilkins.

Venes, D. & Taber, C. W. (2017). *Taber's cyclopedic medical dictionary.* Ed. 23, illustrated in full color/Philadelphia: F.A. Davis.

Wang, S., Ding, C., Xiao, D., Wu, Z., & Wei, L. (2018). Evaluation of a novel general pituitary hormone score to evaluate the function of the residual anterior pituitary (adenohypophysis) in patients following surgery for pituitary adenoma. *Medical Science Monitor*, *24*, 7944–7951. https://doi.org/10.12659/MSM.909925

Wong, L., Hsu, T. H., Perlroth, M. G., Hofmann, L. V., Haynes, C. M., & Katznelson, L. (2008). Reninoma: Case report and literature review. *Journal of Hypertension*, *26*(2), 368–373. https://doi.org/10.1097/HJH.0b013e3282f283f3

CHAPTER 11

Nervous System

The nervous system orchestrates the activity of the other body systems to help maintain **homeostasis** despite changes in the internal and external environment. The major structures of the nervous system include the brain, spinal cord, and nerves. Nerves transmit signals as electrical impulses that can travel at speeds up to 100 meters per second (about 220 miles per hour), allowing rapid responses to regulate body activities. The functions of the nervous system can be classified as sensory, integrative, and motor response. The system receives signals from sensory receptors throughout the body, processes the signals, and coordinates voluntary and involuntary responses. The receptors are specialized. Some sense general stimuli such as pain, pressure, stretch, and temperature, whereas others are dedicated to the special senses of olfaction, taste, vision, hearing, and balance. Coordinated responses

include the regulation of glands, organs, and muscle contraction.

The nervous system has a mass of only 2 kg and is one of the smallest of the body systems, yet it is one of the most complex, providing the ability to think and reason. The two major divisions of the nervous system are the **central nervous system (CNS)** and the **peripheral nervous system (PNS)**. The CNS is made up of the brain and spinal cord and is the site of information processing and integration. The PNS is composed of nerves and lies outside of the brain and spinal cord.

The **brain** is enclosed, and well protected, within the bony cranium. It consists of four sections: the brain stem, the diencephalon, the cerebellum, and the cerebrum. The **brain stem** is the most inferior part of the brain and is made up of the **medulla oblongata**, which controls many autonomic functions such as

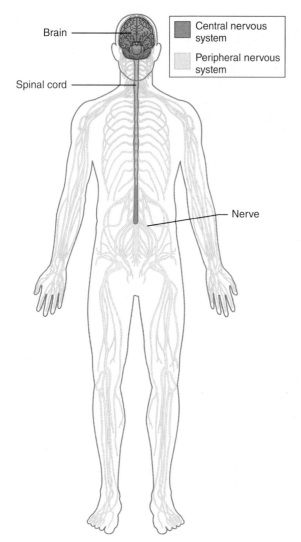

Brain

Spinal cord

Central nervous system

Peripheral nervous system

Nerve

FIGURE 11.1 Location of the central nervous system and the peripheral nervous system

heart rate and breathing, the **pons**, which connects the cerebellum to the rest of the brain, and the **midbrain**, which is associated with vision, hearing, and temperature regulation. The **diencephalon** extends from the brainstem to the cerebrum and includes the **thalamus**, the major relay station for most sensory impulses, and the **hypothalamus**, which controls the release of many hormones and is a major regulator of homeostasis. The **cerebellum**, posterior to the medulla and inferior to the posterior portion of the cerebrum, accounts for about one-tenth of the mass of the brain and is responsible for regulating posture and balance. The **cerebrum** is the largest part of the brain, located in its superior region, and is the "seat of intelligence," responsible for functions such as higher-order thinking, memory, and personality traits. Its right and left halves are called **cerebral hemispheres** and its four lobes are the **frontal**, **parietal**, **temporal**, and **occipital**. An additional lobe, the **insula**, lies deep to the lateral surface of the brain and is included in some references.

The **spinal cord** is continuous with the medulla oblongata and extends inferiorly from it. A series of bony **vertebrae** enclose and protect the spinal cord. Both the brain and spinal cord are protected by connective tissue coverings called **meninges** (singular meninx). In addition, **cerebrospinal fluid (CSF)**, a clear, colorless liquid that continually circulates through cavities in the brain and spinal cord, provides mechanical and chemical protection and facilitates nutrient and waste exchange between the blood and nervous tissue.

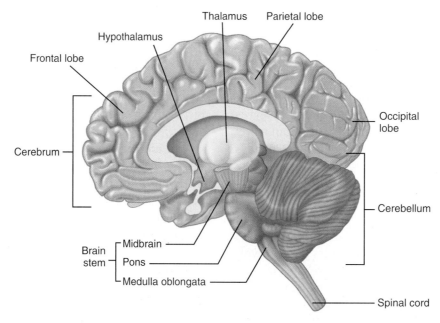

Frontal lobe

Hypothalamus

Thalamus

Parietal lobe

Occipital lobe

Cerebrum

Cerebellum

Brain stem — Midbrain / Pons / Medulla oblongata

Spinal cord

FIGURE 11.2 Midsagittal section of the brain revealing some of the major structures

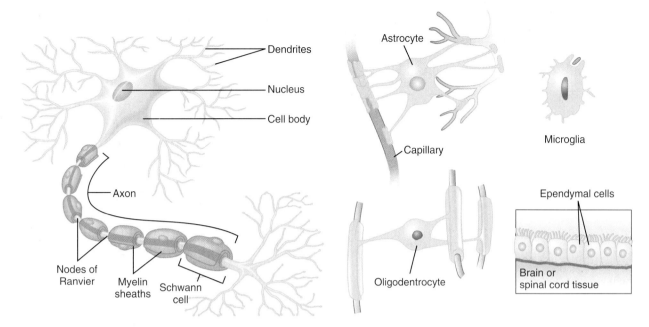

FIGURE 11.3 Components of a neuron and types of neuroglial cells

The PNS is the division that lies outside of the brain and spinal cord. It includes receptors that provide the CNS with information about organ status and the external environment, and mediates responses of muscles and organ function. Twelve pairs of **cranial nerves**, emerging from foramina, or openings in the cranial bones, and 31 pairs of **spinal nerves** that emerge through foramina between adjoining vertebrae in the vertebral column are part of the PNS and facilitate the connection of the CNS to sensory receptors, glands, and muscles throughout the body. Regions of nerves that contain large collections of neuron cell bodies are called **ganglia**. The PNS is divided into the somatic and autonomic nervous systems. The **somatic nervous system (SNS)** relays sensations that are usually consciously perceived such as temperature and pain and stimulates voluntary movement. The **autonomic nervous system (ANS)** is involved with monitoring conditions in the body's internal environment such as CO_2 and blood sugar levels and its responses are involuntary. The two branches of the ANS are the **sympathetic division** and the **parasympathetic division**. The two divisions control antagonistic responses; the sympathetic division dominates during physical or emotional stress and the parasympathetic division dominates during times of rest and recovery.

Both the CNS and PNS are made up of nervous tissue, consisting of **neurons** and various types of **neuroglial cells**. Neurons are the individual nerve cells, which conduct electrical impulses in response to stimuli. Neurons have three parts: **dendrites**, an **axon**, and a **cell body**. Dendrites are short processes that receive information and neurons typically have

multiple dendrites. Axons are long, cylindrical projections that propagate nerve impulses in the form of action potentials, away from a neuron. A neuron has only a single axon ranging in length from a millimeter to longer than a meter. The cell body of a neuron contains a cell nucleus surrounded by cytoplasm, which contains typical cellular organelles.

Neuroglial cells provide physical, metabolic, functional, and immunological support for the nervous system. **Oligodendrocytes** and **Schwann cells** are responsible for forming the myelin sheath, a multilayered lipid and protein sheath that insulates axons in the CNS and PNS, respectively. **Microglia** remove cellular debris and microbes from the CNS and **ependymal cells** produce and assist in the circulation of CSF. **Astrocytes**, so named for their star-like processes, create a blood-brain barrier by isolating neurons of the CNS from potentially harmful substances in the blood. **Satellite cells** surround the cell bodies of PNS neurons to provide nutrients and structural support.

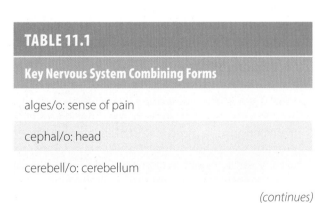

TABLE 11.1
Key Nervous System Combining Forms
alges/o: sense of pain
cephal/o: head
cerebell/o: cerebellum

(continues)

TABLE 11.2	*(continued)*
Key Nervous System Combining Forms	
cerebr/o: cerebrum	
cervic/o: neck; cervix	
clon/o: rapid contracting and relaxing	
concuss/o: to shake violently	
crani/o: skull	
dur/o: dura mater	
dynam/o: force	
electr/o: electric	
embol/o: plug	
encephal/o: brain	
esthesi/o: sensation, feeling	
esthes/o: sensation, feeling	
hemispher/o: hemisphere (of the cerebrum)	
idi/o: unknown	
lamin/o: lamina of vertebral arch	
mening/o: meninges	
meningi/o: meninges	
ment/o: mind	
myel/o: spinal cord; bone marrow	
neur/o: nerve	

Key Nervous System Combining Forms
phon/o: sound
radicul/o: nerve root
thec/o: sheath
thromb/: clot
ton/o: tone

TABLE 11.2
Key Nervous System Suffixes
-arthria: articulation
-asthenia: weakness
-cele: protrusion
-gnosia: knowledge
-grade: to go
-kinesis: movement
-paresis: weakness
-phasia: speech
-plegia: paralysis
-praxia: action
-schisis: split
-taxia: muscle coordination

🔍 STANDARD CASE STUDY

11.1 Spina Bifida

Julianna had just returned from her fetal ultrasound with a devastating diagnosis; the baby she was carrying has spina bifida. When Julianna looked up spina bifida she learned the term had a Latin origin and literally means split spine. She discovered that it could occur in varying degrees of severity including spina bifida occulta, meningocele, and myelomeningocele, all resulting from abnormal myelogenesis. Syringomyelia and agenesis of the corpus callosum are some associated nervous system malformations. Other consequences can be paraplegia, hydrocephalus, and meningitis. Julianna was distraught imagining the life ahead for her baby, until her research turned up a promising treatment advance. Prenatal surgery to correct the neurological defect has been increasingly successful. The neurosurgeon Julianna consulted confirmed that her baby was a candidate for this innovative surgery. Julianna was hopeful for a positive outcome.

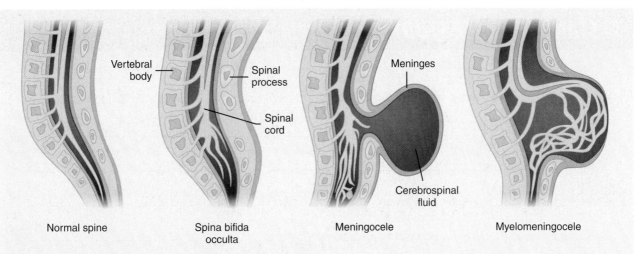

Vertebral body · Spinal process · Spinal cord · Meninges · Cerebrospinal fluid

Normal spine

Spina bifida occulta

Meningocele

Myelomeningocele

CASE FIGURE: The most common forms of spina bifida

1. The meninges are the membranes covering the spinal cord and the brain.

   Define the word parts for *meningocele.*

   Meningocele: Mening/o _____, -cele _____.

   Define the word parts for *meningitis.*

   Meningitis: Mening/o _____, -itis _____.

2. Myel/o is the combining form meaning spinal cord. (Note that myel/o can also mean bone marrow, but in this case refers to spinal cord.) List and define the words in this case study that contain the combining form myel/o, breaking the terms down into their component parts.

3. Use the combining form myel/o to form a medical term meaning splitting of the spinal cord.

4. The corpus callosum connects the left and right side of the brain. Agenesis of the corpus callosum can occur with spina bifida. What does agenesis mean?

(continues)

⌕ STANDARD CASE STUDY (continued)

5. Paraplegia can occur with spina bifida. Depending on context, the prefix para- can mean abnormal, beside, or two like parts of a pair. In the context of paraplegia, para- means _____.

   The suffix -plegia means _____.

   Paraplegia means _____.

   A term that would be used for paralysis of all four limbs would be _____.

   A term that would be used for paralysis of one limb would be _____.

6. Accumulation of cerebrospinal fluid is also known as hydrocephalus. The combining forms that make up this term are _____ and _____. What is the literal meaning of hydrocephalus? _____.

7. When would prenatal surgery be performed?

8. What questions would you recommend Julianna ask before undergoing prenatal surgery for her baby?

⌕ STANDARD CASE STUDY

11.2 Amyotrophic Lateral Sclerosis

Sebastian Emmanuel, a 48-year-old man with no significant past medical history, presents for evaluation of quadriparesis that has worsened over the past month. He is a carpenter and reports that walking distances and performing activities that require him to lift his arms over his head, such as hammering boards on houses, have become challenging. Initial examination reveals muscle atrophy of the hands and feet and difficulty with toe and heel walking. In addition, the patient has mild dysphonia when speaking. Also noticeable are fasciculations in the arms and legs. Electrodiagnostic studies, an MRI, and blood work are ordered, and the patient is instructed to return in 4 weeks.

At the 4-week follow-up visit, Mr. Emmanuel's symptoms have progressed significantly. Myasthenia in his lower limbs has made it necessary for him to ambulate with a cane. He is experiencing mild dyspnea and dysphagia. Diagnostic tests supported by his symptoms indicate a motor neuron disorder. Mr. Emmanuel is diagnosed with amyotrophic lateral sclerosis (ALS).

Prognosis for ALS is poor. Hyperreflexia and clonus can cause myalgia and cramping. Weakness is progressive and patients become wheelchair bound. Dysarthria and dysphasia develop, and it becomes progressively more difficult to eat and breathe. End-stage support is often tracheostomy with ventilator assistance and gastrostomy for nutritional support. Three years following his diagnosis, Sebastian Emmanuel died from respiratory failure secondary to ALS.

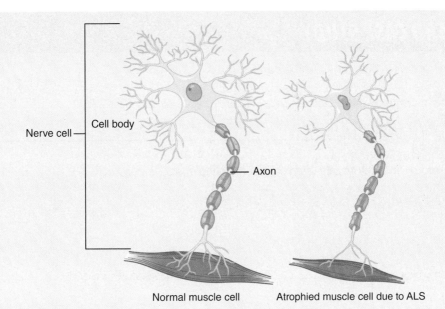

Normal muscle cell   Atrophied muscle cell due to ALS

CASE FIGURE: Atrophied muscle from nerve sclerosis in ALS

1. Define the word parts that make up the diagnosis of ALS, and then explain what ALS is.

    Amyotrophic: A- _____ , my/o _____ , -trophic _____ .

    Lateral: Later/o _____ -al _____ .

    Sclerosis: Scler/o _____ -osis _____ .

2. Mr. Emmanuel initially presents with quadriparesis, which progresses to myasthenia. Define the word parts for *quadriparesis* and *myasthenia* and provide definitions for the terms based on those parts.

    Quadriparesis:

    Myasthenia:

3. The prefix dys- means _____ .

    List and define the words in this case study using the prefix dys-, breaking the terms down into their component parts.

(continues)

🔍 *STANDARD CASE STUDY*   *(continued)*

4. Fasciculations are twitchings of muscle fibers that are classic symptoms of ALS.

    The related term clonus means _____.

    The related term hyperreflexia means _____.

5. The suffixes -otomy and -ostomy are often confused. Define *-otomy* and *-ostomy*.

    A tracheostomy procedure _____ whereas a gastrostomy procedure _____.

🔍 *STANDARD CASE STUDY*

11.3 Spinal Stenosis

Caroline Smith, a 50-year-old woman, visits Dr. Sharp, her primary care physician, with the complaint of bilateral paresthesia of the hands and sporadic cervicodynia. Caroline denies paresis of the brachial or carpal area and also denies any neuralgia. Dr. Sharp thinks Caroline may have carpal tunnel syndrome and refers her for electromyography (EMG). Following normal results from the EMG but progressively worsening paresthesia, Dr. Sharp refers Caroline to Dr. Camber, a neurologist. During Dr. Camber's exam, he notices some slight ataxia. Dr. Camber suspects Caroline may have some spinal myelopathy and orders an MRI of the cervical spine. The results of the MRI indicate radiculopathy caused by a herniated intervertebral disc.

1. Complete the table below for the following terms:

Term	Word Parts	Meaning
bilateral	*bi-; later/o; -al*	*pertaining to two sides*
paresthesia		
cervicodynia		
paresis	N/A	
brachial		
carpal		
neuralgia		
electromyography		
neurologist		
ataxia		
myelopathy		
cervical		
radiculopathy		

2. Circle the correct response for each of the three options in parentheses:

Caroline's symptoms most likely result from (sclerosis, stenosis, ptosis) of the spinal canal. A recommended treatment might be (laminectomy, neurectomy, craniotomy).

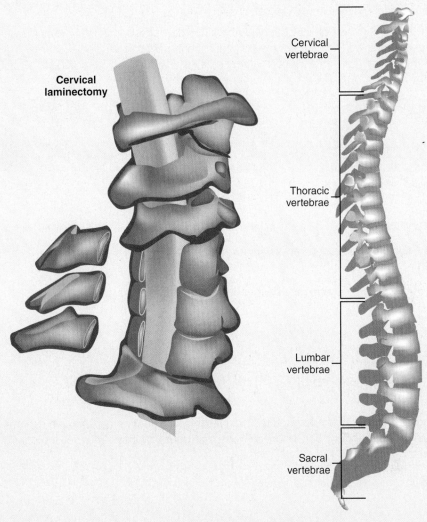

CASE FIGURE: Laminectomy to release pressure on the spinal cord

🔍 *STANDARD CASE STUDY*

11.4 Subdural Hematoma

Current Complaint: Patient is a 21-year-old female brought in by ambulance following head trauma during an ice hockey game. Patient is conscious and oriented to time and place. She has vomited several times and is complaining of vertigo and severe headache.

Past History: Patient has previously been well but apparently suffered a formerly unreported hard fall likely resulting in a concussion 2 days prior to current symptoms.

Signs and Symptoms: The player's coach reports that the player experienced a strike to the head from a hockey stick. After the hit, she skated to the sidelines and appeared confused. She then slumped over in a semiconscious state. While

(continues)

being transported by ambulance, the patient suffered a mild seizure and then regained consciousness. Along with nausea and dizziness, the patient complained of diplopia and photophobia.

Diagnosis: CT scan revealed an acute right-sided subdural hematoma.

Treatment: Surgical intervention to evacuate the hematoma. Ten days after admission to the emergency room, the patient was discharged. Headache and nausea were still present but gradually resolved over time. The patient was unable to recall the ambulance ride or the events that immediately preceded it (anterograde amnesia).

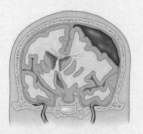 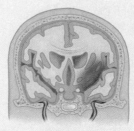 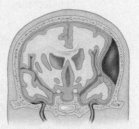

Subdural hematoma   Intracerebral hemorrhage   Epidural hematoma

CASE FIGURE: Types of intracranial hematomas

1. Indicate the word parts for *concussion* and define the term based on those parts.

2. Differential diagnosis of the reported symptoms includes subdural hematoma, epidural hematoma, and intracerebral hemorrhage. Differentiate between these three terms by indicating their word parts and defining them based on those parts:

3. Indicate the word parts for *diplopia* and define the term based on those parts.

4. Indicate the word parts for *photophobia* and define the term based on those parts.

5. What does it mean to be conscious vs. semiconscious?

6. Define the following word parts for the following surgical interventions and then circle the most likely intervention to evacuate the hematoma:

Craniometry: Crani/o _____, -metry _____.

Cranioclasis: Crani/o _____, -clasis _____.

Craniotomy: Crani/o _____, -otomy _____.

Craniectomy: Crani/o _____, -ectomy _____.

7. Amnesia means loss of memory. Indicate the word parts for *anterograde*, define the term based on those parts, and then explain what is meant by *anterograde amnesia*.

8. Why is it relevant that the patient likely suffered a concussion a few days prior to being hit in the head with a hockey stick?

🔍 STANDARD CASE STUDY

11.5 Postherpetic Neuralgia

Pain Clinic Consultation Report

Reason for Consultation: Intractable postherpetic neuralgia (PHN)

History of Present Illness: Patient is an 82-year-old female. She developed shingles, a reactivation of the herpes zoster virus, one year previous, affecting the right chest and upper back. After resolution of the acute shingles rash, she continues to suffer severe pain over the area. The pain is lancinating and constant. Other associated symptoms include allodynia, hyperesthesia, and pruritus, all of the associated area.

Past Medical History: The patient is diabetic.

(continues)

🔍 *STANDARD CASE STUDY*   *(continued)*

Results of Physical Exam: Hyperpigmentation and scarring are present along the T2 and T3 dermatomes. Hyperalgesia is present at the right anterior chest and back regions within these dermatomes.

Assessment: The patient continues to suffer from intractable neuropathic pain despite multiple interventions including pharmacological, topical, psychological, and physical therapies. Pain is interfering with patient's sleep and activities of daily living.

Recommendation: A series of three intrathecal steroid injections, each occurring a week apart with careful monitoring and follow-up.

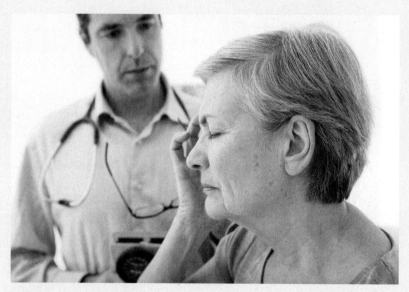

CASE FIGURE: An elderly woman in pain

© Image Point Fr/Shutterstock

1. Define the following word parts:

    Posttherpetic: Post- _____, herpetic _____ *pertaining to herpes* _____

    Neuralgia: Neur/o _____, -algia _____

    Intractable means uncontrollable. Describe what is meant by intractable posttherpetic neuralgia.

2. Complete the following table for the symptoms and physical findings of PHN:

Term	Word Parts	Meaning
allodynia	*allo-; -dynia*	*pain that is different from usual (refers to pain caused by a very light touch)*
hyperesthesia		
pruritus		

Term	Word Parts	Meaning
hyperpigmentation		
hyperalgesia		

3. Indicate the word parts for *dermatome* and define the term based on those parts. Explain what a dermatome refers to.

4. What types of interventions has the patient had?

5. Indicate the word parts for *intrathecal* and define the term based on those parts. Where is an intrathecal injection given?

🔍 *ADVANCED CASE STUDY*

11.6 Rasmussen's Encephalitis

Nine-year-old Adam was playing on the playground with his classmates. "I only have half a brain," he chanted to his friend Damen.

"Oh, I know that!" retorted Damen. "You and Zeke don't even have half a brain!"

"But I'm serious," Adam replied. "I had an operation a few years ago called a hemispherectomy that actually removed half my brain."

"A hemi- what?!!" Damen responded. "What are you talking about?"

Adam's ordeal started when he was 3 years old. Out of nowhere, he began having focal seizures. These increased in frequency and severity to refractory tonic-clonic seizures. The seizures were accompanied by altered mentation, left limb hypodynamia, ipsilateral eye deviations, and posthemiparesis on the left side of his body. Electroencephalography in conjunction with his symptoms led to a diagnosis of Rasmussen's encephalitis, a very rare chronic inflammatory neurological disease. This type of encephalitis is unihemispheric and untreated, leads to progressive atrophy of the affected side of the brain. Long-term consequences can be hemianopia, hemiplegia, aphasia, and cognitive impairment.

Adam was having seizures several times a day, which were uncontrollable with anticonvulsive medication. Surgical intervention seemed to be the only option to stop the seizures and avoid life-long disability. His parents considered hemispherotomy and hemispherectomy and in the end, they opted for the riskier surgery, but the one most likely to result in optimal seizure control.

Adam's right hemispherectomy at age 6 was a success. His seizures were completely eradicated and the amazing plasticity of the nervous system allowed the right side of his brain to take over for his left. With some residual slight paralysis on his left side Adam now lives a normal life.

"You and Zeke may have your whole brains but I'm pretty smart with my half brain," said Adam with a soft undertone as recess ended and he went in to take his math test.

(continues)

🔍 *ADVANCED CASE STUDY* *(continued)*

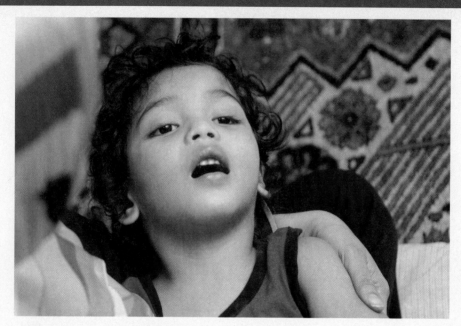

CASE FIGURE: Adam as a toddler having a seizure

© Lens Hitam/Shutterstock

1. What is a focal seizure?

2. What is a tonic-clonic seizure? Use the roots of the terms tonic and clonic to help you define them. What does it mean to be refractory?

3. Indicate the word parts for *encephalitis* and define the term based on those parts.

4. Rasmussen's encephalitis is unihemispheric. Indicate the word parts for *unihemispheric* and define the term based on those parts.

Electroencephalography was used as a diagnostic tool. Define the word parts and meaning for this procedure.

Electroencephalography: Electr/o _____, encephal/o _____,

-graphy _____,

means _____.

5. Complete the table below, listing the symptoms and long-term effects of Rasmussen's encephalitis:

Term	Word Parts	Meaning
mentation (altered)	*ment/o; -ation*	*state of the mind*
hypodynamia		
ipsilateral (eye deviations)		
hemiparesis		
atrophy		
hemianopia		
hemiplegia		
aphasia		

6. Complete the table below, listing treatments of Rasmussen's encephalitis:

Term	Word Parts	Meaning
anticonvulsive		
hemispherotomy		
hemispherectomy		

7. What do you think plasticity is and why did this aid in Adam's recovery?

⌕ *ADVANCED CASE STUDY*

11.7 CSF Rhinorrhea

The patient is a 50-year-old overweight female complaining of progressively worsening clear nasal discharge over the past several months. More recently, she has had some dizziness and nausea accompanied by orthostatic headache. When asked about other pain, she reports discomfort in her interscapular region and in the proximal region of her upper arms. She also mentions an appetite decrease, which she attributes to hyposmia and altered gustation. Laboratory analysis of the leaking fluid identifies it as cerebrospinal fluid. Idiopathic CSF rhinorrhea is not common but appears more frequently in females who are middle-aged and obese. Potential complications of CSF rhinorrhea include meningitis, pneumocephalus, hydrocephalus, and intracranial hypotension. CT and MRI of the head identify the source of the leak and a transnasal endoscopic repair is performed. Symptoms resolve postoperatively and following a six-week period of restricted activity, the patient is completely recovered.

1. Indicate the word parts for *rhinorrhea* and define the term based on those parts.

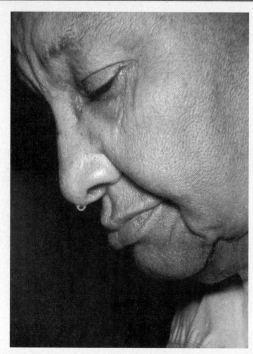

CASE FIGURE: Clear nasal discharge of CSF rhinorrhea

Dr. Thomas Sellers, Emory University, Atlanta, Georgia/Centers for Disease Control and Prevention

2. What is idiopathic CSF rhinorrhea?

3. What is an orthostatic headache?

4. Where is the patient's pain?

5. Circle the correct response: The patient's appetite has decreased due to
   a. decreased thirst and altered taste.
   b. decreased smell and altered taste.
   c. decreased smell and altered glucose metabolism.
   d. offensive breath odor and altered glucose metabolism.

6. Complete the following table for the symptoms of CSF rhinorrhea. It can sometimes be challenging to correlate the literal meaning of the word parts with the actual term definition. Use a medical dictionary to complete the fourth column of this table.

Term	Word Parts	Word Part Meaning	Actual Term Definition
meningitis	mening/o; -itis	inflammation of the meninges	inflammation of the membranes of the spinal cord or brain
pneumocephalus			
hydrocephalus			
intracranial hypotension			

7. What type of procedure is a transnasal endoscopic repair? Indicate and define the component word parts.

🔍 ADVANCED CASE STUDY

11.8 Brachial Plexus Injury

"You came down pretty hard on your shoulder after that tackle," said Dwayne to his buddy Akim in the locker room after the football game. "You'll really feel that tomorrow."

"You're not kidding," responded Akim. When I fell, it felt like an electric shock going down my arm. Now my arm feels numb and weak."

"Oh, that's called a burner or a stinger," said Dwayne. "They're common in defensive players after a hard impact fall on the shoulder. Your arm should feel back to normal pretty quickly."

A week later, Akim's arm was pretty painful and still numb and weak. He headed to the sports medicine clinic for an evaluation. "Your dysesthesia is from a brachial plexus injury," explained Dr. Canfield. "There is a wide range of severity and effects from that type of injury. From your neurological exam, it appears that the injury you sustained is a neurapraxia, the least severe of these types of injury. It is unlikely that you have a nerve rupture or an avulsion or your symptoms would be significantly worse. I'm going to refer you to the physical therapy department and they can help with some stretching and strengthening exercises. In addition, I've had quite a bit of luck having patients use a TENS (transcutaneous electrical nerve stimulation) unit for analgesia. You may not return to football until your symptoms have completely resolved. I'd like to see you back in 4 weeks."

As Dr. Canfield had believed, Akim's injury was relatively minor and by his follow-up visit, he had recovered completely. He was cleared to return to football just in time for their first playoff game.

(continues)

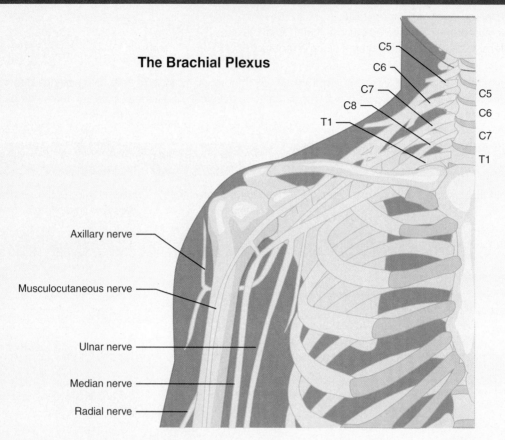

The Brachial Plexus

C5
C6
C7
C8
T1

C5
C6
C7
T1

Axillary nerve

Musculocutaneous nerve

Ulnar nerve

Median nerve

Radial nerve

CASE FIGURE: Nerves of the brachial plexus

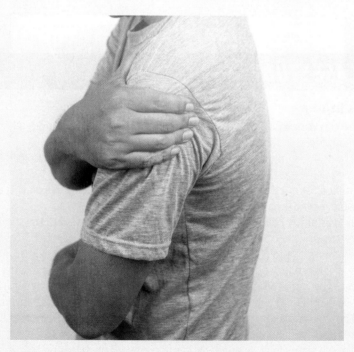

CASE FIGURE: Shoulder pain from a brachial plexus injury

1. What is a plexus? Where would the brachial plexus be located?

2. Indicate the word parts for *neurapraxia* and define the term based on those parts.

3. Nerve rupture and avulsion both refer to tearing of a nerve to different degrees and require surgical intervention. The following suffixes are often confused. Define them and then build a word with the combining form *neur/o* that would refer to an appropriate surgical procedure to repair a torn nerve.

   -rrhexis

   -rrhea

   -rrhaphy

   -rrhagia

4. TENS stands for transcutaneous electrical nerve stimulation and is used for analgesia.

   Indicate the word parts for *transcutaneous* and *analgesia* and define the terms based on their parts.

   How do you think a TENS unit works to relieve pain?

🔍 *ADVANCED CASE STUDY*

11.9 Synkinesis

Mrs. Lomax is a 51-year-old woman who developed a left-sided Bell's palsy 2 years ago. Bell's palsy is an acute mononeuropathy leading to unilateral facial paralysis. Incomplete closure of the eyelid, drooping of the eyebrow and pain around one ear on the same side of the face are common. Onset is sudden, often with an idiopathic origin, although some studies indicate it is related to a viral exposure. Many cases of Bell's palsy resolve completely within a few months, but in some cases, like Mrs. Lomax's, abnormal regrowth of nerve fibers can lead to synkinesis.

Synkinesis refers to involuntary movements accompanying voluntary ones. Mrs. Lomax's synkinesis is ocular-oral; her eye closes each time she attempts to close her lips or smile. She has facial pain, which has worsened over time due to repeated involuntary muscle contractions. Examination reveals significant facial asymmetry and fullness, likely from hypertrophy of hyper-contractile muscles. Physiotherapy and injections of botulinum toxin to block nerve activity to the overworked muscles have had limited success. Today's visit for Mrs. Lomax is to discuss selective neurolysis with Dr. Cambrian, who specializes in this treatment. Mrs. Lomax is hopeful that this surgical procedure will relieve her pain, restore the symmetry of her facial features, and allow her to generate a natural smile.

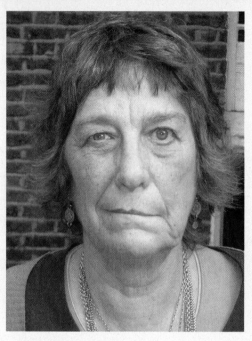

CASE FIGURE: Facial asymmetry from Bell's palsy

© Sally and Richard Greenhill/Alamy Stock Photo

1. Bell's palsy is described as an acute mononeuropathy leading to unilateral facial paralysis. Indicate the word parts, and their definitions, for *acute mononeuropathy* and then describe Bell's palsy in your own words.

2. Circle the correct response: The suffix for drooping is
   a. -ptysis.
   b. -ptosis.
   c. -porosis.
   d. -tocia.

3. Would pain referring to two structures on the same side be ipsilateral or contralateral?

4. Indicate the word parts for *idiopathic* and define the term based on those parts.

5. Complete the following table for possible complications of Bell's palsy:

Term	Word Parts	Meaning
synkinesis	*syn-; -kinesis*	*together movement*
hypertrophy		
asymmetry		

6. Indicate the word parts for *neurolysis* and define the term based on those parts. Then explain why selective neurolysis might be an effective treatment for synkinesis.

7. How might physiotherapy and botulinum toxin (BOTOX®) achieve the same results?

🔍 ADVANCED CASE STUDY

11.10 Transient Ischemic Attack

The patient is a 70-year-old woman accompanied by her husband. She has been a life-long smoker, has hypertension, and has hypercholesterolemia. When asked why she is there she says her "episodes have been happening more often." When asked what episodes she refers to, her husband provides more details. He relates instances over the past year when his wife sees only half an image in both eyes, but just for a brief time. More recently, she has been experiencing periodic bouts of dizziness and what she has called "brain fog." The most recent incident, and the one that made her husband insistent on a visit to the doctor, was a momentary event where she was unable to speak or move.

Based on the signs and symptoms described, the physician suspects a series of transient ischemic attacks (TIAs) due to a blockage causing hypoxia to the brain. During a complete physical exam, a bruit, characteristic of stenosis, is discovered over the carotid artery. Partial occlusion of the left carotid artery is confirmed by ultrasound. Magnetic resonance angiography (MRA) shows a high-grade blockage of 85%. Due to the risk for a major cerebral infarction or stroke, left carotid endarterectomy is recommended as soon as possible. Following recovery from the surgery, the patient will be prescribed anticoagulants and will be counseled to make several lifestyle changes to further decrease her risk for stroke.

1. The medical term for the ocular disturbances experienced by the patient is hemianopia. Indicate the word parts for *hemianopia* and define the term based on those parts.

(continues)

2. Indicate the word parts for *hypoxia* and define the term based on those parts. How does hypoxia relate to the patient's symptoms?

3. A bruit is an abnormal sound heard through a stethoscope. It is an initial, noninvasive way to detect stenosis of an artery, often caused by atherosclerosis. Differentiate between the two like-sounding terms *stenosis* and *atherosclerosis* by indicating their word parts and providing definitions based on those parts.

4. Stroke can be a major life changing and debilitating event. Differentiate the types of stroke listed below by indicating the word parts for *ischemic*, *thrombotic*, *embolic*, and *hemorrhagic*, and provide definitions for the terms based on those parts:

   Transient ischemic attack:

   Thrombotic:

   Embolic:

   Hemorrhagic:

   Stroke is also known as a cerebral infarction. Cerebral means _____.

   Infarction means _____.

5. The following terms, all with different meanings, can be signs of cerebral vascular disease or stroke. Indicate the words parts for the following terms and provide definitions based on those parts:

   Apraxia:

   Agnosia:

Aphasia:

Ataxia:

6. Define the word parts and the meaning for each of the following procedural terms:

Angiography: Angi/o _____, -graphy _____,

means _____

Endarterectomy: Endo-_____, arteri/o _____,

-ectomy _____,

means _____

7. Preventative follow-up is a must following surgery. What risk factors does the patient have that will require lifestyle changes?

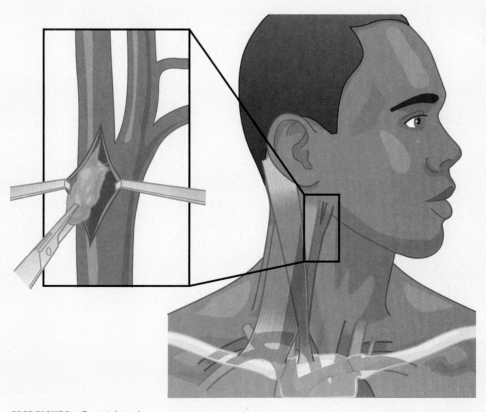

CASE FIGURE: Carotid endarterectomy

References

Dworkin, R. H., O'Connor, A. B., Kent, J., Mackey, S. C., Raja, S. N., Stacey, B. R., Levy, R. M., Backonja, M., Baron, R., Harke, H., Loeser, J. D., Treede, R. D., Turk, D. C., & Wells, C. D. (2013). Interventional management of neuropathic pain: NeuPSIG recommendations. *Pain*, *154*(11), 2249–2261. https://doi.org/10.1016/j.pain.2013.06.004

Fereydooni, A., Gorecka, J., Xu, J., Schindler, J., & Dardik, A. (2019). Carotid endarterectomy and carotid artery stenting for patients with crescendo transient ischemic attacks: A systematic review. *JAMA Surgery*, *154*(11), 1055–1063. https://doi.org/10.1001/jamasurg.2019.2952

Grad, L. I., Rouleau, G. A., Ravits, J., & Cashman, N. R. (2017). Clinical spectrum of Amyotrophic Lateral Sclerosis (ALS). *Cold Spring Harbor Perspectives in Medicine*, *7*(8), a024117. https://doi.org/10.1101/cshperspect.a024117

Heuer, G. G., Moldenhauer, J. S., & Adzick, N. S. (2017). Prenatal surgery for myelomeningocele: Review of the literature and future directions. *Child's Nervous System*, *33*, 1149–1155. doi:10.1007/s00381-017-3440-z

Lobo, B. C., Baumanis, M. M., & Nelson, R. F. (2017). Surgical repair of spontaneous cerebrospinal fluid (CSF) leaks: A systematic review. *Laryngoscope Investigative Otolaryngology*, *2*(5), 215–224. https://doi.org/10.1002/lio2.75

Melancia, J. L., Francisco, A. F., & Antunes, J. L. (2014). Spinal stenosis. *Handbook of Clinical Neurology*, *119*, 541–549. https://doi.org/10.1016/B978-0-7020-4086-3.00035-7g

Pourmomeny, A. A., & Asadi, S. (2014). Management of synkinesis and asymmetry in facial nerve palsy: A review article. *Iranian Journal of Otorhinolaryngology*, *26*(77), 251–256.

Starr, H. M., Jr, Anderson, B., Courson, R., & Seiler, J. G. (2014). Brachial plexus injury: A descriptive study of American football. *Journal of Surgical Orthopaedic Advances*, *23*(2), 90–97. https://doi.org/10.3113/jsoa.2014.0090

Stedman, T. L. (2005). Nath's *Stedman's medical terminology, 2e.* Philadelphia: Lippincott Williams & Wilkins.

Stovits, S. D., Weseman, J. D., Hooks, M. C., Schmidt, R. J., Koffel, J. B., & Patricios, J. S. (2017). What definition is used to describe second impact syndrome in sports? A systematic and critical review. *Current Sports Medicine Reports*, *16*(1), 50–55. doi:10.1249/jsr.0000000000000326

Venes, D. & Taber, C. W. (2017). *Taber's cyclopedic medical dictionary*. Ed. 23, illustrated in full color/Philadelphia: F.A. Davis.

Vining, E. P., Freeman, J. M., Pillas, D. J., Uematsu, S., Carson, B. S., Brandt, Boatman, D., Pulsifer, M. B., & Zuckerberg, A. (1997). Why would you remove half a brain? The outcome of 58 children after hemispherectomy—The Johns Hopkins experience: 1968 to 1996. *Pediatrics*, *100*(2), 163–171. doi:10.1542/peds.100.2.163

CHAPTER 12

Special Senses: Eye and Ear

Special senses are those that have specialized organs devoted to them. The eye, responsible for vision, and the ear, responsible for hearing and balance, are two of these specialized organs. Receptor cells in the eye and ear are excited by external stimuli. Nerve fibers carry these impulses to the brain where they are translated into visual images and sound sensations.

▶ The Eye

The eyes are the organs of vision; they contain more than half the sensory receptors in the human body. Each eyeball measures about 2.5 cm in diameter in an adult, but only one-sixth of it is exposed. The remainder is recessed into a bony cavity of the skull known as the orbit. The wall of the eyeball is made up of three layers: the sclera, the uvea, and the retina.

The outer layer of the eyeball is the **sclera,** or "white of the eye." It is a tough, fibrous layer of dense connective tissue that protects the eye's inner structures. The anterior portion of the sclera is transparent and is known as the **cornea**. The cornea covers the colored **iris**.

The **uvea** is a vascular layer that provides the blood supply for the eye; it is made up of the choroid, the ciliary body, and the iris. The **choroid** lies beneath the sclera. This highly vascularized structure delivers oxygen and nutrients to the retina. The **ciliary body** is found at the anterior of the choroid. It secretes **aqueous humor**, a watery fluid filling the spaces between the cornea and the lens. One function of this fluid is to maintain intraocular pressure, giving the eyeball its roughly spherical shape. Suspensory ligaments of the ciliary body suspend the **lens** behind the iris. The hole in the center of the iris, which allows light rays to enter the eyeball, is called the **pupil**.

The **retina** is the deepest of the three layers of the eye, lining the posterior three-quarters of the eyeball. It contains the photoreceptor sensory cells, the rods, and cones, which respond to light. Rods allow vision in dim light such as moonlight. Bright light stimulates cones, which are sensitive to blue, green, or red light, providing

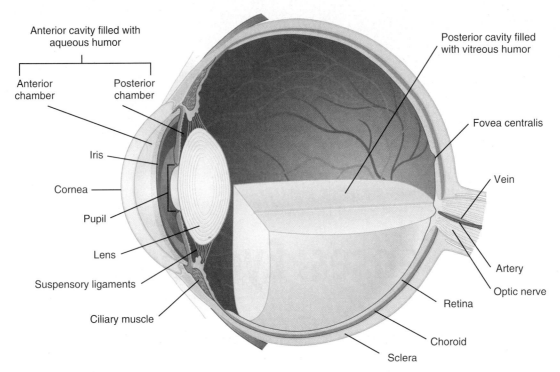

FIGURE 12.1 Sagittal section of the human eye revealing the major tissues and structures

color vision. Interestingly, the surface of the retina is the only place in the body where blood vessels can be viewed directly and observed for pathological changes. The instrument used for this is called an ophthalmoscope. The large space between the lens and the retina is filled with a semisolid gel known as the **vitreous humor**.

Light rays enter the eye at the cornea and then pass through the pupil to the lens, which focuses light on the rods and cones of the retina. The iris muscles control constriction and dilation of the pupil, regulating how much light enters the eye. An upside-down image is formed by the retina and is transmitted as sensory impulses to the optic nerve, which meets the retina at the back of the eye at the optic disc. The impulses are ultimately processed by the primary visual area in the occipital lobe of the cerebral cortex of the brain and the image is translated to one that is right side up. In addition to the components of the eyeball, several accessory structures help protect the eye. The eyelids protect the eye from foreign particles and intense light, the **conjunctiva** is a transparent mucous membrane that covers the outer surface of the eye, and the **lacrimal glands** produce tears to wash and lubricate the eyeball.

▶ The Ear

The ear transduces mechanical sound vibrations into electrical signals that provide the sense of hearing. Interestingly, the human ear continues to function even while sleeping but the brain blocks out the sound. The ear can be divided in three regions: the external or outer ear, the middle ear, and the inner ear.

The external ear is made up of the auricle, external auditory canal, and tympanic membrane. The visible portion of an ear is called the **auricle**, or **pinna**. It is a flap of elastic cartilage attached by ligaments and muscles to the side of the head. Sound waves enter the auditory canal, or external acoustic meatus. The auditory canal is lined with oil glands that secrete a waxy substance called **cerumen**, which lubricates and protects the ear. Sound waves that enter the canal are channeled approximately 2.5 cm to the **tympanic membrane**, also called the eardrum.

The middle ear is a small, air-filled cavity separated from the external ear by the tympanic membrane. The **auditory ossicles**, the smallest bones in the body, extend across the middle ear. These bones, connected by synovial joints, are the **malleus, incus**, and **stapes**. The middle ear is separated from the inner ear by a thin membrane called the oval window and is connected to the nasopharynx by the **auditory tube**, more commonly known as the **eustachian tube**. Air enters this tube during yawning or swallowing to equalize the pressure in the middle ear with atmospheric pressure, thereby preventing damage to the tympanic membrane.

The inner ear is a fluid-filled cavity called the labyrinth because of its maze-like shape. The **vestibule** is the first structure of the inner ear. From the vestibule extend three semicircular canals and the cochlea. The

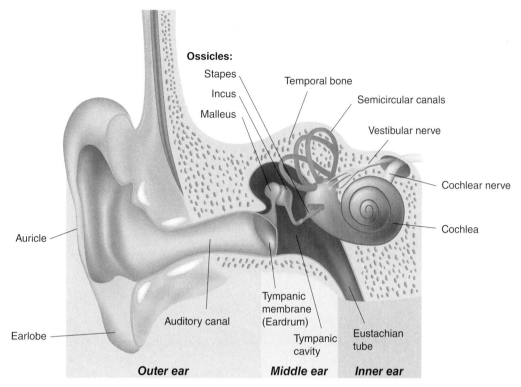

Ossicles:
Stapes
Incus
Malleus
Temporal bone
Semicircular canals
Vestibular nerve
Cochlear nerve
Cochlea
Auricle
Tympanic
membrane
(Eardrum)
Tympanic
cavity
Eustachian
tube
Auditory canal
Earlobe
Outer ear   **Middle ear**   **Inner ear**

FIGURE 12.2 The major structures of the human ear

© Alila Sao Mai/Shutterstock

bony **semicircular canals** are important for balance and equilibrium. The snail shell-shaped **cochlea** contains the receptors for hearing.

Sound waves, originating from vibrating objects, are the input for hearing. These waves are directed by the auricle into the external auditory canal to the tympanic membrane causing it to vibrate. The malleus, connected to the central area of the eardrum, begins to vibrate, and these vibrations are transmitted to the incus, then the stapes, and in turn the oval window. The movement of the oval window generates fluid pressure waves in the cochlea. As the waves travel through the cochlea, they distort long, thread-like stereocilia on the surface of **hair cells**. This activates the hair cells, causing them to send electrical impulses along auditory nerve fibers to the cerebral cortex of the brain, where the impulses are interpreted as sound.

TABLE 12.2
Key Special Senses Combining Forms
acous/o: hearing
aden/o: gland
ambyl/o: dull, dim
audi/o: hearing
audit/o: hearing
aur/o: ear
auricul/o: ear
bar/o: pressure
blephar/o: eyelid
cerumin/o: cerumen
chrom/o: color
chromat/o: color

TABLE 12.1
Key Special Senses Prefixes
eso-: inward
myo-: to shut

(continues)

TABLE 12.2	(continued)
Key Special Senses Combining Forms	
cochle/o: cochlea	
conjunctiv/o: conjunctiva	
corne/o: cornea	
cor/o: pupil	
dacry/o: tear, lacrimal	
dacryoaden/o: tear (lacrimal) gland	
dacryocyst/o: tear (lacrimal) sac	
emmetr/o: correct, proper	
goni/o: angle	
glauc/o: gray	
ir/o: iris	
irid/o: iris	
kerat/o: horny tissue; cornea	
labyrinth/o: labyrinth	
lacrim/o: tears	
laryng/o: larynx	
macul/o: macula lutea	
metr/o: measurement	
mi/o: lessening	
myc/o: fungus	
mydr/o: widening	
myring/o: tympanic membrane	
nyctal/o: night	
ocul/o: eye	
ophthalm/o: eye	
opt/o: eye, vision	

Key Special Senses Combining Forms	
optic/o: eye, vision	
ot/o: ear	
phon/o: sound	
phot/o: light	
presby/o: old age	
pupill/o: pupil	
retin/o: retina	
salping/o: auditory tube, eustachian tube; ovarian tube	
scler/o: sclera; hard	
son/o: sound	
staped/o: stapes	
stigmat/o: point	
ton/o: pressure	
topic/o: specific area	
tympan/o: tympanic membrane	
uve/o: uvea	
vitre/o: glassy	

TABLE 12.3	
Key Special Senses Suffixes	
-acusis: hearing	
-cusis: hearing	
-opia: vision condition	
-opsia: vision condition	
-osmia: olfactory condition	
-otia: ear condition	
-tropia: turned condition	

🔍 *STANDARD CASE STUDY*

12.1 Birdshot Chorioretinopathy

It was a bright summer day when Darcy Cooke, 55, first became aware of the floaters and flashers in front of her eyes. She assumed it was from the sun and didn't think much about it. Over the next year they appeared more frequently, and her vision became blurry as if she were looking through murky water. Darcy also noticed reduced peripheral vision and decreased depth perception. Her family encouraged her to make an appointment with an ophthalmologist.

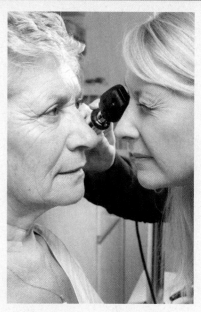

CASE FIGURE: Ophthalmologist examining a patient

© Andrew Bassett/Shutterstock

Dr. Moss questions Darcy about her symptoms, then notes the following visual disturbances: photopsia, photophobia, nyctalopia, dyschromatopsia, and metamorphopsia. She follows with a comprehensive eye exam. Ophthalmoscopy using mydriatic drops reveals mild bilateral vitritis and oval cream-colored posterior choroidal lesions. The ophthalmologist recognizes these spots as indicative of posterior uveitis, also called birdshot chorioretinopathy, so named because the hypopigmented lesions mimic the pattern seen when birdshot pellets are fired from a shotgun. Further imaging with fluorescein angiography reveals evidence of macular edema and retinal vasculitis. Treatment for "birdshot," as it is known, is typically corticosteroids to reduce inflammation and immunomodulating drugs, due to the presumptive autoimmune mechanism of the disease. "Birdshot" is usually progressive, although remission is possible. Monitoring of treatment efficacy for Darcy will be done regularly with perimetry to assess peripheral field loss and electroretinography to evaluate the status of the retina. Long-term, well-monitored treatment can help patients retain visual acuity.

1. Complete the table for the visual disturbances associated with "birdshot." Translate the words directly from their word parts and then use a medical dictionary, if necessary, to write an interpretation of how the term is actually used.

Term	Word Parts	Meaning
photopsia	*phot/o; -opsia*	*vision condition of light (refers to flashes of light in the visual field)*
photophobia		
nyctalopia		
dyschromatopsia		
metamorphopsia		

2. Define the word parts, and meaning, for *vitritis, uveitis, macular edema, and retinal vasculitis*.

Vitritis: Vitre/o _____, -itis _____, means _____.

Uveitis: Uve/o _____, -itis _____, means _____.

Macular edema: Macul/o _____ -ar _____,

edema _____, means _____.

(continues)

Retinal vasculitis: Retin/o _____, -al _____,

vascul/o _____, -itis _____,

means _____.

3. Several diagnostic procedures are mentioned in this case study. List these, indicate and define relevant word parts, and explain their use.

4. What is visual acuity?

🔍 *STANDARD CASE STUDY*

12.2 Otitis Externa

Twelve-year-old Micah Brennan presents to the Urgent Care Clinic with otalgia and otorrhea and aural fullness. Three weeks prior, he was diagnosed with otitis media and prescribed oral antimicrobials and ototopical drops. He has a previous history of tympanostomy tube placement at age 7. His failure to respond to antibiotics raises the suspicion of otomycosis. Examination with an otomicroscope reveals edema and erythema of the auditory canal and a diagnosis of otitis externa is made. Grayish white debris, indicative of the fungal hyphae of *Aspergillus*, is present. Tympanorrhexis, known to make the management of otomycosis more challenging, has not occurred. The boy is a competitive swimmer, an activity known to increase the risk for otomycosis as frequent water exposure removes protective cerumen. The auditory canal is cleared of debris and discharge and antifungal eardrops are prescribed. Micah is instructed to wait at least a week before returning to the pool and to use earplugs while swimming to keep water out of his ears. He is told to dry his ears well after swimming, possibly with a hairdryer set on low, and is directed to avoid putting cotton swabs in his ears.

1. Contrast otitis externa and otitis media.

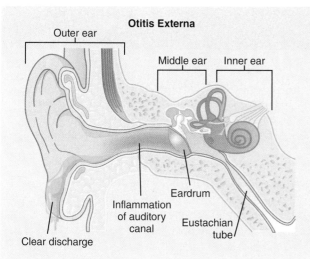

Otitis Externa

CASE FIGURE: Otitis externa, also known as swimmer's ear

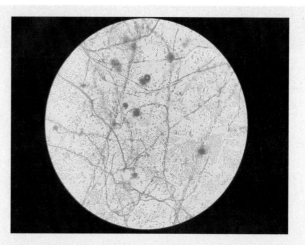

CASE FIGURE: The fungal hyphae of *Aspergillus*, one of the causative agents of otomycosis

© Mohd Firdaus Othman/Shutterstock

2. Complete the following table of terms from the case using the root for ear.

Term	Word Parts	Meaning
otalgia	*ot/o; -algia*	*pain in the ear*
otorrhea		
aural (fullness)		
ototopical		
otomycosis		
otomicroscope		

3. Provide brief definitions of edema, erythema, and cerumen.

4. List the terms in the case using the root for the tympanic membrane (ear drum), indicate their word parts, and define the terms.

Another root used for eardrum is _____

⌕ *STANDARD CASE STUDY*

12.3 Ocular Errors of Refraction

Grant Hunter, 55, was at the optician's office to have his prescription filled for his new eyeglasses. His earlier visit to the optometrist to have his eyesight evaluated included ophthalmoscopy, slit lamp microscopy, reading from a Snellen chart, tonometry, and a visual field test. Grant had worn glasses since he was 12, both to correct an astigmatism and worsening myopia. Now that Grant was getting older, he would need bifocals for correction of presbyopia.

"I hate that I'm getting old," said Grant to Tom the optician, "I'm not ready for bifocals. And I hope I don't have any more painful eye issues like that darn bout with dacryoadenitis last year when I had to visit the ophthalmologist."

"You're not all that old," responded Tom, "and at least the vision in your eyes is relatively equal and your glasses provide you emmetropia. I had a client in here last week who had hyperopia in both eyes, but the eyes were wildly different from each other. Challenging to make glasses for. And several years ago, I had a client near-sighted in one eye and far-sighted in the other eye!"

"Is there such a thing?" asked Grant.

"Rare, but yes there is," said Tom. It's a form of anisometropia, called antimetropia."

"Hmm, interesting," murmured Grant. "OK, I guess I could be much worse off in terms of my vision. I'll be back next week to pick up my new glasses."

1. Define the following word parts for *optometrist*, *optician*, and *ophthalmologist*, the medical professionals in this case study.

   Optometrist: Opt/o _____, -metrist _____.

   Optician: Opt/o _____, -ician _____.

   Ophthalmologist: Ophthalm/o _____, -logist _____.

2. Provide a brief description of the following evaluative procedures. You may need to use a medical dictionary or other reliable resource.

   Ophthalmoscopy:

   Slit lamp microscopy:

   Snellen chart:

   Tonometry:

   Visual field test:

3. Indicate and define the component word parts for *dacryoadenitis*.

4. Refraction refers to the bending of light. Complete the table for the following refractive vision errors.

Term	Word Parts	Meaning
astigmatism	*a-; stigmat/o; -ism*	*state of without a point (light is not sharply focused on the retina)*
myopia		
hyperopia		
presbyopia		
anisometropia		
antimetropia		

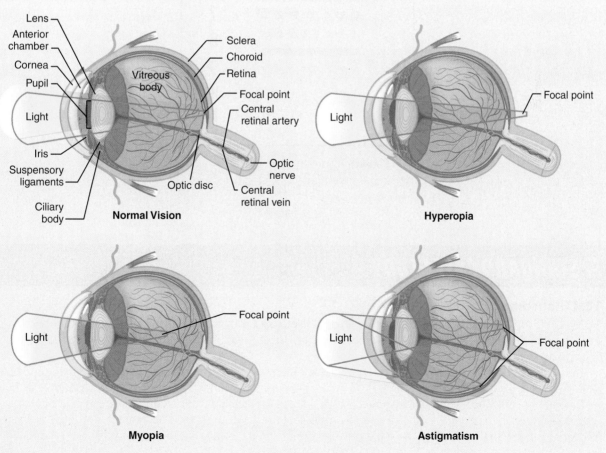

CASE FIGURE: Focal points for various refractive errors of vision

(continues)

🔍 *STANDARD CASE STUDY*   *(continued)*

5. Indicate and define the word parts and meaning for *emmetropia*.

    Emmetropia: Emmetr/o _____, -opia _____,

    means _____.

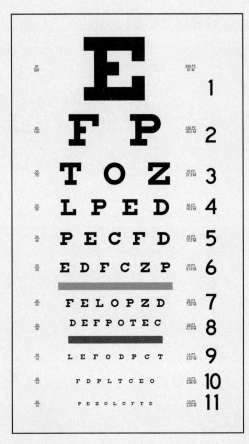

CASE FIGURE: A Snellen chart, used to determine visual acuity

© Germán Ariel Berra/Shutterstock

🔍 *STANDARD CASE STUDY*

12.4 Glaucoma

A 62-year-old African American male presents to an ophthalmologist with complaints of blurred vision, tunnel vision, and headaches. His medical history includes type 2 diabetes, diabetic retinopathy, and uveitis. He reports having an older brother with glaucoma.

   The patient's pupils are dilated to prepare for ophthalmoscopy, which reveals bilateral retinal hemorrhage and optic neuropathy.

   Tonometry results show significant asymmetry in the intraocular pressures supporting a diagnosis of glaucoma. Gonioscopy, used to measure iridocorneal angle, indicates that the glaucoma is likely open-angle, not angle-closure, glaucoma. In open-angle glaucoma, the angle between the iris and the cornea is 20–45 degrees, allowing aqueous humor to migrate from posterior to anterior chamber.

   The patient is prescribed antiglaucoma medication in an effort to reduce the amount of vitreous humor produced.

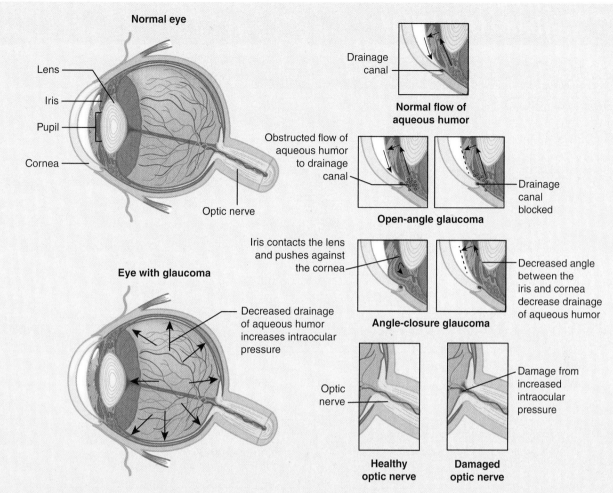

CASE FIGURE: Open-angle glaucoma and angle-closure glaucoma

1. Define the following word parts, meaning, for *ophthalmologist.*

   Ophthalmologist: Ophthalm/o _____, -logist _____,

   means _____.

2. Part of the patient's medical history includes uveitis, an inflammation of the middle layer of the wall of the eye, the uvea. Complete the table below for the following terms related to an inflammation of different tissues of the eye.

Term	Word Parts	Affected Tissue
uveitis	*uve/o; -itis*	*uvea*
keratitis		
scleritis		

(continues)

Term	Word Parts	Affected Tissue
conjunctivitis		
blepharitis		
dacryoadenitis		
dacryocystitis		

3. The patient has type 2 diabetes, with a history of diabetic retinopathy. Type 2 diabetes may be associated with glaucoma, a group of disorders that are characterized by increased intraocular pressure, and can lead to optic nerve damage. Define the following word parts, and meaning, for *retinopathy*, *glaucoma*, and *intraocular*.

Retinopathy: Retin/o _____, -pathy _____,

means _____.

Glaucoma: Glauc/o _____, -oma _____,

means _____.

Note, the word parts of *glaucoma* describe how an affected eye may appear.

Intraocular: Intra- _____, ocul/o _____, -ar _____,

means _____.

4. Gonioscopy is used to measure the iridocorneal angle. Based on the word parts of iridocorneal, between what two anatomical structures is the angle being measured?

5. Define the following word parts, and meaning, for the three diagnostic procedures used in this case; ophthalmoscopy, tonometry, and gonioscopy. Use a medical dictionary, or other reputable resources, if necessary.

Ophthalmoscopy: Ophthalm/o _____, -scopy _____,

means _____.

Tonometry: Ton/o _____, -metry _____,

means _____.

Gonioscopy: Goni/o _____, -scopy _____,

means _____.

🔍 *STANDARD CASE STUDY*

12.5 Myringoplasty

A 45-year-old male is brought to a step-down unit, in stable condition, after being treated for trauma sustained from an accident involving explosives at a quarry. The patient is presenting with otorrhagia and otalgia and is referred to otolaryngology for assessment. Otoscopy reveals bilateral otorrhea and tympanic membrane perforation due to otic barotrauma. The explosion led to a massive pressure discrepancy between the outer and middle ear, resulting in the rupture of the pars tensa, the thinnest region of the tympanic membrane. A tuning fork test and audiometry determined the audiological function was significantly impaired. The ruptured membranes will be repaired with fat graft myringoplasty.

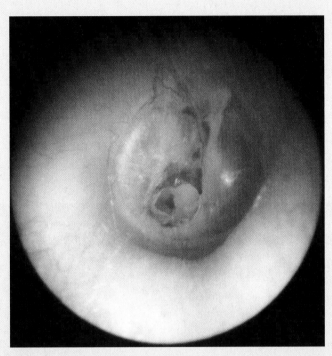

CASE FIGURE: Perforated pars tensa region of the tympanic membrane

© Mikhail V. Komarov/Shutterstock

1. Define the following word parts, and meaning, for *otolaryngology*.

   Otolaryngology: Ot/o _____, laryng/o _____,

   -logy _____, means _____.

2. Complete the table below for the following terms related to the patient's signs and symptoms:

Term	Word Parts	Meaning
otoscopy	ot/o; -scopy	*process of viewing the ear*
otorrhagia		
otalgia		
bilateral		
otorrhea		

(continues)

🔍 STANDARD CASE STUDY   *(continued)*

3. In this case study, the tympanic membranes perforated due to barotrauma. What is meant by barotrauma?

4. Briefly describe two types of procedures: tuning fork tests and audiometry, used to assess audiological function in this case.

5. A fat graft myringoplasty uses adipose tissue transferred from elsewhere in the patient's body to repair small tympanic membrane perforations. Define the word parts of myringoplasty.

   Word: Myring/o _____, -plasty _____.

🔍 ADVANCED CASE STUDY

12.6 Horner Syndrome

Current Complaint: A 4-week-old infant is brought to her pediatrician for evaluation of abnormal ocular features observed by her parents. The baby's pupils are different sizes, one eyelid droops, and oddly, the irises of her eyes are different colors.

Relevant Past History: The infant is recovering from a brachial plexus injury suffered at birth due to shoulder dystocia.

Signs and Symptoms: Anisocoria and heterochromia iridum are present as described by the parents. Mild unilateral blepharoptosis, accompanied by ipsilateral miosis and enophthalmos are apparent. Anhidrosis on the affected side is also observed. Pupillary asymmetry is greater in the dark and is increased by the application of diagnostic eyedrops to each eye.

Diagnosis: Damage to the ipsilateral sympathetic trunk that connect the brainstem to the eyes and face resulting in congenital Horner syndrome, also known as oculosympathetic paresis.

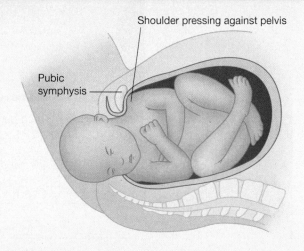

CASE FIGURE: Shoulder dystocia

Data from Robert H Allen, PhD, MS. (2021), Shoulder Dystocia, WebMD LLC. Retrieved from http://emedicine.medscape.com/article/1602970-overview

Plan: Congenital Horner syndrome associated with trauma at birth is not usually associated with severe pathological features. Consultation with a pediatric ophthalmologist to rule out the unlikely possibility of co-existing neuroblastoma. Continue daily physical therapy and therapeutic massage for brachial plexus injury. Regular follow-up to monitor symptoms, which may resolve on their own as the injured nerves heal. Treatment for ptosis may be necessary at a later date to prevent amblyopia.

1. Explain what is meant by oculosympathetic paresis, the other name for Horner syndrome.

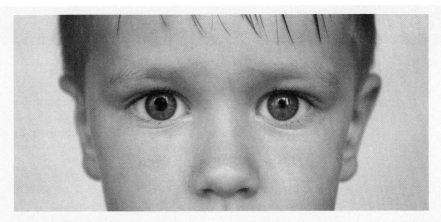

CASE FIGURE: A child with anisocoria

© Logika600/Shutterstock

2. Define the word parts and meaning of *dystocia*. You may need to refer to the chapter on reproduction.

   Dystocia: Dys- _____, -tocia _____

   meaning _____.

3. A plexus is a network of intersecting nerves. Where is the brachial plexus located? Indicate and define the word parts for brachial.

   How can oculosympathetic paresis be explained by a brachial plexus injury?

4. Complete the table for the signs and symptoms of Horner syndrome.

Term	Word Parts	Meaning
anisocoria	*anis/o; cor/o; -ia*	*condition of unequal pupils*
heterochromia iridum		
blepharoptosis		
mioisis		
enophthalmos		
pupillary asymmetry		
anhidrosis		
amblyopia		

(continues)

ADVANCED CASE STUDY

5. Define the word parts for unilateral and ipsilateral and explain their use in the case.

   Unilateral: Uni- _____, later/o _____, -al _____

   Ipsilateral: Ipsi- _____, later/o _____, -al _____

6. Define the word parts and meaning for the two types of physicians mentioned in the case.

   Pediatrician: Ped/o _____, iatr/o _____,

   -ician _____, means _____.

   Ophthalmologist: Ophthalm/o _____, -logist _____,

   means _____.

7. Indicate and define the word parts for *neuroblastoma*.

ADVANCED CASE STUDY

12.7 An Appointment with the Audiologist

Lien Chang has been referred by her primary care physician for an audiology consult to explore the cause of her progressive hearing loss. Lien is 35 and has noticed a deterioration in her hearing over the past year concurrent with increasing tinnitus. It is more challenging for her to distinguish lower tones and frequencies than higher ones. Pneumatic otoscopy and tympanometry indicate a normal tympanic membrane and a mobile malleus. Further audiometric investigation generates an audiogram that shows unilateral low-frequency hearing loss. Otosclerosis is suspected.

The audiologist explains to Lien how hearing works. She tells Lien how sound waves travel through the ear canal to the tympanic membrane, or eardrum, and cause it to vibrate. The vibrations travel to the ossicles in the middle ear, the malleus, the incus, and the stapes. The sound vibrations are then transmitted to the cochlea, the organ of hearing in the inner ear. In otosclerosis, the stapes becomes stuck in place and is unable to transmit vibrations. Thus otosclerosis is conductive, rather than sensorineural, hearing loss. Lien is presented with the option of a hearing aid but is told that this type of hearing loss is typically progressive and usually will affect both ears. A surgical option of stapedectomy or stapedotomy, with the placement of a prosthetic device, is also offered to her. As daunting as this sounds, the audiologist explains to Lien that surgery is a 1-day, minimally invasive procedure and has a high rate of success. Lien schedules an appointment with a surgeon who specializes in the procedure to further discuss her options.

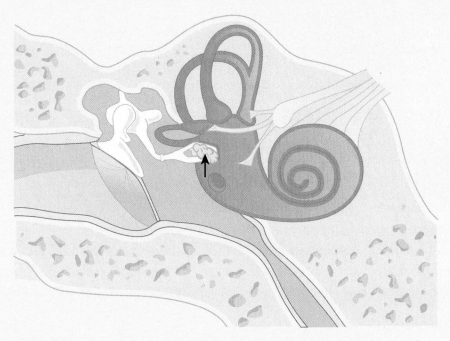

CASE FIGURE: Medical illustration of middle ear. Note the abnormal bone growth (arrow) around the stapes that has caused it to be stuck in place

1. Define the word parts for *audiologist* and *audiology*.

    Audiologist: Audi/o _____, -logist _____

    Audiology: Audi/o _____, -logy _____

2. Define the word parts and meaning for the following terms related to hearing and circle the term most appropriate for the hearing description in this case study.

    Anacusis: An- _____, -acusis _____,

    means _____.

    Hyperacusis: Hyper- _____, -acusis _____,

    means _____.

    Hypoacusis: Hypo- _____, -acusis _____,

    means _____.

    Presbycusis: Presby/o _____, -cusis _____,

    means _____.

    Diplacusis: Dipl/ o _____, -acusis _____,

    means _____.

(continues)

Odynacusis: Odyn/o _____, -acusis _____,

means _____.

3. Provide a brief definition for tinnitus. Use a medical dictionary, if necessary.

4. Complete the table for the diagnostic tests in the case study.

Term	Word Parts	Meaning
pneumatic otoscopy	*pneum/o; -atic ot/o; -scopy*	*process of viewing the ear using air*
tympanometry		
audiometric		
audiogram		
stapedectomy		
stapedotomy		

5. Consult a medical dictionary and contrast sensorineural and conductive hearing loss.

6. Otosclerosis can be due to stapedial ankylosis. Define the word parts and meanings of these terms.

Otosclerosis: Ot/o _____, -sclerosis _____

Stapedial ankylosis: Staped/o _____ ankyl/o _____,

-osis _____.

7. Explain the term prosthetic. Consult a medical dictionary, if necessary.

🔍 *ADVANCED CASE STUDY*

12.8 Ménière's Disease

A 35-year-old female presents to an otorhinolaryngologist with symptoms of hearing loss in her left ear, photophobia, and phonophobia, which have become worse over the past week. She has also had several episodes of vertigo within the last 12 hours. Her medical history is significant for recurring episodes of anacusis, tinnitus, and past episodes of vertigo. The patient's personal history includes smoking approximately 20 cigarettes a day and a poor diet, but she denies alcohol consumption. Audiometry reveals unilateral sensorineural deficits of low and medium frequencies. Magnetic resonance imaging (MRI) reveals endolymphatic hydrops in the affected ear but does not show retrocochlear pathology. The patient meets the minimal criteria for Ménière's disease, a disorder of the inner ear

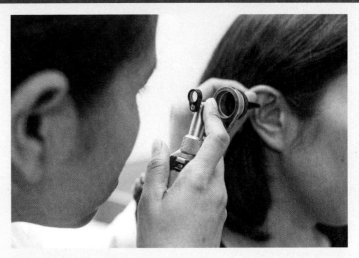

CASE FIGURE: Otorhinolaryngologist examining the patient's ear with an otoscope

© Bangkoker/Shutterstock

that is associated with hearing loss and vertigo. The etiology is unknown, but the disorder is associated with endolymphatic hydrops. The patient is advised to rest, join a smoking cessation program, and reduce salt in her diet. Hormone injections will be prescribed as an initial treatment. Labyrinthectomy, a more aggressive therapeutic option, may also be required.

1. Define the following word parts, and meaning, for *otorhinolaryngologist*.

    Otorhinolaryngologist: Ot/o _____, rhin/o _____,

    laryng/o _____, -logist _____,

    means _____.

2. Define the following word parts, and meanings, for *photophobia* and *phonophobia*.

    Photophobia: Phot/o _____, -phobia _____,

    means _____.

    Phonophobia: Phon/o _____, -phobia _____,

    means _____.

3. Provide a brief definition for anacusis, tinnitus, and vertigo. Use a medical dictionary, if necessary.

    Anacusis:

(continues)

🔍 ADVANCED CASE STUDY

Tinnitus:

Vertigo:

4. Audiometry revealed unilateral sensorineural deficits. Sensorineural refers to hearing, in relation to the cochlea and auditory nerve. Define the following word parts, and meanings, for *audiometry* and *unilateral*, and then describe what is meant by unilateral sensorineural deficits.

Audiometry: Audi/o _____, -metry _____,

means _____.

Unilateral: Uni- _____, later/o _____,

-al _____, means _____.

Unilateral sensorineural deficits:

5. MRI revealed endolymphatic hydrops without retrocochlear pathology. Hydrops refers to abnormal fluctuations in a fluid, endolymph, within the labyrinth of the inner ear. Define the following word parts, and meanings, for *endolymphatic*, *retrocochlear*, and *pathology*.

Endolymphatic: Endo- _____, lymph/o _____,

-ic _____, means _____.

Retrocochlear: Retro- _____, cochle/o _____,

-ar _____, means _____.

Pathology: Path/o _____, -logy _____,

means _____.

6. Define the following word parts, and meaning, of *labyrinthectomy*.

Labyrinthectomy: Labyrinth/o _____, -ectomy _____,

means _____.

🔍 *ADVANCED CASE STUDY*

12.9 Polychondritis

A 35-year-old female presents to her general practitioner (GP) with a fever and erythematous ears with auricular chondritis. She also complains of carpal and metacarpal arthralgia. She reported tinnitus and vertigo the previous day. Her medical history includes celiac disease, hypertension, and previous mild manifestations of auricle and nasal cartilage inflammation. A physical exam shows ocular signs of scleritis, keratitis, and uveitis; although the patient denied eye discomfort. Observation with an otoscope shows external auditory canal stenosis. The patient meets the criteria for relapsing polychondritis, an autoimmune disease that targets cartilage. Relapsing refers to periodic flare ups. A biopsy of the auricular cartilage is taken to confirm the diagnosis. The patient is put on glucocorticoid therapy to treat the inflammation.

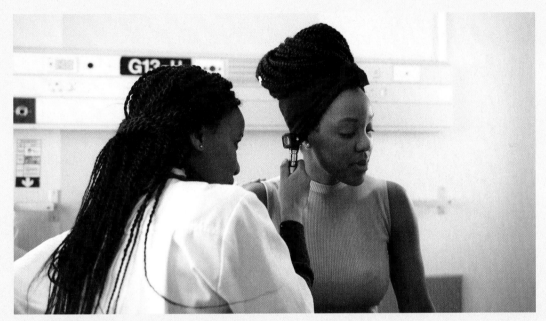

CASE FIGURE: Examination with an otoscope

© StockstudioX/E+/Getty Images

1. Complete the table below for the following terms related to the patient's symptoms:

Term	Word Parts	Meaning
erythematous	*erythr/o; hemat/o; -ous*	*pertaining to blood red (refers to flushing of skin)*
chondritis		
arthralgia		
hypertension		
scleritis		
keratitis		
uveitis		

(continues)

🔍 *ADVANCED CASE STUDY* *(continued)*

2. The case refers to auricular, carpal, metacarpal, and ocular body regions. What is the common name for these body regions?

   Auricular:

   Carpal:

   Metacarpal:

   Ocular:

3. Provide a brief definition for tinnitus and vertigo. Use a medical dictionary, if necessary.

   Tinnitus:

   Vertigo:

4. Observation with an otoscope showed stenosis of the external auditory canal. Define the word parts, and meanings, for *otoscope*, *stenosis*, and *external auditory*.

   Otoscope: Ot/o _____, -scopy _____,

   means _____.

   Stenosis: Sten/o _____, -osis _____,

   means _____.

   External auditory: External _____*outer*_____, audit/o _____,

   -ory _____, means _____.

5. The patient is diagnosed with relapsing polychondritis, an autoimmune disease that targets cartilage; a biopsy was taken to confirm the diagnosis. Define the word parts, and meanings, for *polychondritis*, *autoimmune*, and *biopsy*.

   Polychondritis: Poly- _____, chondr/o _____,

   -itis _____, means _____.

Autoimmune: Auto- _____, immun/o _____,

means _____.

Biopsy: Bi/o _____, -opsy _____,

means _____.

6. Patients with relapsing polychondritis often have comorbid autoimmune disorders. The patient in this case has celiac disease. Provide a simple description of celiac disease; use a medical dictionary, if necessary.

🔍 *ADVANCED CASE STUDY*

12.10 Homonymous Hemianopia

An 85-year-old female recovering from a left cerebral ischemic stroke presents with homonymous right hemianopia. Macular vision is spared. Tonometry and keratometry are normal. The stroke resulted from occlusion of the left posterior cerebral artery and infarction within the occipital lobe. A Goldmann perimetry test was ordered to measure her function visual field; the results reflected the visual deficits that the patient described.

The visual pathway starts with the retina. Photoreceptor rods and cones, interneurons, and retinal ganglion cells respond to, and process, photic information from the environment. This relatively unrefined information leaves the retina through optic nerves, which contain retinal ganglion cell axons. The optic nerves travel anterior and medially and meet at the optic chiasm, where neurons either continue ipsilaterally or contralaterally, such that neurons in each retina dedicated to the left visual fields travel to the left side of the brain, and the right visual fields travel to the right. Each retrochiasmatic pathway then travels to a lateral geniculate nucleus (LGN), an optic radiation, and terminates in the primary visual cortex of the occipital lobe. It is here that information from the retina is ultimately integrated and processed. Lesions to the pathway from prechiasmatic, chiasmatic, and retrochiasmatic ischemia affect the visual fields differently.

The patient will begin rehabilitation to develop strategies to improve reading, and navigate the world, with homonymous hemianopia.

1. The patient was presenting with right homonymous hemianopia during recovery from a cerebral ischemic stroke. Define the word parts, and meanings, for *homonymous*, *hemianopia*, *cerebral*, and *ischemic*.

Homonymous: Homo- _____, -nymous _____,

means _____.

Hemianopia: Hemi- _____, an- _____,

-opia _____, means _____,

Cerebral: Cerebr/o _____, -al _____,

means _____.

Ischemic: Isch/o _____, hem/o _____,

-ic _____, means _____,

(continues)

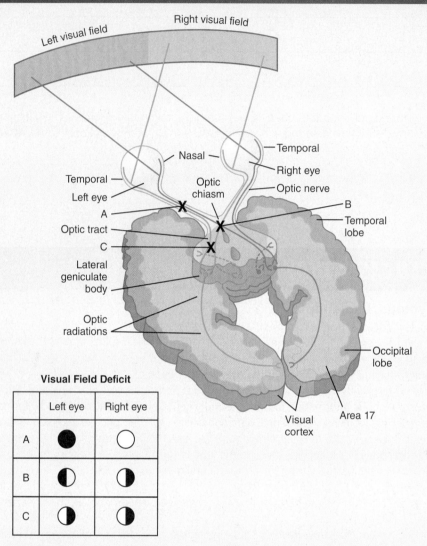

CASE FIGURE: The visual pathway and the effect of lesions at different levels of the pathway. Damage at A would result in blindness in one eye. Damage at B would result in heteronymous hemianopsia. Damage at C would result in homonymous right hemianopsia

2. The patient lost the right half of her vision in both eyes. A Goldmann perimetry test confirmed the hemianopia due to cerebral infarction, but macular vision was spared. Briefly describe a Goldmann perimetry test, infarction, and the macula. Use a medical dictionary, or other reputable resources, if necessary.

Goldmann perimetry test:

Infarction:

Macula:

3. Define the word parts, and meaning, for the two diagnostics used in this case: *tonometry and keratometry*.

   Tonometry: Ton/o _____, -metry _____,

   means _____.

   Keratometry: Kerat/o _____, -metry _____,

   means _____.

4. Define the word parts, and meanings, for *ipsilateral* and *contralateral*.

   Ipsilateral: Ipsi- _____, later/o _____, -al _____,

   means _____.

   Contralateral: Contra- _____, later/o _____,

   -al _____, means _____.

5. The visual pathway can be described in relation to the optic chiasm (crossing of the optic nerves). Define the word parts, and meanings, for *prechiasmatic*, *chiasmatic*, and *retrochiasmatic*.

   Prechiasmatic: Pre- _____, chiasma _____*cross*_____, -tic _____,

   means _____.

   Chiasmatic: Chiasma _____*cross*_____, -tic _____,

   means _____.

   Retrochiasmatic: Retro- _____, chiasma _____*cross*_____,

   -tic _____, means _____.

References

Batson, L., & Rizzolo, D. (2017). Otosclerosis: An update on diagnosis and treatment. *JAAPA*, *30*(2), 17–22. https://doi.org/10.1097/01.JAA.0000511784.21936.1b

Chauhan K, Surmachevska N, Hanna A. Relapsing Polychondritis. [Updated 2020 Jun 4]. In: StatPearls [Internet]. Treasure Island (FL): StatPearls Publishing; 2020 Jan-. Available from: https://www.ncbi.nlm.nih.gov/books/NBK436007/

Dolhi N, Weimer AD. Tympanic Membrane Perforations. [Updated 2020 May 8]. In: StatPearls [Internet]. Treasure Island (FL): StatPearls Publishing; 2020 Jan-. Available from: https://www.ncbi.nlm.nih.gov/books/NBK557887/

Ho, T., Vrabec, J. T., Yoo, D., & Coker, N. J. (2006). Otomycosis: Clinical features and treatment implications. *Otolaryngology—Head and Neck Surgery*, *135*(5), 787–791. https://doi.org/10.1016/j.otohns.2006.07.008

Jeffery, A. R., Ellis, F. J., Repka, M. X., & Buncic, J. R. (1998). Pediatric Horner syndrome. *Journal of the American Association for Pediatric Ophthalmology and Strabismus*, *2*(3), 159–167. https://doi.org/10.1016/s1091-8531(98)90008-8

Koenen L, Andaloro, C. Meniere Disease. [Updated 2020 Jun 25]. In: StatPearls [Internet]. Treasure Island (FL): StatPearls

Publishing; 2020 Jan-. Available from: https://www.ncbi.nlm.nih.gov/books/NBK536955/

Mahabadi N, Foris LA, Tripathy K. Open Angle Glaucoma. [Updated 2020 Jul 4]. In: StatPearls [Internet]. Treasure Island (FL): StatPearls Publishing; 2020 Jan-. Available from: https://www.ncbi.nlm.nih.gov/books/NBK441887/

Minos, E., Barry, R. J., Southworth, S., Folkard, A., Murray, P. I., Duker, J. S., Keane, P. A., & Denniston, A. K. (2016). Birdshot chorioretinopathy: Current knowledge and new concepts in pathophysiology, diagnosis, monitoring and treatment. *Orphanet Journal of Rare Diseases, 11*(61). https://doi.org/10.1186/s13023-016-0429-8

Pula, J. H., & Yuen, C. A. (2017). Eyes and stroke: The visual aspects of cerebrovascular disease. *Stroke and Vascular Neurology, 2*(4), 210–220. https://doi.org/10.1136/svn-2017-000079

Rodrigues, G. B., Abe, R. Y., Zangalli, C., Sodre, S. L., Donini, F. A., Costa, D. C., Leite, A., Felix, J. P., Torigoe, M., Diniz-Filho, A., & de Almeida, H. G. (2016). Neovascular glaucoma: A review. *International Journal of Retina and Vitreous, 2*(26). https://doi.org/10.1186/s40942-016-0051-x

Stedman, T. L. (2005). Nath's *Stedman's medical terminology, 2e.* Philadelphia: Lippincott Williams & Wilkins.

Tomkins-Netzer, O., Taylor S. R. J, & Lightman S. (2014). Long-term clinical and anatomic outcome of Birdshot Chorioretinopathy. *JAMA Ophthalmology, 132*(1), 57–62. doi:10.1001/jamaophthalmol.2013.6235

Teggi, R., Fabiano, B., Recanati, P., Limardo, P., & Bussi, M. (2010). Case reports on two patients with episodic vertigo, fluctuating hearing loss and migraine responding to prophylactic drugs for migraine. Menière's disease or migraine-associated vertigo? *Acta Otorhinolaryngologica Italica, 30*(4), 217.

Venes, D. & Taber, C. W. (2017). Taber's cyclopedic medical dictionary. Ed. 23, illustrated in full color/Philadelphia: F. A. Davis.

Vincent, S. J., & Read, S. A. (2014). Progressive adult antimetropia. *Clinical and Experimental Optometry, 97*(4), 375–378. https://doi.org/10.1111/cxo.12129

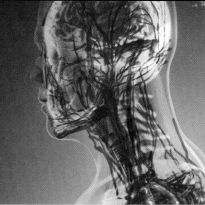

CHAPTER 13

Special Topics

There are many medical specialties within the health-care field. This chapter addresses a few of these including cancer medicine (oncology); mental health (psychiatry and psychology); rehabilitative medicine including physical and occupational therapy, diagnostic imaging, pain management, pharmacology and substance abuse, and dental medicine. In addition, many cases in the chapter integrate all body systems.

TABLE 13.1
Key Mental Health Prefixes
sui-: self

TABLE 13.2
Key Mental Health Combining Forms
depress/o: to press down
electr/o: electricity
hallucin/o: imagined perception
hypn/o: sleep
ment/o: mind

Key Mental Health Combining Forms
pharmac/o: drug
phob/o: irrational fear
pol/o: extreme
pysch/o: mind
schiz/o: split
somat/o: body
somn/o: sleep

TABLE 13.3
Key Mental Health Suffixes
-cide: killing
-mania: frenzy
-orexia: appetite
-phoria: feeling
-therapy: treatment

TABLE 13.4
Key Rehabilitative Medicine Combining Forms
erg/o: work
habilitat/o: ability
orth/o: straight
physi/o: function
prosthet/o: addition

TABLE 13.5
Key Rehabilitation Suffixes
-nomic: pertaining to law

TABLE 13.6
Key Oncology Combining Forms
carcin/o: cancerous
chem/o: chemical
duct/o: to bring; duct
mutat/o: to change
onc/o: tumor

TABLE 13.7
Key Oncology Suffixes
-oma: tumor
-plasia: formation of cells

TABLE 13.8
Key Pharmacology Combining Forms
chem/o: drug
pharmac/o: drug
topic/o: a specific area

TABLE 13.9
Key Dental Combining Forms
dent/o: tooth
gingiv/o: gums
halit/o: breath
odont/o: tooth
or/o: mouth
periodont/o: around the teeth

TABLE 13.10
Key Pain Prefixes
dys-: painful
noci-: pain

TABLE 13.11
Key Pain Combining Forms
alges/o: pain
esthesi/o: sensation
neur/o: neuron; nerve

TABLE 13.12
Key Pain Suffixes
-algia: pain
-ceptor,: receiver
-dynia: pain
-receptor: receiver

TABLE 13.13		Key Alcoholism Combining Forms
Key Alcoholism Combining Forms		hepat/o: liver
bil/i: gallbladder		jaund/o: yellow
cirrh/o: yellow-orange		steat/o: fat
diaphar/o: profuse sweating		toxic/o: poison

⌕ STANDARD CASE STUDY

13.1 Choking Phobia—Mental Health

Palomah Desai is brought to the psychiatrist by her parents upon recommendation of her pediatrician. Palomah, nearly 12 years old and close to 5 feet tall, has lost 20 pounds in the past 3 months, shifting her BMI (body mass index) from the 50th percentile to the 6th percentile. The weight loss was precipitated by Palomah's refusal to eat solid food after seeing her younger sister choking on a piece of hard candy. Since the incident, Palomah has subsisted on milk, juice, soup, and more recently the protein shakes her parents had bought her in an effort to halt the weight loss. Palomah reports that when faced with solid food, her throat closes up and she feels like she will choke. Lately, dreams of choking have kept her up at night. The psychiatrist identifies Palomah's dysphagia as a choking phobia and prescribes the psychotropic medication Xanax, used to treat anxiety and panic disorders. Palomah also participates in several psychotherapy sessions using hypnosis and graduated exposure to solid food. Following a weekly treatment regimen of 4 months' duration, Palomah is again able to enjoy solid foods. Over the 4 months, she shows a gradual weight gain, approaching her BMI before developing her phobia.

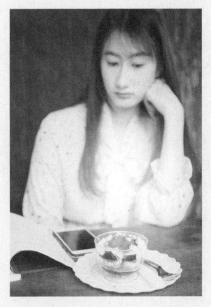

CASE FIGURE: A young woman refusing food

© Pskamn/Shutterstock

1. Define the word parts and meaning of *dysphagia*.

   Dysphagia: Dys- _____, phag/o _____, -ia _____,

   means _____.

(continues)

2. The suffix -phobia means an irrational fear. There are many different types of phobias. Define the word parts for the following phobias and circle the most likely diagnosis for this case.

Hematophobia: Hemat/o _____, -phobia _____,

means _____.

Gynophobia: Gyn/o _____, -phobia _____,

means _____.

Androphobia: Andr/o _____, -phobia _____,

means _____.

Phagophobia: Phag/o _____, -phobia _____,

means _____.

Acrophobia: Acr/o _____, -phobia _____,

means _____.

Pathophobia: Path/o _____, -phobia _____,

means _____.

3. Indicate and define the word parts, then define the following terms related to the mind.

Psychiatrist:

Psychotropic:

Psychotherapy:

4. Define the word parts for *hypnosis* and then explain how this is used therapeutically. You may need to consult a medical dictionary or other reliable resource.

Hypnosis: Hypn/o _____, -osis _____.

🔍 *STANDARD CASE STUDY*

13.2 Bipolar Disorder—Mental Health

Psychiatric Consult

Ismah Knox, a 28-year-old female, presents for a psychiatric consult with her husband Euan. Euan reports that this is his wife's first time out of bed except to go to the bathroom in over 2 weeks. He states that she has barely eaten and has not bathed, combed her hair, or changed her clothes. Scaring Euan the most though, was Ismah's mention of suicide. When Ismah is asked about past episodes of depression, she relates that she has cycled through episodes of depression alternating with excessive euphoria since she was a teenager, but lately the lows have been lower, and the highs have been higher. Euan declares that this was the worst depressive episode he has seen in his wife. When Euan is asked to describe the opposite end of the spectrum, what would constitute a period of euphoria for Ismah, he relays instances of several days when she barely sleeps, staying up nearly all night for several nights in a row to write pages and pages in her journal.

"She'll talk on and on, planning different career changes, unable to focus on any one of them," Euan shares. "During Ismah's last episode, she spent thousands of dollars on clothes to wear to interviews for jobs she never even applied for. It's usually about 4 days of frenzied behavior like this, then a time of being really down. In between though, she's pretty much stable."

Listening to a detailed history of the pattern of Ismah's behavior, the psychiatrist diagnoses her with bipolar disorder, characterized by periods of hypomania alternating with periods of dysphoria. Treatment will be a combination of psychotherapy, antidepressants, and mood stabilizer drugs. Electroconvulsive therapy (ECT) will be considered if Ismah's depression does not respond to medication. Euan will be encouraged to connect with a mental health support group to be an active part of his wife's treatment and to gain coping strategies for himself.

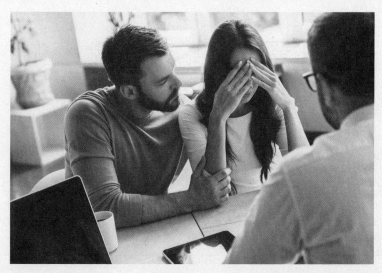

CASE FIGURE: A patient and her husband at a psychiatric consult
© G-Stock Studio/Shutterstock

1. Define the word parts, and meaning, for *psychiatric*.

   Psychiatric: Psych/o _____, -iatric _____,

   means _____

2. Complete the table for the following psychiatric terms used in the case.

Term	Word Parts	Meaning
suicide	*sui-; -cide*	*killing of one's self*
depression		

(continues)

Term	Word Parts	Meaning
euphoria		
hypomania		
dysphoria		

3. Ismah's sleep patterns cycle between insomnia and hypersomnia. Indicate and define the word parts for these terms.

   Insomnia:

   Hypersomnia:

4. Provide brief descriptions of the following treatments mentioned in the case: psychotherapy, antidepressants, mood stabilizer drugs, and electroconvulsive therapy (ECT).

5. Define the word parts, and meaning, of *bipolar*, then describe what is meant by bipolar disorder.

   Bipolar: Bi- _____, pol/o _____, -ar _____,

   means _____.

🔍 *STANDARD CASE STUDY*

13.3 Quality of Life Care in a Cancer Patient—Rehabilitative Medicine

Padma K. is a 30-year-old woman with stage 4 ovarian cancer. She is receiving palliative care and has expressed distress about her ability to manage her physical and emotional needs and states that pain, reduced mobility, and fatigue make it challenging to perform activities of daily living (ADLs). Padma is meeting today with both a physical and an occupational therapist to assess her needs and establish some realistic goals.

Aims of physical therapy at the palliative stage can include nonpharmaceutical relief of pain with treatment modalities such as massage and thermotherapy. Physical therapists can also help with ambulation challenges and therapeutic exercise such as those involving range of motion (ROM), which can help prevent joint contractures, muscle atrophy, and reduce fatigue. Occupational therapists work in conjunction with physical therapists to provide strategies for self-care management and provide guidance on adaptive equipment and creation of ergonomic workspaces. Occupational therapy can also help Padma play an active role in parenting her 6-year-old son, provide strategies for managing the home, and facilitate engagement in leisure activities. Her care team will be coordinated by a physiatrist who will help Padma revise her goals as her needs and health status change, ensuring that she can retain her independence for as long as possible. The team will also support the role of her husband and other caregivers. With this multidisciplinary approach, Padma's physical, cognitive, and emotional needs can be addressed to preserve quality of life (QOL).

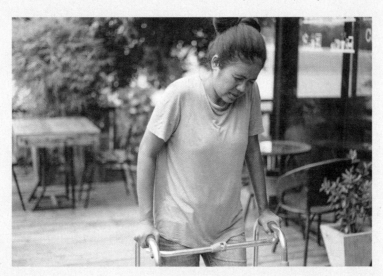

CASE FIGURE: A woman using a walker to provide support

© Anut21ng Stock/Shutterstock

1. Define the word parts, and meaning, of *rehabilitation*.

   Rehabilitation: Re- _____, habilitat/o _____,

   -ion _____, means _____.

2. Use a medical dictionary or other reliable resource to provide descriptions of the following:

   Palliative care:

   Physical therapy:

   Occupational therapy:

   Activities of daily living (ADL):

(continues)

🔍 *STANDARD CASE STUDY* *(continued)*

3. Define the word parts and meaning for *nonpharmaceutical* and then provide a brief explanation of the nonpharmaceutical interventions in this case: massage, thermotherapy.

   Nonpharmaceutical: Non- _____, pharmac/o _____,

           -al _____, means _____

4. Define the word parts and meaning of *ergonomic*.

   Ergonomic: Erg/o _____, -nomic _____,

           means _____.

5. Use a medical dictionary or other reliable resource to explain what is meant by adaptive equipment.

6. Range of motion (ROM) exercises can help preserve flexibility and mobility. These exercises can be active or passive. Use a medical or other reliable resource to distinguish these.

7. Indicate and define the word parts for *physiatrist* and explain the role of this specialist.

8. Maintenance of quality of life (QOL) is an important strategy for a patient with a terminal illness. QOL is subjective and involves the individual's perception of their well-being. Describe the needs that are important to consider in maintaining QOL.

🔍 *STANDARD CASE STUDY*

13.4 Diagnostic Imaging

Gillian, an endoscopy technician, collapsed into a chair at the breakroom table. Her lunch break was much needed, and well-deserved, after preparing the endoscopy unit for a fully-booked morning, a total of five procedures. Two colonoscopies were performed on patients without sedation, and two gastroscopies and a duodenoscopy were performed on patients under general anesthesia. The duodenoscopy was the most challenging; it was performed as an endoscopic retrograde cholangiopancreatography (ERCP) to confirm the presence of gallstones. Unfortunately, the procedure had caused a tear in the duodenum, which led to a flurry of chaos in the unit and made preparing for the afternoon procedures much more involved than was typical. She took a deep breath, and a spoonful of chicken soup, then mentally prepared herself for an afternoon packed with three more procedures.

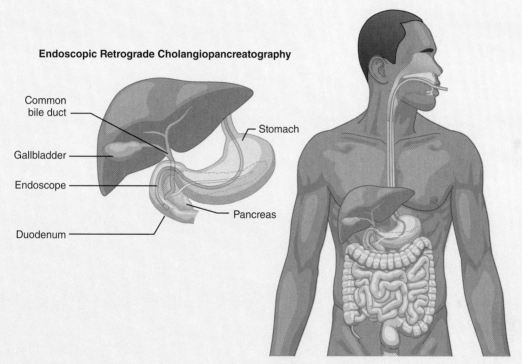

Endoscopic Retrograde Cholangiopancreatography

Common bile duct

Gallbladder

Endoscope

Duodenum

Stomach

Pancreas

CASE FIGURE: Endoscopic retrograde cholangiopancreatography (ERCP)

1. Define the following word parts, and meaning, of *endoscopy*.

   Endoscopy: Endo- _____, -scopy _____,

   means _____.

2. What is an endoscope? Provide a simple description of the instrument. Use a medical dictionary, or other dependable resource, if necessary.

(continues)

⌕ *STANDARD CASE STUDY* *(continued)*

3. Complete the table below for some examples of types of endoscopy that can be performed.

Term	Word Parts	Procedure for Viewing:
angioscopy	*angi/o; -scopy*	*blood vessels*
anoscopy		
arthroscopy		
bronchoscopy		
colonoscopy		
colposcopy		
cystoscopy		
esophagogastroduodenoscopy		
fetoscopy		
gastroscopy		
hysteroscopy		
laparoscopy		
laryngoscopy		
nephroscopy		
otoscopy		
proctosigmoidoscopy		
rhinoscopy		
sigmoidoscopy		

4. The duodenoscopy was performed as part of an endoscopic retrograde cholangiopancreatography (ERCP). The term retrograde in this procedure refers to the injection of a contrast dye back up into the biliary and pancreatic ducts to enhance X-ray imaging. Define the following word parts, and meaning, of *cholangiopancreatography*.

Cholangiopancreatography: Chol/e _____, angi/o _____,

pancreat/o _____, -graphy _____,

means _____.

🔍 *STANDARD CASE STUDY*

13.5 Multiorgan System Response

A 45-year-old Hispanic male with a severe acute respiratory syndrome coronavirus-2 (SARS-CoV-2) infection, confirmed by PCR test, has been in an intensive care unit (ICU) for 4 weeks with severe coronavirus disease 2019 (COVID-19) symptoms. The patient is on a mechanical ventilator due to hypoxemic respiratory failure. Since being admitted, he has sustained renal injury and developed proteinuria. A physical assessment is significant for tachycardia (110 beats per minute) and an erythematous rash on his feet. Blood lab values reveal lymphopenia, and hyperglycemia (190 mg/dL) from new-onset diabetes. Before being placed on ventilation, the patient complained of anosmia, myalgia, arthralgia, and diarrhea. The patient had been treated with antiviral medications (remdesivir), and is now on anti-inflammatory agents (dexamethasone) and anticoagulants (heparin).

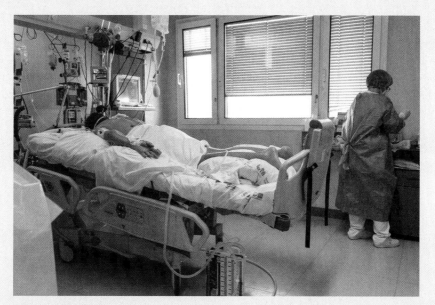

CASE FIGURE: COVID-19 Patient
© David Benito/Getty Images News/Getty Images

1.   Complete the table below for the patient's presenting signs, symptoms, and history:

Term	Word Parts	Meaning
hypoxemic	*hypo-; ox/o; -emic*	*blood condition of insufficient oxygen*
renal		
proteinuria		
tachycardia		
erythematous		
lymphopenia		
hyperglycemia		

(continues)

🔍 *STANDARD CASE STUDY* *(continued)*

Term	Word Parts	Meaning
anosmia		
myalgia		
arthralgia		
diarrhea		

2. SARS-CoV-2 is the virus that causes the disease, COVID-19. SARS-CoV-2 can infect, replicate in, and destroy cells of the respiratory system, but in severe COVID-19 cases, the disease may involve every body system. Fill in the table below with the body system primarily associated with each sign, symptom, or piece of information from the case. Each system will only be used once. The body systems are the integumentary, skeletal, muscular, nervous, endocrine, lymphatic (immune), cardiovascular, respiratory, digestive, urinary, and reproductive systems.

Sign, Symptom, or Information	Body System
The patient is a male. Of patients in the ICU with COVID-19, males are disproportionately affected.	*reproductive system*
hypoxemic respiratory failure	
proteinuria	
tachycardia	
erythematous rash	
lymphopenia	
hyperglycemia from new-onset diabetes	
anosmia	
myalgia	
arthralgia	
diarrhea	

🔍 *ADVANCED CASE STUDY*

13.6 Invasive Ductal Carcinoma—Oncology

Aubrey Berman, 55, had been born with an extra nipple in the inframammary fold of her left breast. Over the past few months she had noticed redness and pain near the nipple and now could feel a mass directly posterior to this area. She made an appointment with her primary care physician, Dr. Carillo, who examined the lesion and palpated a mass approximately 2 cm in diameter in the area of the supernumerary breast. Supraclavicular lymphadenopathy was not apparent; however, a palpable left axillary lymph node was detected. Aubrey was sent for immediate diagnostic mammography, which confirmed a suspicious 2.2 cm mass with spiculated margins. Punch biopsy was performed and histopathology revealed anaplastic cells. Immunohistochemistry showed the tumor to be positive for estrogen receptors. Positron-emission tomography (PET scan) was positive for one left axillary lymph node, with no involvement of supraclavicular, subclavicular, or subpectoral lymph nodes. Aubrey is diagnosed with stage IIb (T2N1M0) invasive ductal carcinoma. After consultation with an oncologist, a treatment protocol is mapped out. Aubrey will undergo a complete mastectomy. She will then receive adjuvant chemotherapy with the hormone antagonist anastrozole to reduce the risk of recurrence. Five-year survival rates of women diagnosed with stage II breast cancer following treatment are about 90%, so Aubrey is hopeful for a positive outcome.

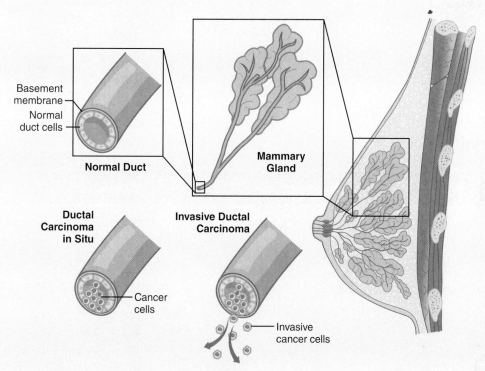

CASE FIGURE: Ductal carcinoma of the breast

1. Using word parts, describe the location of Aubrey's extra nipple and the location of the mass she feels.

2. Aubrey's extra nipple is considered a supernumerary breast. Define the word parts, and meaning, of *supernumerary* and explain what is meant by a supernumerary breast. Another term for this is polymastia. Define the word parts for this term.

Supernumerary: Super/o _____, numer/o _____,

-ary _____, means _____.

Polymastia: Poly- _____, mast/o _____, -ia _____,

means _____.

(continues)

🔍 **ADVANCED CASE STUDY**   *(continued)*

3. Complete the table for the terms used in the case used to describe the lymph nodes.

Term	Word Parts	Meaning
supraclavicular	*supra-; clavicul/o; -ar*	*pertaining to above the clavicle (collarbone)*
subclavicular		
axillary		
subpectoral		
lymphadenopathy		

4. Complete the table below for procedural terms in the case.

Term	Word Parts	Meaning
mammography	*mamm/o; -graphy*	*process of recording the breast*
biopsy		
histopathology		
immunohistochemistry		
mastectomy		
chemotherapy		
oncologist		

5. Aubrey is diagnosed with stage IIb (T2N1M0) cancer. Use a medical dictionary or other reliable resource to explain what staging of cancer means and what the TNM system indicates.

6. Use a medical dictionary to describe invasive ductal carcinoma. Contrast this to ductal cell carcinoma in situ, an earlier stage of the same type of cancer.

7. Explain the terms spiculated and anaplastic.

8. Aubrey will receive adjuvant chemotherapy with a hormone antagonist to reduce the risk of recurrence of her cancer. Explain, using a medical dictionary or other reliable resource.

🔍 *ADVANCED CASE STUDY*

13.7 A Class in Pharmacology

"Hey Gemma, how are you? Are you feeling better?" Hiraku asked.

"Yes, much better, thank you," answered Gemma. "What did I miss in pharmacology class?" she asked.

"You missed a fair amount," Hiraku sighed. "There's so much information. Do you want to grab a cup of coffee and I can go over some of it with you? Reviewing it will help me make sure I understand it all."

"That would be great!" Gemma responded. "With our exam right around the corner, I would really appreciate that."

Hiraku pulled out his notes and told Gemma they had started off talking a little about pharmacokinetics. Then their professor had told them how the same drug can have multiple names: a chemical name, a generic name, and a brand name.

"There are so many different ways drugs can be given," Hiraku went on. "Some drugs must be administered by a particular route to be effective. Others can be administered by a variety of routes."

"I looked at these," said Gemma. "I know drugs can be administered orally, sublingually, rectally, buccally, or topically. Many I know are administered parenterally. What else did Professor Sosa talk about?"

"She talked a lot about essential medical information to be aware of before administering a drug such as actions and interactions, potential side effects, and any contraindications for administration."

"Wow, that was a lot of information to miss," sighed Gemma. "You've helped a lot though. Now I know what to study and I will definitely be ready for next week's exam. Thank you—you're a lifesaver!"

1. The root pharmac/o means drug. Explain what is meant by pharmacology and pharmacokinetics. Then build a term for someone who specializes in drugs.

2. Use a medical dictionary or other reliable resource to distinguish the chemical name, generic name, and brand name of a drug.

(continues)

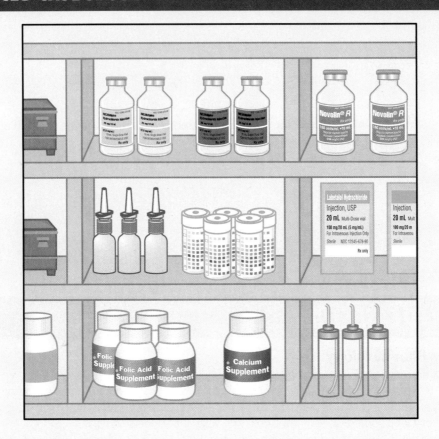

3. Complete the table for the routes of drug administration used in the case.

Term	Word Parts	Meaning
oral	or/o; -al	pertaining to mouth
sublingual		
rectal		
buccal		
topical		

4. Parenteral (para-; enter/o; -al) literally means pertaining to near the intestine. Parenteral drugs need to be injected and there are several forms of parenteral administration. Complete the table to describe types of parenteral administration.

Term	Word Parts	Meaning
intradermal	intra-; derm/o; -al	pertaining to within the skin
subcutaneous		

Term	Word Parts	Meaning
intravenous		
intramuscular		
intrathecal		

5. Provide brief definitions of the following terms related to pharmacology. Use a medical dictionary or other reliable resource, if needed.

   Drug action:

   Drug interaction:

   Drug side effect:

   Drug contraindication:

🔍 ADVANCED CASE STUDY

13.8 Periodontitis—Dental Medicine

A 65-year-old male presents to his dentist with severely inflamed gums that are quick to bleed and a history of gingivitis. An oral exam reveals halitosis, significant dental plaque, supragingival and subgingival calculus, and a periodontal abscess between the left maxillary bicuspids. Periodontal probing causes bleeding and identifies periodontal pockets up to 6 mm deep and significant tooth mobility. Bite-wing X-rays show significant alveolar bone loss. The patient is diagnosed with severe periodontitis. He is scheduled for a scaling, root planing, and consultation with a periodontist to discuss pocket reduction surgery.

1. Define the word parts, and meaning, of *dentist*.

   Dentist: Dent/o _____, -ist _____,

   means _____.

2. Define the following word parts, and meaning, of *gingivitis* and *halitosis*.

   Gingivitis: Gingiv/o _____, -itis _____,

   means _____.

(continues)

🔍 *ADVANCED CASE STUDY* *(continued)*

Halitosis: Halit/o _____, -osis _____,

means _____.

3. What does plaque refer to in dental medicine? Use a medical dictionary, or other reputable source, if needed.

4. A calculus (plural calculi) translates from Latin to English as stone, or pebble. What does a calculus refer to in dental medicine? Use a medical dictionary, or other reputable source, if needed.

5. Define the following word parts, and meaning, of *supragingival, subgingival,* and *periodontal.*

Supragingival: Supra- _____, gingiv/o _____,

-al _____, means _____.

Subgingival: Sub- _____, gingiv/o _____,

-al _____, means _____.

Periodontal: Periodont/o _____, -al _____,

means _____.

6. An abscess is a painful pocket containing pus. The dentist found one between the left maxillary bicuspid (premolar) teeth. Based on the description, was the abscess found on gums of the upper or lower jaw?

7. Probing and bite-wing X-rays (which provided a side view of the teeth and jaw) show open pockets in the gums around the teeth and deterioration of the alveolar bone sockets that hold the teeth. This confirms a diagnosis of periodontitis. Scaling and root planing were scheduled to clean and correct the surface of the teeth, and roots, respectively. The pockets will also be surgically reduced by a periodontist. Define the following word parts, and meaning, of *periodontitis* and *periodontist.*

Periodontitis: Periodont/o _____, -itis _____,

means _____.

Periodontist: Periodont/o _____, -ist _____,

means _____.

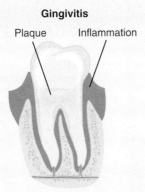
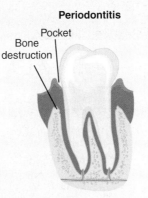
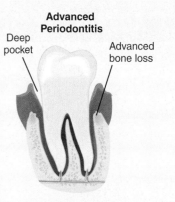

Healthy Gums and Tooth

Gingivitis
Plaque   Inflammation

The early stage of periodontal disease. Plaque inflame the gums and bleed easily.

Periodontitis
Bone destruction   Pocket

Pockets and moderate bone loss.

Advanced Periodontitis
Deep pocket   Advanced bone loss

Severe bone loss and deep pockets. Tooth is in danger of falling out.

CASE FIGURE: Normal gums; and gums with gingivitis, periodontitis, or severe periodontitis

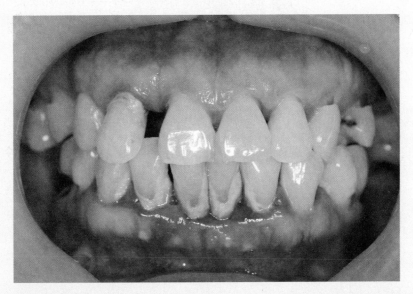

CASE FIGURE: Advanced periodontitis

🔍 *ADVANCED CASE STUDY*

13.9 Fibromyalgia—Pain Management

Jason, a 45-year-old male, has a 5-year history of enduring failed pain management strategies for suspected fibromyalgia syndrome. His chief complaints are persistent allodynia, hyperalgesia, and paresthesia. He reports that he has also been experiencing days-long depressive episodes. Prior treatments to manage the patient's pain have included nonsteroidal anti-inflammatory drugs (NSAIDs) and opioids, but these have not been effective. Functional magnetic resonance imaging (fMRI) is ordered and reveals decreased brain volume and patterns confirming fibromyalgia. The antidepressive drug the patient is currently taking will be changed in an effort to better treat both the depression and centralized pain. If the pain continues, motor cortex stimulation (MCS) or deep brain stimulation (DBS) may be considered.

(continues)

🔍 *ADVANCED CASE STUDY*   *(continued)*

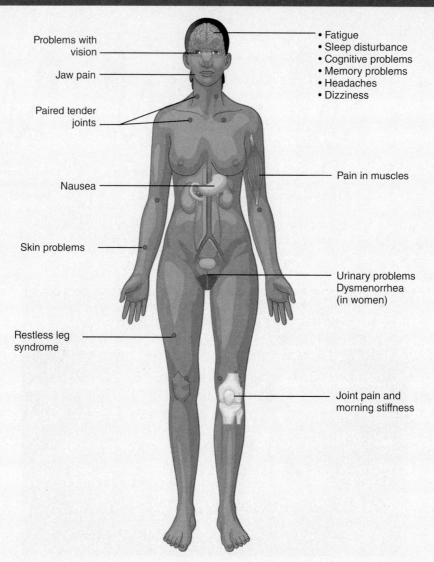

Problems with vision

Jaw pain

Paired tender joints

Nausea

Skin problems

Restless leg syndrome

• Fatigue
• Sleep disturbance
• Cognitive problems
• Memory problems
• Headaches
• Dizziness

Pain in muscles

Urinary problems
Dysmenorrhea
(in women)

Joint pain and
morning stiffness

CASE FIGURE: Signs and Symptoms of Fibromyalgia

1. Fibromyalgia syndrome is characterized by stiffness and pain throughout the body. In the name of the syndrome, the word part *fibr/o* means fibers, referring to connective tissue fibers. Define the following word parts, and meaning, of *fibromyalgia*.

    Fibromyalgia: Fibr/o _____, my/o _____,

    alges/o _____, -ia _____,

    means _____.

2. The patient complains of allodynia, hyperalgesia, and paresthesia. Define the following word parts, and meaning, of *allodynia*, *hyperalgesia*, and *paresthesia*.

    Allodynia: All/o _____, -dynia _____,

    means _____.

Hyperalgesia: Hyper- _____, alges/o _____,

-ia _____, means _____.

Paresthesia: Para- _____, esthes/o_____, -ia _____,

means _____.

3. Complete the table below for the following terms related to pain or pain relief:

Term	Word Parts	Meaning
analgesia	*an-; -algesia*	*without pain*
anesthesia		
dysesthesia		
hyperalgesia		
hyperesthesia		
hypoalgesia		
hypoesthesia		
neuralgia		
nociceptor		

4. Define the following word parts, and meaning, of *neuropathy*.

Neuropathy: Neur/o _____, -pathy _____,

means _____.

5. NSAIDs and opioids have not been effective in treating the pain from Jason's neuropathy. Using a medical dictionary, or other reputable source, provide a brief description of NSAIDs and opioids.

NSAIDs:

Opioids:

(continues)

🔍 *ADVANCED CASE STUDY* (continued)

6. Using a medical dictionary, or other reputable source, provide a brief description of motor cortex stimulation (MCS) and deep brain stimulation (DBS).

   MCS:

   DBS:

🔍 *ADVANCED CASE STUDY*

13.10 Alcoholism—Substance Abuse

A 65-year-old male was brought to the emergency department after collapsing and falling down a set of stairs. The patient appeared intoxicated with a laceration above his right eye and had manifestations of jaundice and facial telangiectasia. His medical history included hypertension and hepatobiliary disease. He denied smoking cigarettes but reported drinking the equivalent of 5–10 drinks each day. Hepatomegaly was suggested from palpation of his right upper abdominal quadrant. His vital signs were remarkable for tachycardia (110 beats per minute) and hypertension (160/95 mm Hg). A computed tomography (CT) scan provided radiographic evidence of fatty liver. Lab tests were ordered to measure biomarkers of alcoholic liver disease. The patient was given an alcohol screening questionnaire, which determined that his alcohol intake was physically and behaviorally problematic. He was transferred to a rehabilitation center to monitor for signs and symptoms of delirium tremens, including tachycardia, hypertension, hyperthermia, and diaphoresis.

The notable findings from his blood tests are included in the table below.

Test	Result	Reference Range
CDT: carbohydrate deficient transferrin	75 mg/L	<6.0 mg/dL
GGT: gamma-glutamyl transferase	85 U/L	<38 U/L
AST: aspartate aminotransferase	85 U/L	7–27 U/L
ALT: alanine aminotransferase	40 U/L	1–21 U/L
MCV: mean corpuscular volume	95 μm^3/RBC	86–98 μm^3/RBC

1. Define the following word parts, and meaning, of *intoxication*.

   Intoxication: In- _____ , toxic/o _____ ,

   -ation _____ ,

   means _____

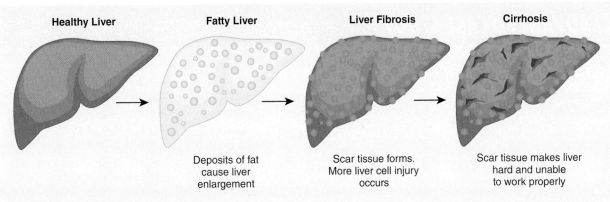

Healthy Liver

Fatty Liver

Deposits of fat
cause liver
enlargement

Liver Fibrosis

Scar tissue forms.
More liver cell injury
occurs

Cirrhosis

Scar tissue makes liver
hard and unable
to work properly

CASE FIGURE: Stages of liver disease

2. Complete the table below for the patient's presenting signs, symptoms, and history:

Term	Word Parts	Meaning
jaundice	*jaund/o; -ice*	*condition of yellowing (refers to a yellow cast of the skin and eyes)*
telangiectasias		
hypertension		
hepatobiliary		
hepatomegaly		
tachycardia		

3. A CT scan provided radiographic evidence of a condition commonly referred to as fatty liver. Define the following word parts, and meaning, for different types of liver conditions and then circle the one that the patient has.

Cirrhosis: Cirrh/o _____, -osis _____,

means _____.

Hepatic fibrosis: Hepat/o _____, -ic _____,

fibr/o _____, -osis _____,

means _____.

Hepatic steatosis: Hepat/o _____, -ic _____,

steat/o _____, -osis _____,

means _____.

(continues)

🔍 ADVANCED CASE STUDY   *(continued)*

4. A blood test was performed to look for biomarkers of alcohol abuse. These include measuring specific enzymes (e.g., GGT, AST, and ALT) that are more abundant in the serum of alcoholics. Moreover, an AST/ALT ratio of >2 is highly suggestive of alcoholic liver disease. Increased red blood cell size (i.e., mean corpuscular volume) is also common in alcoholics. Are this patient's lab values consistent with alcoholism and liver damage?

5. Severe alcohol withdrawal can result in delirium tremens. Using a medical dictionary, or other dependable resource, briefly describe delirium tremens and the signs and symptoms included in this case.

Delirium tremens:

Tachycardia:

Hypertension:

Hyperthermia:

Diaphoresis:

References

Agrali, O. B., & Kuru, B. E. (2015). Periodontal treatment in a generalized severe chronic periodontitis patient: A case report with 7-year follow-up. *European Journal of Dentistry, 9*(2), 288–292. https://doi.org/10.4103/1305-7456.156844

Barawid, E., Covarrubias, N., Tribuzio, B., & Liao, S. (2015). The benefits of rehabilitation for palliative care patients. *American Journal of Hospice and Palliative Medicine, 32*(1), 34–43. https://doi.org/10.1177/1049909113514474

Bhatraju, P. K., Ghassemieh, B. J., Nichols, M., Kim, R., Jerome, K. R., Nalla, A. K., Greninger, A. L., Pipavath, S., Wurfel, M. M., Evans, L., Kritek, P. A., West, T. E., Luks, A., Gerbino, A., Dale, C. R., Goldman, J. D., O'Mahony, S., & Mikacenic, C. (2020). Covid-19 in critically ill patients in the Seattle region — case Sseries. *The New England Journal of Medicine, 382*(21), 2012–2022. https://doi.org/10.1056/NEJMoa2004500

Dydyk, A. M., Givler, A. Central Pain Syndrome. [Updated 2020 Apr 12]. In: StatPearls [Internet]. Treasure Island (FL): StatPearls Publishing; 2020 Jan-. Available from: https://www.ncbi.nlm.nih.gov/books/NBK553027/

Fernandez, J. M., Collier, E. K., Foshee, J. P., Davis, T., Hsiao, J. L., & Shi, V. Y. (2020). Invasive ductal carcinoma arising from an accessory nipple. *JAAD Case Reports, 6*(6), 540–542. https://doi.org/10.1016/j.jdcr.2020.04.028

Gendler, L. S., & Joseph, K. A. (2005). Breast cancer of an accessory nipple. *New England Journal of Medicine, 353*(17), 1835–1835. doi:10.1056/nejmicm050728

McCormick, U., Murray, B., & McNew, B. (2015). Diagnosis and treatment of patients with bipolar disorder: A review for advanced practice nurses. *Journal of the American Association of Nurse Practitioners, 27*(9), 530–542. https://doi.org/10.1002/2327-6924.12275

McNally R. J. (1994). Choking phobia: A review of the literature. *Comprehensive Psychiatry, 35*(1), 83–89. https://doi.org/10.1016/0010-440x(94)90174-0

Newman, R. K., Stobart Gallagher M. A., Gomez, A. E. Alcohol withdrawal. [Updated 2020 Mar 2]. In: StatPearls [Internet]. Treasure Island (FL): StatPearls Publishing; 2020 Jan-. Available from: https://www.ncbi.nlm.nih.gov/books/NBK441882/

Pergolotti, M., Bailliard, A., McCarthy, L., Farley, E., Covington, K. R., & Doll, K. M. (2020). Women's experiences after ovarian cancer surgery: Distress, uncertainty, and the need for occupational therapy. *The American Journal of Occupational Therapy, 74*(3), 7403205140p1–7403205140p9. https://doi.org/10.5014/ajot.2020.036897

Reid D. B. (2016). A case study of hypnosis for phagophobia: It's no choking matter. *The American Journal of Clinical Hypnosis, 58*(4), 357–367. https://doi.org/10.1080/00029157.2015.1048544

Rubino, F., Amiel, S. A., Zimmet, P., Alberti, G., Bornstein, S., Eckel, R. H., Mingrone, G., Boehm, B., Cooper, M. E., Chai, Z., Del Prato, S., Ji, L., Hopkins, D., Herman, W. H., Khunti, K., Mbanya, J. C., & Renard, E. (2020). New-Onset Diabetes in Covid-19. *New England Journal of Medicine, 383*, 789–790 doi: 10.1056/NEJMc2018688

Smith, B.T. & Pacitti, D.F. (2020). Pharmacology for nurses. Ed. 2, Burlington: Jones and Bartlett Learning.

Spiegel, D. R., Dhadwal, N., & Gill, F. (2008). I'm sober, Doctor, really': Best biomarkers for underreported alcohol use. *Current Psychiatry, 7*(9), 15–27.

Stedman, T. L. (2005). Nath's *Stedman's medical terminology, 2e.* Philadelphia: Lippincott Williams & Wilkins.

Venes, D. & Taber, C. W. (2017). Taber's cyclopedic medical dictionary. Ed. 23, illustrated in full color/Philadelphia: F.A. Davis.

Wiersinga, W. J., Rhodes, A., Cheng, A. C., Peacock, S. J., & Prescott, H. C. (2020). Pathophysiology, transmission, diagnosis, and treatment of coronavirus disease 2019 (COVID-19): A review. *JAMA, 324*(8), 782–793. 10.1001/jama.2020.12839. [Advance online publication.] https://doi.org/10.1001/jama.2020.12839

Appendix A

Word Part Definitions

▶ Prefix

a-	without, not
ab-	away from
acid-	acidic
acro-	extremity; top; point
ad-	toward
alkal-	basic
allo-	other, different from usual
an-	without
ana-	up; backward
ante-	before, in front of
anti-	against
apo-	off, away
asthen-	weaknesss
auto-	self
bi-	two
brady-	slow
circum-	around
co-	together, with
con-	together, with
contra-	against, opposite
de-	without
di-	aside, two
dia-	complete, through; apart
dis-	apart
dys-	painful; abnormal; difficult
e-	outward
ec-	out, outside
echo-	reflected sound
ecto-	out, outside
en-	inward, within
endo-	within
epi-	above
eso-	inward
eu-	normal
ex-	outward
exo-	outward
extra-	outside of
febri-	fever
hemi-	half
hetero-	different
homeo-	same, unchanging
homo-	same
hyper-	above, excessive
hypo-	below, deficient, insufficient
in-	inward; not
infra-	below, beneath
inter-	between
intra-	within
ipsi-	same
juxta-	near
macro-	large
mal-	bad
malign-	harmful
meso-	middle
meta-	beyond
micro-	small
mono-	one
multi-	many
myo-	to shut
neo-	new
noci-	pain
non-	not
nulli-	none
opac-	obscure
opistho-	backward; behind
pachy-	heavy, thick
pan-	all
para-	beside; two like parts of a pair; abnormal
per-	through
peri-	around
poly-	many, much
post-	after
pre-	before
primi-	first
pro-	before, forward
pseudo-	false
quadri-	four

re-	back; again
retro-	back, behind
semi-	partial
sub-	under
supra-	above, upper
sym-	together, with
syn-	together, with
tachy-	fast
tetra-	four
trans-	across, through
tri-	three
ultra-	beyond
un-	not
uni-	one

▶ Combining Form

abdomin/o	abdomen
acous/o	hearing
acr/o	extremity
actin/o	ray
aden/o	gland
adenoid/o	adenoid
adenotonsill/o	adenoid
adip/o	fat
adren/o	adrenal gland
adrenal/o	adrenal gland
aer/o	air
agglutin/o	clumping
albin/o	white
albumin/o	albumin
alges/o	pain
all/o	other
alveol/o	alveolus, small sac
ambly/o	dull, dim
amni/o	amnion
amyl/o	starch
an/o	anus
andr/o	male
angi/o	vessel
anis/o	unequal
ankyl/o	stiffening
anter/o	front
anthrac/o	coal
aort/o	aorta
appendico/o	appendix
aque/o	water
arter/o	artery
arteri/o	artery
arthr/o	joint
asbest/o	asbestos

astr/o	star
atel/o	incomplete
ather/o	fatty substance
atri/o	atrium
audit/o	hearing
aur/o	ear
auricul/o	ear
axill/o	armpit
axon/o	axon
azot/o	nitrogenous waste
bacteri/o	bacteria
balan/o	glans penis
bar/o	pressure
bi/o	life
bil/i	bile; gallbladder
bilirubin/o	bilirubin, bile pigment
blast/o	immature
blephar/o	eyelid
bronch/o	bronchus
bronchi/o	bronchus
bronchiol/o	bronchiole
bucc/o	cheek
burs/o	sac
calc/o	calcium
calcane/o	heel
calciton/o	calcitonin
calcul/o	little stone
capillar/o	capillary
capn/o	carbon dioxide
carcin/o	cancer
cardi/o	heart
carotid/o	carotid artery
carp/o	wrist
caud/o	tail
cephal/o	head
cerebell/o	cerebellum
cerebr/o	cerebrum
cerumin/o	cerumen
cervic/o	cervix; neck
cheil/o	lip
chem/o	chemical
chem/o	drug
chlor/o	green
chol/e	bile, gall
cholangi/o	bile duct
cholecyst/o	gallbladder
choledoch/o	common bile duct
cholesterol/o	cholesterol
chondr/o	cartilage
chori/o	chorion
chorion/o	chorion
chrom/o	color

chromat/o	color	duoden/o	duodenum
chron/o	time	dur/o	dura mater
chyl/o	chyle (mixture of lymph and fats)	dynam/o	force
cili/o	cilia	edemat/o	swelling
cirrh/o	yellow-orange	electr/o	electric
clon/o	rapid contracting and relaxing	embol/o	plug
clavicul/o	clavicle	emmetr/o	correct, proper
coagul/o	clotting	encephal/o	brain
cochle/o	cochlea	enter/o	small intestine
col/o	colon	eosin/o	rosy
colon/o	colon	epididym/o	epididymis
colp/o	vagina	epiglott/o	epiglottis
concuss/o	to shake violently	episi/o	vulva
coni/o	dust	epitheli/o	epithelium
conjunctiv/o	conjunctiva	erg/o	work
constrict/o	narrow	erythr/o	red
contine/o	hold back, restrain, keep in	esophag/o	esophagus
cor/o	pupil	esthesi/o	sensation, feeling
corne/o	cornea	esthes/o	sensation, feeling
coron/o	heart	estr/o	female
corpor/o	body	extens/o	to stretch out
cortic/o	outer layer	faci/o	face
cost/o	rib	fasci/o	fascia
crani/o	skull	femor/o	femur
cricothyr/o	ligament between the cricoid and thyroid cartilages	fet/o	fetus
		fibr/o	fiber
crin/o	secreting	fistul/o	tube, pipe
cry/o	cold	flex/o	to bend
crypt/o	hidden	follicul/o	follicle
cutane/o	skin	gen/o	beginning; birth
cyan/o	blue	gastr/o	stomach
cycl/o	circle	gingiv/o	gums
cyst/o	urinary bladder; sac	glanul/o	glans penis
cyt/o	cell	glauc/o	gray
dacry/o	tear; lacrimal gland	globin/o	protein
dacryoaden/o	tear; lacrimal gland	glomerul/o	glomerulus
dacryocyst/o	tear; lacrimal gland	gloss/o	tongue
dactyl/o	digit, finger, toe	gluc/o	sugar
defec/o	evacuation of feces	glyc/o	sugar
dent/o	tooth	glycos/o	sugar
dentin/o	tooth	gnath/o	jaw, mandible
depress/o	to press down	gonad/o	sex gland; gonad
derm/o	skin	goni/o	angle
dermat/o	skin	gynec/o	woman, female
diaphar/o	profuse sweating	habilitat/o	ability
dilat/o	widen	halit/o	breath
dipl/o	double	hallucin/o	imagined perception
dips/o	thirst	hem/o	blood
dist/o	away from	hemat/o	blood
diverticul/o	pouch	hemispher/o	hemisphere (of the cerebrum)
dors/o	back	hepat/o	liver
duct/o	to bring; duct	hidr/o	sweat

hirsut/o	hairy	mamm/o	breast
histi/o	tissue	man/o	pressure
hist/o	tissue	mast/o	breast
hydr/o	water	maxill/o	maxilla, upper jaw
hypn/o	sleep	meat/o	meatus
hyster/o	uterus	medi/o	middle
iatr/o	physician, medicine, treatment	medull/o	inner region
ichthy/o	scaly	melan/o	black
icter/o	jaundice	men/o	menstruation
idi/o	unknown	meningi/o	meninges
ile/o	ileum	mening/o	meninges
immun/o	immune, protection	ment/o	mind
infer/o	below	metacarp/o	metacarpal, hand bone
inguin/o	groin	metr/o	measurement; uterus
iod/o	iodine	metri/o	uterus
ir/o	iris	mineral/o	mineral, electrolyte
irid/o	iris	mi/o	lessening
isch/o	to hold back	morph/o	shape
is/o	same, equal	muc/o	mucus
jaund/o	yellow	muscul/o	muscle
jejun/o	jejunum	mutat/o	to change
kal/i	potassium	myc/o	fungus
kary/o	nucleus	my/o	muscle
kel/o	tumor	mydr/o	widening
kerat/o	horny tissue; cornea	myel/o	bone marrow; spinal cord
ket/o	ketone	myocardi/o	heart muscle, myocardium
keton/o	ketone	myomat/o	muscular tumor
kinesi/o	movement	myring/o	tympanic membrane
klept/o	stealing	myx/o	mucin, mucus
kyph/o	hump	nas/o	nose
labyrinth/o	labyrinth	nat/o	birth
lacrim/o	tears	natr/o	sodium
lact/o	milk	necr/o	death
lamin/o	lamina of vertebral arch	nephr/o	kidney
lapar/o	abdomen	neur/o	nerve; neuron
laps/o	slip, slide	neutr/o	neutral
laryng/o	larynx	noct/i	night
later/o	side	noct/o	night
lei/o	smooth	nocturn/o	night
leuk/o	white	norm/o	normal
levat/o	levator ani muscle	numer/o	number
ligat/o:	binding	nyctal/o	night
lingu/o	tongue	obstetr/o	pregnancy; childbirth
lip/o	fat	ocul/o	eye
lith/o	stone	odont/o	tooth
lob/o	lobe	odyn/o	pain
lord/o	curve	olig/o	scanty
lumb/o	lower back	onc/o	tumor
lymph/o	lymph	onych/o	nail
lymphaden/o	lymph node	o/o	egg
lymphangi/o	lymph vessel	oophor/o	ovary
macul/o	macula lutea	ophthalm/o	eye

optic/o	eye, vision	protein/o	protein
opt/o	eye, vision	proxim/o	near to
or/o	mouth	prurit/o	itchy
orch/o	testicle, testis	psor/o	itchy
orchid/o	testicle, testis	pub/o	pubis
orchi/o	testicle, testis	pulmon/o	lung
orth/o	straight	pupill/o	pupil
oste/o	bone	pustul/o	pustule
ot/o	ear	py/o	pus
ov/o	egg, ovum	pyel/o	renal pelvis
ovari/o	egg, ovum	pyr/o	fire
ovul/o	egg, ovum	pysch/o	mind
ox/i	oxygen	radi/o	radiation
ox/o	oxygen	radicul/o	nerve root
palat/o	palate	rect/o	rectum
pancreat/o	pancreas	ren/o	kidney
parathyroid/o	parathyroid gland	reticul/o	network
path/o	disease	retin/o	retina
ped/o	child; foot	rhabdomy/o	skeletal muscle
pedicul/o	lice	rheumat/o	watery flow
pelv/o	pelvis	rhin/o	nose
pen/o	penis	roentgen/o	unit of X-ray exposure
periodont/o	around the teeth	rotat/o	rotation
peripher/o	away from center	rrhythm/o	rhythm
peritone/o	peritoneum	sacr/o	sacrum
phag/o	eat, swallow	salping/o	auditory tube, eustachian tube; uterine tube
phalang/o	phalange, finger, toe		
pharmac/o	drug	scapul/o	scapula
pharyng/o	pharynx, throat	sarc/o	flesh; connective tissue
phleb/o	vein	schiz/o	split
phob/o	irrational fear	scint/i	spark
phon/o	voice, sound	scler/o	hard; sclera
phot/o	light	scoli/o	crooked
physi/o	function	scrot/o	scrotum
pil/o	hair	seb/o	oil
pineal/o	pineal gland	sect/o	to cut
pituit/o	pituitary gland	segment/o	piece
pituitar/o	pituitary gland	semen/o	semen, seed
plei/o	more, many; varied	sept/o	wall
pleur/o	pleura	sial/o	saliva
pneumat/o	air	sialaden/o	salivary gland
pneum/o	lung; air	sigmoid/o	sigmoid colon
pneumon/o	lung; air	silic/o	glass
poikil/o	varied, irregular	sinus/o	sinus
pol/o	extreme	somat/o	body
polyp/o	polyp	somn/o	sleep
poster/o	back	son/o	sound
presby/o	old age	spermat/o	sperm cells, semen
proct/o	anus, rectum	sperm/o	sperm cells, semen
prosencephal/o	forebrain	sphygm/o	pulse
prostat/o	prostate gland	spir/o	breathing
prosthet/o	addition	splen/o	spleen

spondyl/o	vertebra
squam/o	scale
staped/o	stapes
steat/o	fat
sten/o	narrowed
steth/o	chest
stigmat/o	point
stomat/o	mouth
super/o	above
syncop/o	cut off; faint
syring/o	cavity, tube
system/o	system
systol/o	contraction
tele/o	distant
ten/o	tendon
tendin/o	tendon
tend/o	tendon
tens/o	pressure
terat/o	monster
testicul/o	testis
thec/o	sheath
therm/o	heat
thorac/o	chest
thromb/o	clot
thryoid/o	thyroid gland
thym/o	thymus gland
thyr/o	thyroid cartilage; thyroid gland;
tom/o	to cut
ton/o	pressure, tone
tonsill/o	tonsils
topic/o	specific area
toxic/o	poison
tox/o	poison
trache/o	trachea
trich/o	hair
troph/o	nourishment
tympan/o	tympanic membrane
ulcer/o	erosion
ungu/o	nail
ur/o	urine
ureter/o	ureter
urethr/o	urethra
urin/o	urine
uve/o	uvea
vagin/o	vagina
valv/o	valve
valvul/o	valve
varic/o	dilated vein
vas/o	vas deferens, vessel
vascul/o	vessels
ven/o	vein
ventr/o	belly

ventricul/o	ventricle
vers/o	to turn
vertebr/o	vertebra
vesic/o	vesicles
vesic/o	urinary bladder
vesicul/o	vesicles
viscos/o	sticky
vitre/o	glassy
vulv/o	vulva
xanth/o	yellow
xen/o	foreign
xer/o	dry
zo/o	animal life

▶ Suffix

-a	pertaining to
-ac	pertaining to
-aceous	characterized by
-acusis	hearing
-agogue	bringer of
-al	pertaining to
-algesia	sensitivity to pain
-algia	pain
-an	pertaining to
-ant	that is
-apharesis	removal, carry away
-ar	pertaining to
-arche	beginning
-arity	relating to
-arthria	articulation
-ary	pertaining to
-ase	enzyme
-asthenia	weakness
-ated	process, condition
-atic	pertaining to
-ation	process, condition
-atory	pertaining to
-blast	immature
-capnia	carbon dioxide
-cardia	heart condition
-cele	protrusion
-centesis	puncture to withdraw fluid
-ceptor	receiver
-chezia	defecation, elimination of waste
-cide	killing
-clast	to break
-constriction	narrowing
-crine	secretion
-crit	separation of
-cusis	hearing

-cyesis	state of pregnancy	-ive	tendency
-cyte	cell	-ization	process of making
-cytic	pertaining to cells	-kinesis	movement
-cytosis	more than the normal number of cells	-lepsy	seizure
-derma	skin condition	-listhesis	slipping
-desis	surgical fusion	-lithiasis	condition of stones
-dipsia	condition of thirst	-lithotomy	incision for removing a stone
-dynia	pain	-lithotripsy	surgical crushing of stones
-eal	pertaining to	-logic	pertaining to study of
-ectasia	dilation	-logist	one who studies
-ectasis	dilation	-logy	study of
-ectomy	surgical removal	-lysis	to breakdown, destroy
-edema	swelling	-lytic	destruction
-emesis	vomiting	-malacia	softening
-emia	blood condition	-mania	frenzy
-emic	blood condition	-manometer	instrument to measure pressure
-esis	condition, state of	-megaly	enlarged
-esthesia	nervous condition	-meter	instrument to measure
-eurysm	widening	-metric	pertaining to measuring
-gen	that which produces	-metrist	specialist in measuring
-genesis	producing, forming	-metry	measuring
-genic	produced by or in	-nic	pertaining to
-genous	producing	-nomic	pertaining to law
-globin	protein	-nuclear	nucleus
-globulin	protein	-nymous	name
-gnosia	knowledge	-oid	resembling
-grade	to go	-oma	tumor, mass
-gram	record or picture	-opia	vision condition
-graphy	recording	-opsia	vision condition
-gravida	pregnancy	-opsy	view of
-ia	condition	-or	one that is; condition of
-iac	pertaining to	-orexia	appetite
-iasis	abnormal condition	-ory	pertaining to
-iatric	pertaining to medical treatment	-ose	pertaining to
-iatrist	physician	-osis	abnormal condition
-iatry	medical treatment	-osmia	olfactory condition
-ic	pertaining to	-ostomy	surgically create an opening
-ical	pertaining to	-ostosis	bone development
-ice	condition	-otia	ear condition
-ician	specialist	-otomy	cutting into
-id	pertaining to	-ous	pertaining to
-ification	process of becoming	-para	to bear, bring forth offspring
-ile	pertaining to	-paresis	weakness; paralysis
-ine	pertaining to	-parous	bearing, bringing forth
-ion	process	-partum	childbirth
-ior	pertaining to	-pathy	disease
-ism	condition of	-penia	abnormal decrease
-ist	specialist	-pepsia	digestion
-istry	specialty of; pertaining to	-pexy	surgical fixation
-itis	inflammation	-phage	to eat
-ity	condition	-phagia	eating
		-phasia	speech

-phil	attracted to	-static	pertaining to stopping, standing still
-phobia	irrational fear		
-phoresis	carrying	-statin	to stop
-phoria	feeling	-stenosis	narrowing
-phyte	plant-like growth	-stomia	condition of the mouth
-plasia	development; formation of cells	-taxia	muscle coordination
-plasm	growth, formation	-tension	pressure
-plasty	surgical repair	-therapy	treatment
-plegia	paralysis	-thorax	pleural cavity, chest
-pnea	breathing	-tic	pertaining to
-poiesis	formation	-tocia	labor, childbirth
-poietic	pertaining to formation	-tome	instrument to cut
-porosis	porous	-tonia	tone
-prandial	meal	-tory	pertaining to
-praxia	action	-tous	pertaining to
-pressin	to press down	-tresia	opening
-ptosis	drooping, drooping eyelid	-tripsy	surgical crushing
-ptysis	spitting	-trophic	pertaining to development; stimulation
-receptor	receiver		
-rrhage	abnormal flow	-trophy	development
-rrhagia	abnormal flow condition	-tropia	turned condition
-rrhaphy	surgical suturing	-tropic	pertaining to stimulating
-rrhea	discharge	-tropin	to stimulate
-rrhexis	rupture	-tropin	to act on, stimulate
-salpinx	uterine tube	-tubation	putting a tube within
-schisis	split	-ule	small
-sclerosis	hardening	-um	structure
-scope	instrument for viewing	-uria	urine condition
-scopic	pertaining to visually examining	-us	structure, thing
-scopy	visually examining	-version	act of turning
-spadia	cut, tear	-volemia	blood volume
-spasm	sudden contraction	-y	condition, process
-spermia	condition of sperm		
-stasis	standing still		

Appendix B

Word Parts Listed by Definitions

▶ Prefix

abnormal	dys-, para-
above	epi-, hyper-, supra-
acidic	acid-
across	trans-
after	post-
again	re-
against	anti-, contra-
air	pneum/o, pneumon/o,
all	pan-
apart	dis-, dia-
area	topic/o
around	circum-, peri-
aside	di-
away from	ab-, apo-
back	re-, retro-
backward	opistho-, ana-
bad	mal-
basic	alkal-
before	ante-, pre-, pro-
behind	retro-, opistho-
below	infra-, hypo-
beneath	infra-
beside	para-
between	inter-
beyond	meta-, ultra-
complete	dia-
deficient	allo-, hypo-
different	hetero-
difficult	dys-
excessive	hyper-
extremity	acro-
false	pseudo-
fast	tachy-
fever	febri-
first	primi-
foreword	pro-
four	quadri-, tetra-
half	hemi-
harmful	malign-
heavy	pachy-
in front of	ante-
insufficient	hypo-
inward	en-, eso-, in-
large	macro-
many	multi-, poly-
middle	meso-
much	poly-
near	juxta-
new	neo-
none	nulli-
normal	eu-
not	a-, in-, non-, un-
obscure	opac-
off	apo-
one	mono-, uni-
opposite	contra-
other	allo-
out	ec-, ecto-
outside	ec-, ecto-, extra-
outward	e-, ex-, exo-
pain	noci-
painful	dys-
paired	para-
partial	semi-
point	acro-
same	homeo-, homo-, ipsi-
self	auto-
slow	brady-
small	micro-
sound (reflected)	echo-
thick	pachy-
three	tri-
through	dia-, per-, trans-
together	co-, con-, sym-, syn-
top	acro-
toward	ad-
two	bi-, di-
under	sub-

up	ana-	bronchiole	bronchiol/o
upper	supra-	bronchus	bronchi/o, bronch/o
weakness	asthen-	calcitonin	calciton/o
with	co-, con-, sym-, syn-	calcium	calc/o
within	en-, endo-, intra-	cancer	carcin/o
without	a-, an-, de-	capillary	capillar/o
		carbon dioxide	capn/o
		carotid artery	carotid/o

▶ Combining Form

abdomen	abdomin/o, lapar/o	cartilage	chondr/o
ability	habilitat/o	cavity	syring/o
above	super/o	cell	cyt/o
addition	prosthet/o	cerebellum	cerebell/o
adenoid	adenoid/o, adenotonsill/o	cerebrum	cerebr/o
adrenal gland	adrenal/o, adren/o	cerumen	cerumin/o
air	aer/o, pneumat/o	cervix	cervic/o
albumin	albumin/o	change	mutat/o
alveolus	alveol/o	cheek	bucc/o
amnion	amni/o	chemical	chem/o
angle	goni/o	chest	steth/o, thorac/o
anus	an/o, proct/o	child	ped/o
aorta	aort/o	childbirth	obstetr/o
appendix	appendic/o	cholesterol	cholesterol/o
armpit	axill/o	chorion	chori/o, chorion/o
artery	arteri/o, arter/o	chyle	chyl/o
asbestos	asbest/o	cilia	cili/o
atrium	atri/o	circle	cycl/o
auditory tube	salping/o	clavicle	clavicul/o
away from	dist/o	clot	thromb/o
axon	axon/o	clotting	coagul/o
back	dors/o, poster/o	clumping	agglutin/o
bacteria	bacteri/o	coal	anthrac/o
beginning	gen/o	cochlea	cochle/o
belly	ventr/o	cold	cry/o
below	infer/o	colon	col/o, colon/o
bend	flex/o	color	chromat/o, chrom/o
bile	bil/i, chol/e	common bile duct	choledoch/o
bile duct	cholangi/o	conjunctiva	conjunctiv/o
bilirubin	bilirubin/o	connective tissue	sarc/o
binding	ligat/o	contraction	systol/o
birth	gen/o, nat/o	cornea	corne/o, kerat/o
black	melan/o	correct	emmetr/o
blood	hemat/o, hem/o	crooked	scoli/o
blue	corpor/o, cyan/o, somat/o	curve	lord/o
bone	oste/o	cut	sect/o, tom/o
bone marrow	myel/o	death	necr/o
brain	encephal/o	depress	depress/o
breast	mamm/o, mast/o	digit	dactyl/o
breath	halit/o	dim	ambly/o
breathing	spir/o	disease	path/o
bring	duct/o	distance	tele/o
		double	dipl/o
		drug	chem/o, pharmac/o

dry	xer/o	gonad	gonad/o
duct	duct/o	gray	glauc/o
dull	ambly/o	green	chlor/o
duodenum	duoden/o	groin	inguin/o
dura mater	dur/o	gums	gingiv/o
dust	coni/o	hair	pil/o, trich/o
ear	auricul/o, aur/o, ot/o	hairy	hirsut/o
eat	phag/o	hard	scler/o
egg	o/o, ovari/o, ov/o, ovul/o	head	cephal/o
electric	electr/o	hearing	acous/o, audit/o
epididymis	epididym/o	heart	cardi/o, coron/o
epiglottis	epiglott/o	heart muscle	myocardi/o
epithelium	epitheli/o	heat	therm/o
equal	is/o	heel	calcane/o
erosion	ulcer/o	hemisphere	
esophagus	esophag/o	(of the cerebrum)	hemispher/o
eustachian tube	salping/o	hidden	crypt/o
defecate	defec/o	hold back	contine/o, isch/o
extreme	pol/o	horny tissue	kerat/o
extremity	acr/o	hump	kyph/o
eye	ocul/o, ophthalm/o,	ileum	ile/o
	optic/o, opt/o	hallucination	hallucin/o
eyelid	blephar/o	immature cell	blast/o
face	faci/o	immune	immun/o
faint	syncop/o	incomplete	atel/o
fascia	fasci/o	inner region	medull/o
fat	adip/o, lip/o, steat/o	iodine	iod/o
fatty substance	ather/o	iris	irid/o, ir/o
feeling	esthesi/o, esthes/o	irrational fear	phob/o
female	estr/o, gynec/o	itchy	prurit/o, psor/o
femur	femor/o	jaundice	icter/o
fetus	fet/o	jaw	gnath/o
fiber	fibr/o	jejunum	jejun/o
finger	dactyl/o, phalang/o	joint	arthr/o
fire	pyr/o	ketone	ket/o, keton/o
flesh	sarc/o	kidney	nephr/o, ren/o
follicle	follicul/o	labyrinth	labyrinth/o
foot	ped/o	larynx	laryng/o
force	dynam/o	lessening	mi/o
forebrain	prosencephal/o	levator ani muscle	levat/o
foreign	xen/o	lice	pedicul/o
front	anter/o	life	bi/o
function	physi/o	life (animal)	zo/o
fungus	myc/o	light	phot/o
gall	chol/e	lip	cheil/o
gallbladder	bil/i, cholecyst/o	liver	hepat/o
gland	aden/o	lobe	lob/o
glans penis	balan/o, glanul/o	lower back	lumb/o
glass	silic/o	lung	pneum/o, pneumon/o,
glassy	vitre/o		pulmon/o
glomerulus	glomerul/o	lymph	lymph/o
glucose	gluc/o, glyc/o	lymph node	lymphaden/o

lymph vessel	lymphangi/o	parathyroid gland	parathyroid/o
macula lutea	macul/o	pelvis	pelv/o
male	andr/o	penis	pen/o
mandible	gnath/o	peripheral	peripher/o
many	plei/o	peritoneum	peritone/o
maxilla	maxill/o	phalange	phalang/o
measurement	metr/o	pharynx	pharyng/o
meatus	meat/o	physician	iatr/o
medicine	iatr/o	piece	segment/o
meninges	meningi/o, mening/o	pineal gland	pineal/o
menstruation	men/o	pituitary gland	pituitar/o, pituit/o
metacarpal	metacarp/o	pleura	pleur/o
middle	medi/o	plug	embol/o
milk	lact/o	point	stigmat/o
mind	ment/o, pysch/o	poison	toxic/o, tox/o
mineral	mineral/o	polyp	polyp/o
monster	terat/o	potassium	kal/i
more	plei/o	pouch	diverticul/o
mouth	or/o, stomat/o	pregnancy	obstetr/o
movement	kinesi/o	pressure	bar/o, man/o, tens/o, ton/o
mucus	muc/o, myx/o	profuse sweating	diaphar/o
muscle	muscul/o, my/o	proper	emmetr/o
muscular tumor	myomat/o	prostate gland	prostat/o
myocardium	myocardi/o	protection	immun/o
nail	onych/o, ungu/o	protein	globin/o, protein/o
narrow	constrict/o, sten/o	pubis	pub/o
near	proxim/o	pulse	sphygm/o
neck	cervic/o	pupil	cor/o, pupill/o
nerve	neur/o	pus	py/o
nerve root	radicul/o	pustule	pustul/o
network	reticul/o	radiation	radi/o
neuron	neur/o	ray	actin/o
neutral	neutr/o	rectum	proct/o, rect/o
night	noct/i, noct/o, nocturn/o, nyctal/o	red	erythr/o
		renal pelvis	pyel/o
nitrogenous waste	azot/o	restrain	contine/o
normal	norm/o	retina	retin/o
nose	nas/o, rhin/o	rhythm	rrhythm/o
nourishment	troph/o	rib	cost/o
nucleus	kary/o	rosy	eosin/o
number	numer/o	rotation	rotat/o
oil	seb/o	sac	burs/o, cyst/o
old age	presby/o	sacrum	sacr/o
other	all/o	saliva	sial/o
outer layer	cortic/o	salivary gland	sialaden/o
ovary	oophor/o	same	is/o
ovum	ovari/o, ov/o, ovul/o	scapula	scapul/o
oxygen	ox/i, ox/o	scale	ichthy/o, squam/o
pain	alges/o, odyn/o	scanty	olig/o
palate	palat/o	sclera	scler/o
pancreas	pancreat/o	scrotum	scrot/o

secreting	crin/o	thymus gland	thym/o
semen	semen/o, spermat/o, sperm/o	thyroid cartilage	thyr/o
		thyroid gland	thryoid/o, thyr/o
sensation	esthes/o, esthesi/o	time	chron/o
shake violently	concuss/o	tissue	histi/o, hist/o
shape	morph/o	toe	dactyl/o, phalang/o
sheath	thec/o	tone	ton/o
side	later/o	tongue	gloss/o, ingu/o
sigmoid colon	sigmoid/o	tooth	dentin/o, dent/o
sinus	sinus/o	tonsils	tonsill/o
skeletal muscle	rhabdomy/o	tooth	odont/o
skin	cutane/o, dermat/o, derm/o	trachea	trache/o
		treatment	iatr/o
skull	crani/o	tube	fistul/o, syring/o
sleep	hypn/o, somn/o	tumor	kel/o, onc/o
slip	laps/o	turn	vers/o
small intestine	enter/o	tympanic membrane	myring/o, tympan/o
smooth	lei/o	unequal	anis/o
sodium	natr/o	unknown	idi/o
sound	phon/o, son/o	ureter	ureter/o
spark	scint/i	urethra	urethr/o
sperm cells	spermat/o, sperm/o	urinary bladder	cyst/o, vesic/o
spinal cord	myel/o	urine	urin/o, ur/o
spleen	splen/o	uterine tube	salping/o
split	schiz/o	uterus	hyster/o, metri/o, metr/o
stapes	staped/o	uvea	uve/o
star	astr/o	vagina	colp/o, vagin/o
starch	amyl/o	valve	valv/o, valvul/o
stealing	klept/o	varied	plei/o, poikil/o
sticky	viscos/o	vas deferens	vas/o
stiffening	ankyl/o	vein	phleb/o, ven/o
stomach	gastr/o	vein (dilated)	varic/o
stone	calcul/o, lith/o	ventricle	ventricul/o
straight	orth/o	vertebra	spondyl/o, vertebr/o
stretch out	extens/o	vesicles	vesic/o, vesicul/o
sugar	gluc/o, glyc/o, gylcos/o	vessel	angi/o, vascul/o, vas/o
swallow	phag/o	vision	optic/o, opt/o
sweat	hidr/o	voice	phon/o
swelling	edemat/o	vulva	episi/o, vulv/o
system	system/o	wall	sept/o
lacrimal gland	dacryoaden/o, dacryocyst/o	water	aque/o, hydr/o
		watery flow	rheumat/o
tail	caud/o	white	albin/o, leuk/o
tear	dacry/o, lacrim/o	widen	dilat/o, mydr/o
tendon	tendin/o, tend/o, ten/o	woman	gynec/o
testicle	orchid/o, orchi/o, orch/o, testicul/o	work	erg/o
		wrist	carp/o
testis	orchid/o, orchi/o, orch/o, testicul/o	X-ray (unit)	roentgen/o
		yellow	jaund/o, xanth/o
thirst	dips/o	yellow-orange	cirrh/o
throat	pharyng/o		

▶ Suffix

act on	-tropin
action	-praxia
appetite	-orexia
articulation	- arthria
attracted to	-phil
bearing	-para, -parous
becoming	-ification
beginning	-arche
blood (condition)	-emia, -emic
blood (volume condition)	-volemia
bone development	-ostosis
break	-clast
breakdown	-lysis
breathing	-pnea
bringer of	-agogue
bringing forth	-parous
carbon dioxide (condition)	-capnia
carrying	-phoresis
cell	-cyte, -cytic
cells (excessive number)	-cytosis
characterized by	-aceous
chest	-thorax
childbirth	-partum
condition	-esis, -ia, -ice, -ism, -ity, -or, -y
condition (abnormal)	-iasis, -osis
contraction	-spasm
cut	-spadia
cutting into	-otomy
cutting instrument	-tome
decrease (abnormal)	-penia
defecation (condition)	-chezia
destruction	-lytic
development	-plasia, -trophic, -trophy
digestion (condition)	-pepsia
dilation	-ectasia, -ectasis
discharge	-rrhea
disease	-pathy
drooping (drooping eyelid)	-ptosis
ear (condition)	-otia
eat	-phage, -phagia
enlarged	-megaly
enzyme	-ase
feeling (condition)	-phoria
flow (abnormal)	-rrhage, -rrhagia
formation	-poiesis, -poietic
frenzy (condition)	-mania
go	-grade
growth	-plasm

hardening	-sclerosis
hearing	-acusis, -cusis
heart (condition)	-cardia
immature	-blast
inflammation	-itis
irrational fear (condition)	-phobia
killing	-cide
knowledge (condition)	-gnosia
labor	-tocia
law (pertaining to)	-nomic
making	-ization
mass	-oma
meal	-prandial
measuring	-metric, -metry
measuring instrument	-meter
medical treatment	-iatric, -iatry
mouth (condition)	-stomia
movement	-kinesis
muscle coordination	-taxia
name	-nymous
narrowing	-constriction, -stenosis
nervous condition	-esthesia
nucleus	-nuclear
olfactory condition	-osmia
one that is	-or
one who studies	-logist
opening	-tresia
opening created by surgery	-ostomy
pain	-algia, -dynia
pain (sensitivity)	-algesia
paralysis	-plegia, -paresis
pertaining to	-a, -ac, -al, -an, -ar, -ary, -atic, -atory, -eal, -iac, -ic, -ical, -id, -ile, -ine, -ior, -istry, -nic, -ory, -ose, -ous, -tic, -tory, -tous
physician	-iatrist
plant-like growth	-phyte
porous	-porosis
pregnancy	-gravida
pregnancy (state of)	-cyesis
press down	-pressin
pressure	-tension
pressure measuring instrument	-manometer
process	-ated, -ation, -ion, -y
producing	-genesis, -gen, -genic, -genous
protein	-globin, -globulin

protrusion	-cele	stop	-statin
puncture to withdraw fluid	-centesis	structure	-um, -us
putting a tube within	-tubation	study of	-logic, -logy
receiver	-ceptor, -receptor	surgical crushing	-tripsy
record	-gram, -graphy	surgical crushing of stones	-lithotripsy
relating to	-arity	surgical fixation	-pexy
removal	-apharesis	surgical fusion	-desis
resembling	-oid	surgical removal	-ectomy
rupture	-rrhexis	surgical repair	-plasty
secretion	-crine	surgical suturing	-rrhaphy
seizure	-lepsy	swelling	-edema
separation of	-crit	tear	-spadia
skin condition	-derma	tendency	-ive
slipping	-listhesis	that is	-ant
small	-ule	thirst (condition)	-dipsia
softening	-malacia	tone	-tonia
specialist	-ician, -ist	treatment	-therapy
specialist in measuring	-metrist	tumor	-oma
specialty of	-istry	turning	-tropia, -version
speech	-phasia	urine (condition)	-uria
sperm (condition)	-spermia	uterine tube	-salpinx
spitting	-ptysis	view of	-opsy
split	-schisis	viewing instrument	-scope
standing still	-stasis, -static	vision (condition)	-opia, -opsia
state of	-esis	visually examining	-scopy, -scopic
stimulation	-trophic, -tropic, -tropin	vomiting	-emesis
		weakness	-asthenia, -paresis
stone (surgical removal)	-lithotomy	widening	-eurysm
stones (condition)	-lithiasis		

Appendix C

Abbreviations

AAA: abdominal aortic aneurysm
AB: abortion
ABGs: arterial blood gas
ac: before meals
ACE: angiotensin-converting enzyme
ACh: acetylcholine
ACTH: adrenocorticotropic hormone
AD: Alzheimer's disease
ADH: antidiuretic hormone
ad lib: freely, as desired
ADD: attention deficit disorder
ADHD: attention deficit hyperactivity disorder
ADL: activities of daily living
AFP: alpha fetoprotein
Ag: antigen
AIDS: acquired immunodeficiency syndrome
AKI: acute kidney injury
ALS: amyotrophic lateral sclerosis
ALT: alanine transaminase
AMI: acute myocardial infarction
ANA: antinuclear antibody test
AP: anteroposterior
ARDS: acute respiratory distress syndrome
ARF: acute renal failure
ASHD: arteriosclerotic heart disease
AS: arteriosclerosis
ASD: atrial septal defect
AST: aspartate transaminase
AV: arteriovenous, atrioventricular
BAL: bronchoalveolar lavage
basos: basophils
BBB: bundle branch block
BCC: basal cell carcinoma
BDT: bone density testing
BE: barium enema
bid.: twice a day (*bis in die*)
BM: bowel movement
BMA: bone marrow aspiration
BMI: body mass index
BMR: basal metabolic rate

BMT: bone marrow transplant
BP: blood pressure
BPH: benign prostatic hyperplasia; benign prostatic hypertrophy
BT: blood transfusion
BUN: blood urea nitrogen
Bx: biopsy
C: Celsius
C&S: culture and sensitivity
C-section: cesarean section
C1-C7: cervical vertebrae 1-7
Ca: calcium
Ca^{2+}: calcium ion
CA: cancer, carcinoma
CABG: coronary artery bypass graft
CAD coronary artery disease
CAPD: continuous ambulatory peritoneal dialysis
cath: catheter, catheterization
CBC: complete blood count
cc: cubic centimeter
C. diff: *Clostridium difficile*
CF: cystic fibrosis
CHF: congestive heart failure
CK: creatine kinase
Cl: chlorine
Cl^-: chlorine ion
cm: centimeter
CMG: cystometrogram
CNS: central nervous system
CO_2: carbon dioxide
COPD: chronic obstructive pulmonary disease
COVID-19: coronavirus disease 2019
CP: cerebral palsy; chest pain
CPAP: continuous positive airway pressure
CPK: creatine phosphokinase
CPR: cardiopulmonary resuscitation
CRF: chronic renal failure
crit: hematocrit
CSF: cerebrospinal fluid
CT: calcitonin; computed tomography

CTE: chronic traumatic encephalopathy
CTS: carpal tunnel syndrome
CVA: cerebrovascular accident
CVS: chorionic villus sampling
CXR: chest X-ray
dB: decibel
DCIS: ductal carcinoma in situ
DCT: distal convoluted tubule
DEXA, DXA: dual-energy X-ray absorption
DI: diabetes insipidus; diagnostic imaging
DM: diabetes mellitus
DOB: date of birth
DOE: dyspnea on exertion
DPT: diphtheria, pertussis, tetanus vaccine
DRE: digital rectal exam
DTR: deep tendon reflex
DVT: deep vein thrombosis
Dx: diagnosis
EBV: Epstein-Barr virus
ECG, EKG: electrocardiogram
ECHO: echocardiography
ECT: electroconvulsive therapy
ED: erectile dysfunction
ED&C: electrodesiccation and curettage
EDC: estimated date of confinement
EDD: estimated date of delivery
EEG: electroencephalogram
EENT: eyes, ears, nose, and throat
EGD: esophagogastroduodenoscopy
eGFR: estimated glomerular filtration rate
EGFR: epidermal growth factor receptor
EMG: electromyogram
ENT: ears, nose, and throat
eos, eosins: eosinophils
EPO: erythropoietin
ER, ED: emergency room, emergency department
ERCP: endoscopic retrograde
    cholangiopancreatography
ESR: erythrocyte sedimentation rate
ESRD: end-stage renal disease
ERV: expiratory reserve volume
ESWL: extracorporeal shock wave lithotripsy
EUS: endoscopic ultrasound
F: Fahrenheit
Fe: iron
FNA: fine-needle aspiration
FS: frozen section
FSH: follicle-stimulating hormone
Fx, FX: fracture
g, gm: gram
GBS: group B streptococcus
GCT: germ cell tumor

GERD: gastroesophageal reflux disease
GFR: glomerular filtration rate
GH: growth hormone
GI: gastrointestinal
GIST: gastrointestinal stromal tumor
grav I: first pregnancy
GTT: glucose tolerance test
GU: genitourinary
GXT: graded exercise test
GYN: gynecology
H_2O: water
H&P: history and physical
HBV: hepatitis V virus
hCG: human chorionic gonadotropin
HCl: hydrochloric acid
HCO_3: bicarbonate, bicarbonate ion
HCT, Hct, ht: hematocrit
HCV: hepatitis C virus
HEENT: head, eyes, ears, nose, and throat
HEV: hepatitis E virus
HGB, Hb, Hgb: hemoglobin
HIDA: hepatobiliary iminodiacetic acid
HIV: human immunodeficiency virus
HM: Holter monitor
H. pylori: *Helicobacter pylori*
HPV: human papillomavirus
HRT: hormone replacement therapy
HSG: hysterosalpingogram
HSV-1: herpes simplex virus type 1
Ht: height
HTN: hypertension
Hx: history
Hz: hertz
I&D: incision and drainage
I&O: input and output
IBS: irritable bowel syndrome
IC: inspiratory capacity
ICP: intracranial pressure
ICU: intensive care unit
ID: intradermal
IDDM: insulin-dependent diabetes mellitus
Ig: immunoglobulin
ILD: interstitial lung disease
IM: intramuscular
inj: injection
IOL: intraocular lens
IOP: intraocular pressure
IPD: intermittent peritoneal dialysis
IRDS: infant respiratory distress syndrome
IRV: inspiratory reserve volume
ITP: idiopathic thrombocytopenic
    purpura

IU: international units (avoid using abbreviation as it can be mistaken for IV)

IUD: intrauterine device

IV: intravenous (avoid using abbreviation as it can be mistaken for IU)

IVF: in vitro fertilization

IVP: intravenous pyelogram

IVU: intravenous urogram

K: potassium

K^+: potassium ion

kg: kilogram

KS: Kaposi's sarcoma

KUB: kidneys, ureters, and bladder

L: liter

L1-L5: lumbar vertebrae 1-5

Lab: laboratory

LASIK: laser-assisted in situ keratomileusis

LBW: low birth weight

LES: lower esophageal sphincter

LH: luteinizing hormone

LLQ: left lower quadrant

LMP: last menstrual period

LP: lumbar puncture

LUP: left upper quadrant

lymphs: lymphocytes

m: meter

mcg: microgram

MD: Doctor of Medicine; muscular dystrophy

mEq: milliequivalent

MEN: multiple endocrine neoplasia

MERS: Middle East respiratory syndrome

mg: milligram

Mg: magnesium

Mg^{2+}: magnesium ion

MG: myasthenia gravis

MI: myocardial infarction, mitral insufficiency

mL: milliliter

mm: millimeter

mm Hg: millimeters of mercury

Mono: mononucleosis

MRA: magnetic resonance angiography

MRCP: magnetic resonance cholangiopancreatography

MRI: magnetic resonance imaging

MS: multiple sclerosis (avoid using for morphine sulfate or magnesium sulfate)

MSH: melanocyte-stimulating hormone

MTF: male to female

Na: sodium

Na^+: sodium ion

NG: nasogastric

NHL: non-Hodgkin's lymphoma

NICU: neonatal intensive care unit

NK: natural killer cells

noc: night

NPO, npo: nothing by mouth (*non per os*)

NSAID: nonsteroidal anti-inflammatory drug

O_2: oxygen

OA: osteoarthritis

OB: obstetrics

OB/GYN: obstetrics/gynecology

OCD: obsessive-compulsive disorder

od: overdose (avoid abbreviation for once daily)

OD: right eye (*oculus dexter*)

OR: operating room

OS: left eye (*oculus sinister*)

OT: occupational therapy

OTC: over the counter

OU: both eyes (*oculus uterque*)

oz: ounce

P: pulse rate; phosphorus

pc: after metals (*post cibum*)

prn: as needed (*pro re nata*)

PA: physician's assistant; posteroanterior; pernicious anemia

PAD: peripheral arterial disease

PCT: proximal convoluted tubule

PCV: packed cell volume

PDA: patent ductus arteriosus

PE: pulmonary embolism

PET: pediatric emission tomography

PFT: pulmonary function test

PharmD: registered pharmacist

PID: pelvic inflammatory disease

PLT: platelet count

PNS: peripheral nervous system

po: by mouth (*per os*)

POC: products of conception

polys: polymorphonuclear neutrophil

postop: postoperative

preop: preoperative

PPD: purified protein derivative

PRK: photorefractive keratectomy

PSA: prostate-specific antigen

pt: patient

PT: physical therapy

PTCA: percutaneous transluminal coronary angioplasty

PTH: parathyroid hormone

PTSD: post-traumatic stress disorder

PUD: peptic ulcer disease

PVC: premature ventricular contraction

Px: prognosis

q: take

qh: every hour (*quaque hora*)

qid: four times a day (*quarter in die*; avoid using abbreviation for daily)

R: respiratory rate

RA: rheumatoid arthritis

RAI: radioactive iodine

RBC: red blood cell, red blood cell count

REM: rapid eye movement

RF: rheumatoid factor, respiratory failure

RIA: radioimmunoassay

RLQ: right lower quadrant

RP: retrograde pyelogram

ROM: range of motion

RUQ: right upper quadrant

RV: reserve volume

Rx: prescription; take

S1, S2: first and second heart sound

SA: sinoatrial

SAB: spontaneous abortion

SAD: seasonal affective disorder

SARS: severe acute respiratory syndrome

SBS: shaken baby syndrome

SCC: squamous cell carcinoma

SG: skin graft; specific gravity

SK: streptokinase

sl: sublingual

SLE: systemic lupus erythematosus

SOB: shortness of breath

SOM: serous otitis media

SPP: suprapubic prostatectomy

SPECT: single photon emission computed tomography

STAT, stat: immediately

STD: sexually transmitted disease

STI: sexually transmitted infection

Subc, Subq: subcutaneous (avoid using SC as it can be mistaken for SL)

SUI: stress urinary incontinence

Sx: symptom

T: temperature; tablespoon

t: teaspoon

T&A: tonsillectomy and adenoidectomy

T1-T12: thoracic vertebrae 1-12

T_3: tri-iodothyronine

T_4: thyroxine

TAB: therapeutic abortion

TAH: total abdominal hysterectomy

TAH-BSO: total abdominal hysterectomy-bilateral salpingo-oophorectomy

TB: tuberculosis

TBI: traumatic brain injury

TEE: transesophageal echocardiography

TENS: transcutaneous electrical nerve stimulation

TFT: thyroid function test

TIA: transient ischemic attack

tid: three times a day (*ter in die*)

TO: telephone order

top: topical application

tPA: tissue plasminogen activator

TPN: total parenteral nutrition

Tr: treatment

TRUS: transrectal ultrasound

TSH: thyroid-stimulating hormone

tsp: teaspoon

TSS: toxic shock syndrome

TUIP: transurethral incision of the prostate

TURB: transurethral resection of bladder tumor

TUPR: transurethral resection of the prostate

TV: tidal volume

Tx: treatment

U: unit (avoid using abbreviation as it can be mistaken for "0", "4", or "cc")

UA: urinalysis

UGI: upper gastrointestinal

URI: upper respiratory infection

UTI: urinary tract infection

UV: ultraviolet

V fib: ventricular fibrillation

VA: visual acuity

VATS: video-assisted thoracoscopic surgery

VCUG: voiding cystourethrogram

VD: venereal disease

VF: visual field

VO: verbal order

VS: vital signs

VSD: ventricular septal defect

VT: ventricular tachycardia

vWD: von Willebrand disease

WBC: white blood cell, white blood cell count

Wt, wt: weight

Appendix D

Vital Signs and Laboratory Test Values

TABLE D.1

Vital Signs

Blood Pressure	90/60 mm Hg to 120/80 mm Hg
Body Temperature	97.8°F to 99.1°F (36.5°C to 37.3°C)
Heart Rate (Pulse)	60–100 beats/min
Breathing Rate	12–18 breaths/min

TABLE D.2

Blood (B), Plasma (P), or Serum (S) Laboratory Values

Amino Acids (P)	2.3–5.0 mg/dL
Ammonia (P)	12–55 µmol/L
Bicarbonate, HCO_{3-} (P)	20–28 mEq/L
Bilirubin (S)	<0.4 mg/dL
Calcium (S)	8.5–10.5 mg/dL
Carbon dioxide, CO_2 (Arterial Blood)	35–48 mm Hg (male) 32–45 mm Hg (female)
Chloride (P)	100–106 mEq/L
Cholesterol (S)	<200 mg/dL
Creatinine (P)	0.6–1.5 mg/dL
Glucose (B)	70–100 mg/dL
Iron (S)	65–175 µg/dL (male) 50–170 µg/dL (female)

Blood (B), Plasma (P), or Serum (S) Laboratory Values

Ketones (B)	<0.6 mmol/L
Lactic Acid (Venous Blood)	8.1–15.3 mg/dL
Magnesium (S)	1.5–2.0 mEq/L
Oxygen, O_2 (Arterial Blood)	75–100 mm Hg
pH (Arterial Blood)	7.35–7.45
Phosphorus (S)	3.0–4.5 mg/dL
Potassium (S)	3.5–5.0 mEq/L
Sodium (S)	135–145 mEq/L
Urea nitrogen, BUN (S)	8–25 mg/dL
Uric Acid (S)	3.0–7.0 mg/dL

TABLE D.3

Serum Proteins Laboratory Values

Albumin	35–52 g/L
Alkaline Phosphatase, ALK	36–92 U/L
Alanine Aminotransferase, ALT	1–21 U/L
Aspartate Aminotransferase, AST	7–27 U/L
Creatine Kinase, CK	15–105 U/L (male) 10–80 U/L (female)
Carbohydrate Deficient Transferrin, CDT	<6.0 mg/dL

(continues)

TABLE D.3 (continued)

Serum Proteins Laboratory Values

Gamma-glutamyl Transferase, GGT	<38 U/L
Fibrinogen (P)	2.0–4.0 g/L
Ig (Total)	10.0–22.0 g/L
IgG	7.0–16.0 g/L
IgA	0.7–3.8 g/L
IgM	0.5–2.6 g/L
IgD	0–0.08 g/L
IgE	3–423 U/mL
Protein (Total)	60–84 g/L

TABLE D.4

Complete Blood Count (CBC)

Red Blood Cell (RBC) Count	$4.7–6.1 \times 10^6/mm^3$ (male) $4.2–5.4 \times 10^6/mm^3$ (female)
Hemoglobin (Hb)	14.0–18.0 g/dL (male) 12.0–16.0 g/dL (female) 11.2–16.5 g/dL (children) 17.0–23.0 g/dL (newborn)
Hematocrit (Hct) or Packed Cell Volume (PCV)	42–52% (male) 37–47% (female) 30–43% (children) 53–65% (newborn)
Mean Corpuscular Volume (MCV)	86–98 μm^3/RBC
Mean Corpuscular Hemoglobin	27–32 pg/RBC
Platelets	$150–400 \times 10^3/mm^3$
Total White Blood Cell (WBC) Count	$4,800–10,800/mm^3$

Complete Blood Count (CBC)

Neutrophils	$150–400/mm^3$ (Band; Immature) $3,000–5,800/mm^3$ (Segmented; mature)
Lymphocytes	$1,200–3,400/mm^3$
Monocytes	$110–590/mm^3$
Granulocytes	$1,400–6,500/mm^3$
Eosinophils	$<700/mm^3$
Basophils	$<200/mm^3$

TABLE D.5

Endocrine Test Laboratory Values

Adrenocorticotropic Hormone (ACTH)	4.7–48.8 ng/L
Growth Hormone (GH)	0–1 µg/L (men) 0–10 µg/L (women)
Insulin	6-26 µU/mL
Follicle-Stimulating Hormone (FSH)	1.4–18.1 mU/mL (men) 2.5–10.2 mU/L (women in the follicular phase) 3.4–33.4 mU/mL (women in the ovulatory period) 1.5–9.1 mU/mL (women in the luteal phase) 23–116 mU/mL (menopausal women)
Luteinizing Hormone (LH)	1.5–9.3 mU/mL (men) 1.9–12.5 mU/mL (women in the follicular phase) 8.7–76.3 mU/mL (women in the ovulatory period) 0.5–16.9 mU/mL (women in the luteal phase) 15.9–54 mU/mL (menopausal women)
Parathyroid Hormone (PTH)	<25 pg/mL

Endocrine Test Laboratory Values

Prolactin (PRL)	2.1–17.7 µg/L (men)
	2.8–29.2 µg/L (nonpregnant women)
	9.7–208 µg/L (pregnant women)
	1.8–20.3 µg/L (menopausal women)
Tri-iodothyronine (T_3)	75–195 ng/dL
Thyroxine (T_4)	4–12 µg/dL
Thyroid-Stimulating Hormone (TSH)	0.35–5.5 µU/mL

TABLE D.6

Urinalysis Laboratory Values

Calcium	<300 mg/day
Creatine	<100 mg/day
Creatinine	15–25 mg/kg of body weight per day
Glucose	negative
Potassium	25–125 mEq per day
Protein	<150 mg/day
Sodium	40–220 mEq per day

Appendix E

Metric Measurements

TABLE E.1
Common Base Units and Derived Units

Quantity	Unit (symbol)
Length	Meter (m)
Area	Square meter (m²)
Volume	Cubic meter (m³)
Mass	Kilogram (kg)
Time	Second (s)
Temperature	Celsius (C)

Prefixes and Multiples

Prefix	Symbol	Power	Multiple or Portion of a Multiple
deci-	d	10^{-1}	0.1
centi-	c	10^{-2}	0.01
milli-	m	10^{-3}	0.001
micro-	μ	10^{-6}	0.000001
nano-	n	10^{-9}	0.000000001
pico-	p	10^{-12}	0.000000000001

TABLE E.2
Prefixes and Multiples

Prefix	Symbol	Power	Multiple or Portion of a Multiple
tera-	T	10^{12}	1,000,000,000,000
giga-	G	10^{9}	1,000,000,000
mega-	M	10^{6}	1,000,000
kilo-	k	10^{3}	1,000
hecto-	h	10^{2}	100
deca-	da	10^{1}	10
unity			1

TABLE E.3
Commonly Used Lengths

Length	Meters
1 kilometer (1 km)	1,000
1 hectometer (hm)	100
1 decameter (dam)	10
1 meter (m)	1
1 decimeter (dm)	0.1
1 centimeter (cm)	0.01
1 millimeter (mm)	0.001

(continues)

TABLE E.3   (continued)

Commonly Used Lengths

Length	Meters
1 micrometer (μm)	10^{-6}
1 nanometer (nm)	10^{-9}
1 picometer (pm)	10^{-12}

TABLE E.4

Commonly Used Masses

Mass	Grams
1 kilogram (1 kg)	1,000
1 hectogram (hg)	100
1 decagram (dag)	10
1 gram (g)	1
1 decigram (dg)	0.1
1 centigram (cg)	0.01
1 milligram (mg)	0.001
1 microgram (μg, mcg)	10^{-6}
1 nanogram (ng)	10^{-9}
1 picogram (pg)	10^{-12}

TABLE E.5

Conversions

Metric Equivalent	U.S. Equivalent
1 km	0.62 miles
1 m	39.4 inches, 1.1 yards
1 cm	0.39 inches
1 kg	2.2 lb
1 g	0.035 oz
1 L	1.06 qt
1 mL	0.034 oz

Glossary

A

Actin A protein that makes up the thin filaments of the contractile myofibrils of muscle.

Adenohypophysis The anterior lobe of the pituitary gland; responsible for the synthesis and release of several hormones that regulate many physiological processes. Also called the anterior pituitary.

Adrenal cortex The outer layer of the adrenal gland that secretes cortisol, aldosterone, and supplemental androgens.

Adrenal gland One of two paired endocrine glands lying superior to each kidney. Also called suprarenal gland.

Adrenal medulla The inner portion of the adrenal gland that secretes epinephrine and norepinephrine.

Adrenaline See epinephrine.

Adrenocorticotropic hormone (ACTH) One of the hormones synthesized by the adenohypophysis. It is produced in response to stress and controls the release of hormones from the adrenal cortex.

Agranulocyte A white blood cell that lacks conspicuous cytoplasmic granules when stained. Lymphocytes and monocytes are agranulocytes.

Albumin A protein produced by the liver and the most abundant plasma protein. It helps transport steroid hormones and fatty acids through the bloodstream.

Aldosterone A hormone secreted by the adrenal cortex that affects blood pressure by regulating salt and water balance.

Alveolus A microscopic air sac at the ends of the respiratory bronchioles in the lungs where gas exchange occurs. Plural is alveoli.

Amnion The innermost of two membranes surrounding the fetus. It forms the amniotic sac, which is filled with amniotic fluid.

Androgens Steroid hormones secreted by the testes and the adrenal cortex that have a masculinizing effect.

Aneurysm A weakness in an arterial wall that leads to a widening.

Angina A constricting pain caused by reduced blood flow to the heart. Also called angina pectoris.

Anterior pituitary See adenohypophysis.

Antidiuretic hormone (ADH) A hormone produced by the hypothalamus and stored and released by the neurohypophysis. It helps regulate water balance and blood pressure.

Anus The distal end of the rectum; opens to the exterior through which feces are evacuated.

Aorta The largest artery in the body through which the left ventricle pumps oxygenated blood.

Aortic valve The semilunar valve between the left ventricle of the heart and the aorta.

Apex of lung The tip, or superior end, of the lung.

Appendicular skeleton The bones that support the appendages, including the bones of the upper and lower limbs and the bones of the shoulder and pectoral girdle.

Aqueous humor A watery fluid that fills the anterior cavity of the eye between the lens and cornea.

Areola A ring of pigmented skin surrounding the nipple of the breast.

Arrector pili muscle A bundle of smooth muscle attached to the base of a hair follicle; its contraction pulls the hair into a vertical position, leading to the phenomenon of "goosebumps."

Arteriole The smallest branch of an artery; branches to form capillaries.

Artery A large, thick-walled blood vessel that carries blood away from the heart.

Articular cartilage Hyaline cartilage covering the ends of bones where they articulate at joints.

Ascending colon The first part of the colon; extends upward from the cecum.

Astrocyte A star-shaped neuroglial cell of the central nervous system that helps form the blood-brain barrier.

Atom The smallest unit of a chemical element; made up of protons, neutrons, and electrons.

Atrioventricular (AV) valve A valve between an atrium and ventricle of the heart. The bicuspid (mitral) valve and the tricuspid valve are both atrioventricular valves.

Atrium A superior chamber of the heart. The left atrium receives blood from the lungs and the right atrium receives blood from the body. Plural is atria.

Auditory ossicles The three tiny bones of the middle ear: the malleus, the incus, and the stapes.

Auditory tube See eustachian tube.

Auricle The visible portion of the external ear. Also called the pinna.

Autonomic nervous system (ANS) The branch of the nervous system involved in monitoring the body's internal environment; its two branches are the sympathetic and parasympathetic divisions.

Axial skeleton The bones along the body's long axis including the bones of the head and trunk.

Axon The long, cylindrical projection of a neuron that propagates impulses toward the synapse.

B

Basophil A type of granulocytic white blood cell that secretes heparin and histamine.

Bicarbonate ion (HCO$_3$-) A polyatomic ion critical for maintaining acid-base homeostasis in the body.

Bicuspid valve See mitral valve.

Bile An alkaline fluid containing bile salts produced by the liver. It is stored in the gallbladder and emulsifies fats to aid in their digestion.

Blastocyst The stage of embryonic development that begins at about day 5 or 6, when cells begin to differentiate into either cells of the inner cell mass which forms the embryo, or into an outer layer of trophoblast cells, which forms extraembryonic structures.

Blood The fluid of the circulatory system that consists of plasma, blood cells, and thrombocytes. It is the chief means of transporting materials throughout the body.

Blood pressure The force exerted by the blood against the walls of blood vessels.

Bolus A chewed up mass of food ready to be swallowed.

Brain The part of the central nervous system that is enclosed in the cranial cavity. It integrates sensory information, coordinates motor output, and is the center for thought, memory, emotion, and judgement.

Brain stem The portion of the brain immediately superior to the spinal cord, made up of the medulla oblongata, the pons, and the midbrain. It controls many autonomic functions such as breathing and heartbeat.

Bronchial tree The extensive network of airways branching from the trachea.

Bronchiole Small airways in the lung; branch of a tertiary bronchus.

Bulbourethral gland One of two small glands located on either side of the male urethra near the prostate gland. They secrete an alkaline fluid to neutralize the acidity of the urethra and the female vagina. Also called Cowper's glands.

C

Cachexia Extreme weight loss and generalized wasting from a severe, chronic illness.

Calcitonin A hormone secreted by the thyroid gland that lowers the amount of plasma calcium and phosphate by storing them in bone or inhibiting their reabsorption in the kidneys, so they are eliminated in the urine.

Calcium/calcium ion (Ca^{2+}) An element found in plasma, bone, and teeth that is important for blood clotting, enzyme activation, and nerve and muscle function.

Calyx A chamber in the kidney through which urine passes. Urine flows from renal papillae to numerous minor calyces (plural), which drain into a few major calyces and then to a single renal pelvis.

Capillary A microscopic blood vessel that connects an arteriole to a venule. It facilitates gas, nutrient, and waste exchange between blood and tissue.

Cardiac muscle The involuntary striated muscle that makes up the walls of the heart.

Carina A projection of the last tracheal cartilage at which the trachea divides into right and left primary bronchi.

Catheter A flexible tube inserted into the body to drain, or inject, fluids.

Cecum The first part of the colon; receives digested material from the ileum. The appendix originates off of it.

Cell The smallest unit of life. All living things are composed of one or more cells.

Cell body The portion of a neuron containing the cell nucleus.

Central nervous system (CNS) The portion of the nervous system consisting of the brain and spinal cord.

Cerebellum The portion of the brain lying posterior to the medulla oblongata and responsible for controlling balance and equilibrium.

Cerebral hemisphere The right and left halves of the cerebrum.

Cerebrospinal fluid (CSF) A clear, colorless liquid that circulates through cavities in the brain and spinal cord. It provides protection from shock.

Cerebrum The largest part of the brain; the part responsible for higher order thinking.

Cerumen A thick, waxy substance produced by glands in the auditory canal. Also called ear wax.

Ceruminous gland A gland of the integumentary system that secretes cerumen in the external ear.

Cervix Neck; any constricted portion of an organ but most often refers to the cylindrical part of the uterus that joins to the vagina.

Chlorine/chloride ion (Cl$^-$) One of the most important ions in the blood. It has a key role in maintaining electrolyte, acid-base, and fluid balance, and is critical for neuronal signaling.

Chordee A congenital defect of the penis where it usually curves downward. It is often associated with an abnormal opening of the urethra.

Chorion The outer of two membranes surrounding a developing fetus; helps to form the placenta.

Choroid The middle vascular layer of the eyeball.

Chyme A soupy liquid of partially digested food that moves from the stomach to the duodenum of the small intestine.

Ciliary body A part of the eye that changes the shape of the lens and secretes aqueous humor.

Circulatory system The system that transports blood throughout the body; consists of the heart and blood vessels. Also called the cardiovascular system.

Claudication Pain in the extremities caused by inadequate blood flow to the muscles.

Clitoris A small organ that is part of the female vulva; contains sensitive erectile tissue.

Cochlea The snail-shaped portion of the inner ear containing hearing receptors.

Common bile duct The duct that carries bile from the gallbladder to the duodenum.

Compact bone The hard exterior of bones.

Complete blood count (CBC) A combination of blood tests that includes counts of red blood cells and thrombocytes, types of white blood cells, a hematocrit, and measure of hemoglobin content.

Conjunctiva A protective, transparent mucous membrane that covers the outer surface of the eye

Connective tissue The tissue that supports and connects organs; includes bone, tendon, cartilage, fat, and blood.

Cornea The transparent anterior portion of the sclera that allows light to enter the interior of the eye.

Coronary artery An artery that branches off the aorta to carry blood to the myocardium.

Cortisol A hormone secreted by the adrenal cortex that plays a role in the body's response to stress.

Cowper's gland See bulbourethral gland.

Cranial nerves The 12 pairs of nerves that arise from the brain.

Cyanotic A bluish color of the lips and skin due to a deficiency of oxygen in the blood.

D

Deep fascia A layer of tough, fibrous connective tissue that holds muscles with similar functions together and lines the body wall.

Dendrite A process of a neuron that carries impulses toward the cell body.

Dermis The layer of the integument between the epidermis and the subcutaneous layer.

Descending colon The part of the colon that extends downward from the transverse colon to the sigmoid colon.

Diaphragm The dome-shaped muscle that separates the thoracic from the abdominal cavity and is the major muscle of breathing.

Diaphysis The central shaft of a long bone.

Diastolic pressure The lower arterial blood pressure during relaxation of the heart ventricles.

Diencephalon The part of the brain extending from the brainstem to the cerebrum; contains the thalamus and hypothalamus.

DNA The genetic information of a cell contained within its nucleus and mitochondria. Stands for deoxyribonucleic acid.

Ductus deferens See vas deferens.

Duodenum The first portion of the small intestine; connects the stomach to the jejunum.

E

Ear drum See tympanic membrane.

Ejaculation The expulsion of semen from the penis.

Ejaculatory duct The tube that transports sperm from the vas deferens to the urethra.

Electrolyte A chemical that separates into charged particles when dissolved in an aqueous solution.

Embryo The stage of human development between the blastocyst and fetal stages; from two weeks postfertilization to the end of the eighth week.

Emesis The process of vomiting.

Endocardium The innermost layer of the wall of the heart; it lines its chambers and covers its valves.

Eosinophil A type of granulocytic white blood cell responsible for the destruction of parasites. It also plays a role in allergic reactions.

Ependymal cell A neuroglial cell responsible for the production of cerebrospinal fluid.

Epicardium The outermost layer of the wall of the heart. Also called the visceral pericardium.

Epidermis The superficial layer of the skin; composed of keratinized stratified squamous epithelium.

Epididymis A coiled tube on the posterior and superior aspect of the testis where sperm are stored and mature. Plural is epididymides.

Epiglottis A flap of cartilage that covers the larynx when swallowing, preventing food from entering the larynx and trachea.

Epinephrine A hormone secreted by the adrenal medulla during the fight or flight response. Also called adrenaline.

Epiphysis The wide end of a long bone.

Epistaxis A nosebleed.

Epithelial tissue Sheets of cells that cover organs and line tubular or hollow structures throughout the body.

Eponychium The narrow band of tissue at the proximal border of the nail. Also called a cuticle.

Erythema Flushing or reddening of the skin.

Erythrocyte A red blood cell. It contains hemoglobin, the protein that binds oxygen to transport it to body cells.

Esophagus The hollow muscular tube that carries ingested material from the pharynx to the stomach.

Estrogen A hormone produced by the ovaries. It works with progesterone to control the menstrual cycle and is responsible for female secondary sex characteristics.

Eustachian tube The canal that connects the middle ear with the nasopharynx and allows for balance of pressure between the middle and outer ear. Also called the auditory tube.

Exhalation See expiration.

Expiration The expelling of air from the lungs to the atmosphere; breathing out. Also called exhalation.

External nares The openings into the nasal cavity on the underside of the nose. Also called nostrils.

F

Fascia The fibrous membranes that cover, support, and separate muscles.

Fascicle A bundle of muscle fibers (cells).

Feces The waste discharged from the rectum that contains undigested food and bacteria. Also called stool.

Fetus The stage of human development following the embryonic stage from the end of the eighth week until birth.

Fibrinogen A type of protein found in plasma that plays an essential role in blood clotting.

Fibrous pericardium The superficial layer of the membrane that surrounds the heart, anchoring it to the mediastinum.

Fistula A tube that is usually an abnormal connection between two hollow organs.

Flat bone A plate-shaped bone that provides significant protection and extensive area for muscle attachment.

Follicle-stimulating hormone (FSH) A hormone secreted by the adenohypophysis that stimulates the development of follicles in females and sperm in males.

Free edge A nail part, such as a fingernail or toenail, that extends beyond the skin of the finger or toe.

Frequency (urinary) Urinating more often than usual without an increase in the total daily volume of urine.

Frontal lobe One of four pairs of lobes of the cerebral cortex. Responsible for voluntary movement, speech, personality development, and higher-order executive functions.

G

Gallbladder A small organ located on the posterior aspect of the liver. It stores bile and releases it into the duodenum via the common bile duct.

Gamete A male or female reproductive sex cell an egg or sperm.

Ganglion A group of neuronal cell bodies found outside of the central nervous system. Plural is ganglia.

Gland An organ that releases secretions. Exocrine glands release their substances into ducts; endocrine glands release their substances directly into the bloodstream.

Glans penis The soft tip of the distal end of the penis.

Glial cells See neuroglial cells.

Globulins Proteins found in blood plasma that play a role in immunity.

Glomerular filtration rate (GFR) A test to measure kidney function that estimates how much blood is filtered within kidney glomeruli each minute.

Glomerulus A ball of capillaries within a renal corpuscle where blood is filtered; the site of filtrate production. Plural is glomeruli.

Glucagon A hormone released by the pancreas that increases blood glucose levels.

Gonad An organ that produces gametes and hormones. The male gonads are the testes and the female gonads are the ovaries.

Granulocyte White blood cells that contain visible cytoplasmic granules when stained. Neutrophils, eosinophils, and basophils are granulocytes.

Gray matter Nervous tissue that contains neurons that do not have a myelin sheath.

H

Hair A thread-like structure of the integumentary system. Also called a pilus.

Hair cells The sensory receptors of the inner ear responsible for hearing and balance.

Hair follicle A structure in the dermis of the integument that surrounds the root of a hair.

Hair papilla A structure within a hair follicle that is the site of cell division responsible for hair growth.

Hair shaft The superficial portion of a hair that extends out from the epidermal surface.

Hematocrit (HCT) The percentage of red blood cells within the total volume of blood.

Hematopoiesis The formation of blood cells and thrombocytes; occurs in red bone marrow.

Hemoglobin The most abundant protein of red blood cells; transports much of the oxygen, and a small fraction of the carbon dioxide in the blood; composed of four protein subunits that each have an iron-containing heme group.

Hilum A depression in an organ where blood vessels and nerves enter and exit the organ.

Homeostasis The maintenance of a relatively stable internal environment of the body within physiological limits.

Hormone A chemical substance secreted by an endocrine gland that alters the physiological activity of its target cells.

Human growth hormone (hGH) A hormone secreted by the adenohypophysis that stimulates the growth of body tissue and has other metabolic functions. Also called somatotropin.

Hyaline cartilage A glossy connective tissue made of collagen found on many joint surfaces to assist in their movement.

Hydrogen ion (H⁺) The ion that defines the pH of an aqueous solution, or how acidic or alkaline it is. The greater the concentration of free H^+ in solution, the lower the pH and the more acidic it is.

Hymen A thin membrane that covers the external vaginal opening.

Hypodermis See subcutaneous layer.

Hyponychium The thickened region of epithelial tissue underlying the free edge of the nail securing it to the finger.

Hypophysis A small pea-sized gland that is frequently referred to as the pituitary gland. It is located at the base of the brain and controls the function of many other endocrine glands. The term hypophysis may also be used more generally to describe an outgrowth.

Hypothalamus A part of the diencephalon of the brain. It has important roles in emotion, maintaining homeostasis, and regulates the release of several hormones from the pituitary gland.

I

Ileum The third part of the small intestine, terminating at the cecum of the colon.

Incontinence A lack of voluntary control over urination or defecation.

Incus One of three auditory ossicles; transmits vibrations from the malleus to the stapes.

Inferior vena cava The vein that carries deoxygenated blood from the lower body to the right atrium of the heart. It is the largest vein in the human body.

Infundibulum The stalk-like structure that connects the pituitary to the hypothalamus in the brain. Also called the pituitary stalk.

Inhalation See inspiration.

Inspiration The drawing of air into the lungs from the atmosphere; breathing in. Also called inhalation.

Insula A small triangular region of the cerebral cortex that lies deep within the fissure separating the temporal lobe from the parietal and frontal lobes. Some references include it as one of the lobes of the cerebral cortex. It is thought to play a role in the processing of emotions and may play a role in addictive behavior.

Insulin A hormone released by the pancreas that functions to lower blood glucose levels.

Integument The skin and its accessory structures.

Interatrial septum The wall that divides the left and right atria of the heart.

Intercalated discs The double membrane layers in between cardiac muscle cells that facilitate signaling between the cells.

Intercostal muscles The muscles between the ribs that participate in normal, or quiet, breathing.

Interstitial fluid The fluid that fills the microscopic spaces between the cells of tissues.

Interventricular septum The wall that divides the left and right ventricles of the heart.

Intussusception The slipping of one part of the intestine into another like a telescope.

Iris The colored portion of the eye that controls the amount of light reaching the retina by dilating or constricting the pupil.

Irregular bones Bones that cannot be grouped as long, short, flat, or sesamoid bones because of their atypical form.

J

Jaundice A yellowing of the skin, whites of the eyes, and mucous membranes that results from a buildup of bilirubin in the blood.

Jejunum The middle portion of the small intestine between the duodenum and the ileum.

K

Keratin An insoluble protein found in the epidermis, hair, and nails.

Keratinocyte A cell of the epidermis that produces keratin. Keratinocytes are the most numerous of the cells in the epidermis.

Kidney One of the paired organs in the lumbar region of the back. Kidneys are responsible for producing urine and regulating blood volume and pressure.

L

Labia majora The large outer folds of skin that enclose and protect the external female genitalia.

Labia minora The paired folds of skin underlying the labia majora that surround the opening to the vagina and urethra.

Lacrimal gland The gland in the lateral corner of each eyelid that produces tears.

Lactation The secretion of milk from the mammary glands following childbirth.

Langerhans cell A macrophage cell in the epidermis of the integument that is part of the innate immune system.

Laryngopharynx The inferior section of the pharynx. It is the point at which the pharynx divides into the larynx and the esophagus.

Larynx A short passageway that connects the pharynx to the trachea. Also called the voice box.

Lavage The irrigation or therapeutic washing of an organ or body cavity.

Lens The transparent, biconvex body separating the posterior chamber and the vitreous body of the eye.

Leukocyte A white blood cell. A group of several different types of cells that provide protection against microbes and other foreign material. Neutrophils, eosinophils, basophils, monocytes, and lymphocytes are leukocytes.

Liver A large organ located in the upper right quadrant of the abdomen. It serves many functions including producing bile, detoxifying harmful substances, and synthesizing vitamin D.

Long bone Bones that are longer than they are wide. They provide structure and allow mobility.

Lung One of two organs that lie on either side of the heart in the thoracic cavity; the major organ of breathing.

Lunula The half-moon shaped white area at the base of a nail.

Luteinizing hormone (LH) A hormone secreted by the adenohypophysis. It stimulates the production of testosterone in males and in females it helps regulate the menstrual cycle and triggers progesterone secretion from the corpus luteum.

Lymph A clear fluid, similar to blood plasma in composition, that flows through the lymphatic system until it is returned to blood.

Lymph node A bean-shaped structure located along lymphatic vessels that filters and screens lymphatic fluid.

Lymphatic capillary The smallest of the lymphatic vessels. A blind-end structure that collects fluid from between cells.

Lymphatic duct The largest vessel in the lymphatic system. The right lymphatic duct drains lymph from the right side of the head, the right arm, and the right side of the chest. The left lymphatic duct, also called the thoracic duct, drains lymph from the rest of the body.

Lymphatic vessels The extensive network of vessels throughout the body that conducts lymph from tissue to the subclavian veins.

Lymphocyte An agranulocyte white blood cell that helps carry out cell-mediated and antibody-mediated immune responses.

M

Macromolecule A large molecule such as protein, carbohydrate, or nucleic acid.

Macrophage A phagocytic cell derived from a monocyte and found in body tissues; engulfs microbes and debris.

Malaise A general sense of being unwell.

Malleus One of three auditory ossicles; transmits vibrations from the eardrum to the incus.

Mammary gland A female exocrine gland that produces milk for infants.

Mammary papilla The small projection near the center of the mammary gland; a nipple.

Mastication The process of crushing and grinding food; chewing.

Mediastinum The membranous partition between the pleurae of the lungs, extending from the sternum to the vertebral column.

Medulla oblongata The inferior part of the brainstem that connects with the spinal cord. It contains control centers for respiration, blood pressure, and cardiac function.

Medullary cavity The cavity within the diaphysis of long bones that contains yellow bone marrow.

Melanin A dark pigment in hair and in the skin; helps protect against UV damage.

Melanocyte A cell of the epidermis that produces the pigment melanin.

Melatonin A hormone secreted by the pineal gland that helps regulate sleep-wake cycles.

Melena Black, tarry stools that contain blood. May also refer to the process of passing of melena.

Meninges The three protective membranes covering the brain and spinal cord. Singular is meninx.

Merkel cell A cell deep in the epidermis that functions in touch sensation.

Mesentery A heavily vascularized sheet-like organ that attaches the small intestine to the posterior abdominal wall.

Microglia Neuroglial cells that remove cellular debris and microbes from the central nervous system by phagocytosis.

Micturition The act of releasing urine from the urinary bladder. Also called urination.

Midbrain The superior part of the brainstem that is important for visual and auditory processing.

Mitral valve The atrioventricular valve with two cusps between the left atrium and left ventricle of the heart. Also called the bicuspid valve.

Molecule Two or more atoms held together by covalent bonds.

Monocyte An agranulocyte white blood cell that can differentiate into a macrophage and is important in phagocytosis.

Mons pubis The pad of fatty tissue that covers the pubic bone and is covered with pubic hair.

Mucosa associated tissue (MALT) Unencapsulated lymphoid tissue not penetrated by lymphatic vessels and found behind the mucosal membranes of the respiratory, urogenital, and gastrointestinal tracts.

Muscle fiber An individual muscle cell. Also called a myocyte.

Muscle tissue Groups of contractile cells that produce movement. The three types are cardiac, smooth, and skeletal.

Myocardium The middle layer of the heart composed of cardiac muscle tissue.

Myofibril The microscopic filaments that run parallel to each other through a muscle cell; made up of repeating units called sarcomeres.

Myosin A protein that makes up the thick filaments of the contractile myofibrils of muscle.

N

Nail An accessory structure of the integumentary system. A hard plate on the dorsal surface at the distal end of fingers and toes.

Nail body The flat plate of keratin that forms most of a nail.

Nail free edge The part of the nail that extends past the distal end of fingers and toes.

Nasal septum The flexible wall of cartilage that divides the nasal cavity into left and right halves.

Nasopharynx The superior portion of the pharynx that receives air from the nose.

Nephron The functional, microscopic unit of the kidney that filters blood and produces urine. Each kidney contains about 500,000.

Nervous tissue Groups of neurons and neuroglial cells in the brain, spinal cord, and nerves throughout the body that conduct electrical impulses.

Neuroglial cell One of several types of cell that performs support functions for neurons in the nervous system. Also called glial cells.

Neurohypophysis The posterior lobe of the pituitary gland; stores and releases oxytocin and antidiuretic hormone produced in the hypothalamus. Also called the posterior pituitary.

Neuron An individual nerve cell made up of a cell body, axon, and one or more dendrites.

Neutrophil The most abundant of the granulocytic white blood cells; responsible for phagocytosis of microbes.

Noradrenaline See norepinephrine.

Norepinephrine A hormone secreted by the adrenal medulla during the fight or flight response. Also called noradrenaline.

Nose A triangular-shaped protuberance in the center of the face that is the entrance to the respiratory tract.

Nostrils See external nares.

O

Occipital lobe One of the four pairs of lobes of the cerebral cortex; the lobe responsible for vision.

Oligodendrocyte A neuroglial cell that produces myelin in the central nervous system.

Oogenesis A complex differentiation process within ovarian tissue resulting in the production of functional oocytes.

Oral cavity The cavity through which food, drink, and air enter the body; also known as the mouth.

Organ A group of one or more types of tissue performing coordinated functions.

Organ system Groups of organs that work together to perform complex functions.

Organelle A structure within a cell that serves a specific function during cellular activity; examples are the nucleus, endoplasmic reticulum, and mitochondria.

Oropharynx The middle part of the pharynx that is both a respiratory and digestive pathway.

Ovary The female gonad, one of a pair of reproductive glands in women.

Ovulation The rupture of a mature ovarian follicle to release a secondary oocyte into the pelvic cavity.

Ovum The female gamete that is produced by the process of meiosis.

Oxytocin A hormone secreted by the neurohypophysis that stimulates uterine contractions during labor and delivery and the release of milk from mammary glands.

P

Palpate To touch gently.

Pancreas An endocrine and exocrine organ that extends laterally to the left of the duodenum. The pancreas secretes the endocrine hormones insulin, glucagon, and somatostatin and pancreatic juice, which contains digestive enzymes and bicarbonate.

Papilla A small, rounded, nipple-like projection from the body. Plural is papillae.

Papule A small elevated solid circular skin lesion, usually less than 5 mm in diameter.

Paranasal sinuses A group of four paired air-filled spaces that surround the nasal cavity. They produce mucus and increase resonance of the voice.

Parasympathetic division The part of the autonomic nervous system responsible for "rest and digest" responses, including decreasing heart rate, lowering blood pressure, and stimulating digestion.

Parathyroid gland One of three or four endocrine glands located on the posterior surface of the thyroid gland; secretes parathyroid hormone, which raises plasma calcium.

Parathyroid hormone A hormone secreted by the parathyroid gland that increases plasma calcium by releasing it from bone, increasing dietary absorption, and reabsorbing it from the kidneys before it is lost in urine.

Parietal layer The outer layer of the thin cavity that surrounds the heart, lungs, and abdominal viscera.

Parietal lobe One of two lobes located laterally in the brain that is important for sensory perception and integration.

Pectoralis minor One of two paired sets of muscles in the chest that have an origin on ribs 3, 4, and 5, and insert on the scapula. The action of the muscle is to draw the scapula forward and downward, acting as an accessory muscle of respiration. Plural is pectorales minores.

Penis The male copulatory organ, consisting largely of erectile tissue. The penis passes ejaculate and urine.

Pericardial space (cavity) The thin, fluid-filled cavity that surrounds the heart.

Pericardium A covering of the heart that folds back onto itself to form a two-layered membrane cavity filled with serous fluid.

Perineum The body region between the anus and the vulva or scrotum.

Periosteum A connective tissue that surrounds bones with the exception of articular surfaces.

Peripheral nervous system The part of the nervous system that is located outside of the skull and vertebral column.

Peristalsis The rhythmic contraction of muscles in the walls of hollow organs, especially in the gastrointestinal tract, that move contents in one direction.

Petechiae Purple pinpoint skin spots that appear when capillaries bleed, releasing blood under the skin.

Pharynx The posterior portion of the nasal and oral cavities. It has three regions, the nasopharynx, oropharynx, and laryngopharynx. Plural is pharynges.

Phosphate ion (PO_4^{3-}) An ion found in plasma, and abundant within cells, that is an important building block of ATP, cell membranes, RNA, and DNA.

Pilus See hair.

Pineal gland An endocrine gland located near the center of the brain that secretes the hormone melatonin, which regulates sleep.

Pinna See auricle. Plural is pinnae.

Pituitary gland See hypophysis.

Placenta A temporary organ in the uterus composed of fetal and maternal tissue that allows for the exchange of blood gasses, nutrients, and wastes between fetal and maternal blood.

Plaque A broad, raised skin lesion.

Plasma The liquid fraction of blood, which includes water, electrolytes, proteins, and other soluble chemicals. Plasma does contain clotting proteins and does not contain blood cells or thrombocytes.

Platelets See thrombocytes.

Pleura A serous membrane surrounding the lungs, which folds back onto itself to form a two-layered membrane cavity filled with serous fluid. Plural is pleurae.

Pons The middle part of the brain stem, anterior to the cerebellum; important for regulating breathing and the functions of some cranial nerves.

Posterior pituitary See neurohypophysis.

Potassium (K^+) An element found in plasma, and abundant within cells, that is important for regulating fluid balance and cell membrane potential.

Prepuce A fold of skin that surrounds the head of the penis or clitoris. In males, it is also referred to as the foreskin.

Primary bronchus One of two large tubes that conduct air into the lungs; there is a left and right primary bronchus; sometimes referred to as a main bronchus. Plural is bronchi.

Progesterone A steroid hormone produced by the corpus luteum of the ovary and has a role in regulating the female reproductive cycle.

Prolactin A hormone secreted by the adenohypophysis that stimulates milk production by the mammary glands.

Prone The body position when lying horizontal, face down.

Prostate gland The male reproductive endocrine gland located at the base of the bladder that produces a milky, enzyme-rich fluid that composes about one-third of the semen volume.

Protein One of hundreds of thousands of types of amino acid polymers that is encoded in the DNA and performs a wide range of functions in all cells and body tissues.

Pulmonary artery The large vessel that passes deoxygenated blood from the right ventricle to the lungs.

Pulmonary valve The semilunar valve found between the right atrium and the pulmonary trunk.

Pulmonary vein One of four veins that pass oxygen-rich blood from the lungs into the left atrium.

Pulmonary ventilation The process of air moving into, and out of, the lungs.

Pulse The heart rate, or the number of times the heart beats per minute.

Pupil The opening in the center of the iris through which light passes.

Purpura A condition of having pinpoint hemorrhages visible on the skin.

Purulent An adjective that describes the presence of pus, or a structure that contains or discharges pus.

Pustule A small, raised, pus-containing skin lesion.

R

Rales A crackling sound produced by the lungs during inspiration and are usually a sign of the presence of mucus in the small airways.

Rectum A hollow organ of the gastrointestinal tract that stores fecal material collected from the sigmoid colon, which is then eliminated through the anus.

Red bone marrow The tissue found in the cavities of spongy bone that contains stem cells that produce blood cells and thrombocytes, a process called hematopoiesis.

Renal capsule The tough, fibrous layer that surrounds the kidney and is covered in adipose tissue.

Renal cortex The outer layer of the kidney between the renal medulla and capsule that contains nephrons and glomeruli, which filter blood and balance blood chemistry.

Renal medulla The innermost part of the kidney that contains renal pyramids and blood vessels that transport blood to and from the renal cortex. Plural is renal medullae.

Renal papilla The opening at the tip of a renal pyramid that passes urine into a minor calyx.

Renal pelvis The kidney chamber that collects urine from major calyces, which then leaves the kidney through a ureter.

Renal pyramid One of many cone-shaped structures in the renal medulla that contain nephron collecting ducts, which empty filtrate through papillae into minor calyces.

Retina The light-sensitive tissue layer at the back of the eyeball.

Rhonchi Low-pitched wheezing lung sounds that are often an indication of obstruction or secretions in larger airways.

RNA A class of single-stranded nucleic acid polymers that encode proteins, regulate gene expression, and make up ribosomes. There are three major types of RNA: messenger RNA (mRNA), ribosomal RNA (rRNA), and transfer RNA (tRNA). Stands for ribonucleic acid.

S

Salivary gland One of three pairs of exocrine glands that secrete saliva into the oral cavity. The pairs of salivary glands are the parotid, submandibular, and sublingual glands.

Sarcomeres The contractile units of cardiac and skeletal muscle tissue; composed of thin and thick filaments that give the tissue its striated appearance under a microscope.

Satellite cell A microglial cell associated with ganglia of the peripheral nervous system that support and provide nutrients for neurons.

Scalene One of two paired sets of muscles in the neck with origins on cervical vertebrae that insert on the first rib and act as accessory muscles of respiration.

Schwann cell A microglial cell type that forms a myelin sheath around some neurons of the peripheral nervous system, increasing the speed of nerve impulses.

Sclera The tough outermost layer of the eyeball, commonly referred to as the "white of the eye." Plural is sclerae.

Scrotum The skin and connective tissue pouch that contains the testes.

Sebaceous gland An exocrine gland typically associated with hair follicles that secretes an oily substance called sebum.

Sebum An oily substance that coats hair; secreted by sebaceous exocrine glands of the skin.

Semen A fluid that contains sperm and glandular secretions of the male reproductive system.

Semicircular canal The region of the inner ear responsible for detecting movement and imbalance.

Semilunar valve One of two heart valves; the aortic and pulmonary valves.

Seminal vesicle One of two glands located at the base of the bladder; produces a nutrient-rich secretion that contributes to more than half of the volume of semen.

Seminiferous tubule The complex network of ducts within a testis that produces sperm.

Serous fluid The watery secretion of serous membranes.

Serous pericardium A serous membrane surrounding the heart that folds back onto itself to form a two-layered membrane cavity filled with serous fluid.

Serum The liquid fraction of blood without clotting factors. Serum contains water, electrolytes, proteins (except clotting proteins), and other soluble chemicals. Serum does not contain cells or thrombocytes.

Sesamoid bone A classification of bone type that forms within a tendon.

Short bone A bone that is of approximately equal length in all dimensions.

Sigmoid colon The final part of the colon that extends from the descending colon to the rectum.

Skeletal muscle A striated muscle type that attaches to bones by tendons and controls voluntary body movements.

Skin The largest organ of the body, serving as a barrier between the internal and external environment. It is the first line of defense against pathogens.

Small intestine The longest portion of the gastrointestinal tract, connecting the stomach to the colon, and the primary site of digestion and nutrient absorption.

Smooth muscle An involuntary muscle type found in the walls of hollow organs and vessels.

Sodium/sodium ion (Na$^+$) An element that is abundant in plasma and interstitial fluid that is important for regulating blood volume and cell membrane potential.

Somatic nervous system (SNS) The efferent division of the nervous system that innervates skeletal muscles and controls voluntary body movements.

Somatotropin See human growth hormone.

Sperm The male gamete that is produced by the process of meiosis.

Spermatic cord One of two structures that suspends a testis in the scrotum; contains vascular, nervous, and lymphatic tissues and a vas deferens.

Spermatogenesis The process of sperm production by differentiation of spermatogonia in the seminiferous tubules of the testes.

Spinal cord The part of the central nervous systems that descends from the brain stem through the vertebral column to the second lumbar vertebra.

Spinal nerve One of 31 pairs of nerves of the peripheral nervous system that originate from the spinal cord.

Spleen The largest organ of the lymphatic system, located in the upper left abdominal quadrant and responsible for lymphocyte production, blood filtration, and breaking down of old red blood cells.

Spongy bone The trabecular portion of bones that contains red bone marrow; the site of hematopoiesis.

Sprain A painful traumatic injury to a joint that may result in a torn ligament.

Sputum A thick mucus that is coughed up from the lower airway.

Stapes One of three auditory ossicles; transmits vibrations from the incus to the inner ear.

Sternocleidomastoid The long skeletal muscle in the neck with an origin on the clavicle and sternum and insertion on the mastoid process. The action of the muscle is the turning of the head from side to side and flexion of the neck. It acts as an accessory muscle of respiration.

Stomach The hollow muscular organ below the diaphragm that stores ingested material, mixing it with hydrochloric acid and digestive enzymes and transforming it to chyme, before passing it to the duodenum.

Stool See feces.

Strain A muscle injury from excessive stretching.

Striae Linear red marks on the skin that result from rapid weight gain. Singular is stria.

Subcutaneous layer The layer of tissue deep to the dermis that is rich in adipose tissue. Also called the hypodermis.

Sudoriferous gland An exocrine gland of the integument that produces sweat.

Superficial fascia The connective tissue located deep to the dermis.

Superior vena cava The large vein that drains blood into the right atrium from the chest and upper body. Plural is venae cavae.

Supine The body position when lying horizontal, face up, with palms facing anterior.

Suprarenal gland See adrenal gland.

Sympathetic division The part of the autonomic nervous system responsible for "fight or flight" responses, including increasing heart rate and blood pressure, dilating airways, and suppressing digestion.

Systolic pressure The higher arterial blood pressure during contraction of the heart ventricles.

T

Temporal lobe One of two lateral lobes of the brain that contains the primary auditory cortex.

Tendons The connective tissue bands that attach skeletal muscle to bone.

Terminal bronchiole Microscope airways that branch into respiratory bronchioles, which contain some alveoli.

Testicles See testis.

Testis The male gonads, which produce testosterone and sperm in males after puberty. Plural is testes. Also called testicles.

Testosterone The primary androgen secreted by the interstitial cells of the testes.

Thalamus A region of the diencephalon in the brain that acts as a relay station in sensory pathways of the ears, eyes, and skin.

Thick filament A cytoskeletal protein polymer composed mostly of myosin that makes up part of the contractile units in cardiac and skeletal muscle cells.

Thin filament A cytoskeletal protein polymer composed mostly of actin that makes up part of the contractile units in cardiac and skeletal muscle cells.

Thoracic cavity The body cavity superior to the diaphragm that houses the lungs and heart.

Thrombocyte Small cell fragments that contribute to the blood clotting process. Also called platelets.

Thymosin A class of hormones secreted by the thymus that cause the maturation of T lymphocytes.

Thymus gland An endocrine gland located in the mediastinum; important for immunity and the maturation of T lymphocytes.

Thyroid gland A butterfly-shaped endocrine gland located inferior and lateral to the larynx that secretes thyroxine, tri-iodothyronine, and calcitonin.

Thyroid-stimulating hormone (TSH) A hormone secreted by the adenohypophysis that regulates release of the thyroid hormones thyroxine and tri-iodothyronine from the thyroid gland.

Thyroxine (T_4) One of two thyroid hormones, which are important for regulating metabolism, growth, and development.

Tinnitus A ringing in the ears.

Tissue A group or layer of cells that perform specific functions.

Tonsil Soft masses of lymphatic tissue found at the back of the nasal and oral cavities. There are four sets of tonsils pharyngeal (adenoids), tubal, palatine, and lingual.

Trachea The tube that extends from the larynx to the bronchi; conveys air to and from the lungs. Also called the windpipe.

Transverse colon The longest part of the colon, traveling across the abdomen from the hepatic flexure near the liver to the splenic flexure near the spleen.

Tricuspid valve The atrioventricular valve with three cusps between the right atrium and right ventricle of the heart.

Triiodothyronine (T_3) One of two thyroid hormones; important for regulating metabolism, growth, and development.

Tympanic membrane The thin layer of tissue, separating the outer and inner ear, that converts soundwaves into vibrations which are then transmitted to the auditory ossicles in the middle ear. Also called the **eardrum**.

U

Umbilical cord A vascular cord that connects a developing fetus to the placenta, allowing for the exchange of blood gasses, nutrients, and waste products between the fetal and maternal circulatory systems.

Ureter One of two muscular tubes that pass urine produced in the kidneys to the urinary bladder.

Urethra The muscular tube that connects the urinary bladder to the external environment.

Urgency A sudden strong feeling of needing to urinate that may be difficult to control.

Urinalysis A series of physical, chemical, and microscopic laboratory tests that measure urine contents to aid diagnosis or management of a wide range of disorders.

Urinary bladder A hollow muscular organ that temporarily stores urine.

Urinary meatus The external opening of the urethra through which the body discharges urine.

Urination See micturition.

Urine A fluid, typically yellow in color, produced by the kidneys and temporarily stored in the urinary bladder. Urine contains excess water and electrolytes, and also waste products that are eliminated from the body through the urethra.

Urticaria Itchy red raised elevations on the skin; hives.

Uterus The hollow muscular organ in the female pelvis that is superior to the vagina and posterior to the urinary bladder.

Uvea The vascular layer of the eyeball that is beneath the sclera. It includes the choroid, ciliary body, and iris.

V

Vagina The muscular canal that extends from the uterine cervix to the external environment.

Vas deferens The duct that carries sperm from the epididymis to the prostate gland. Plural is vasa deferentia. Also called the ductus deferens.

Vein A vessel that carries blood toward the heart.

Ventricle One of two major chambers of the heart that receive blood from an atrium; also one of a series of chambers in the brain.

Venule A small vein that collects blood from capillary beds.

Vertebra One of a series of bones that forms the spinal column. Plural is vertebrae.

Vertigo A sensation that makes one feel as though they are spinning.

Vestibule The part of the vulva between the labia minora; also the central cavity of the bony labyrinth of the inner ear.

Vitreous body See vitreous humor.

Vitreous humor A clear, gelatinous structure that fills the posterior chamber of the eye between the lens and the retina. Also called the vitreous body.

Vocal cords The folds of tissue in the larynx that add vibrations to air coming from the lungs to produce sounds and speech.

Volvulus An obstruction caused by the bowel twisting on itself.

Vulva The external structures of the female genitalia.

W

White blood cell (WBC) count A diagnostic test to determine the number of different types of white blood cells in a volume of blood.

White matter Nervous tissue that contains myelinated neurons.

Windpipe See trachea.

Y

Yellow bone marrow A soft tissue found in the center of hollow bones that aids in the storage of fats.

Z

Zygote A single diploid cell formed from the fusion of a haploid ovum (egg) and sperm.

Index

Note: Page numbers followed by *f* or *t* indicate materials in figures or tables respectively.